COLLABORATIVE BRIEF THERAPY WITH CHILDREN

Collaborative Brief Therapy with Children

MATTHEW D. SELEKMAN

THE GUILFORD PRESS
New York   London

© 2010 The Guilford Press
A Division of Guilford Publications, Inc.
72 Spring Street, New York, NY 10012
www.guilford.com

Printed in the United States of America

This book is printed on acid-free paper.

Last digit is print number: 9 8 7 6 5 4 3 2 1

Library of Congress Cataloging-in-Publication Data
is available from the publisher.

ISBN 978-1-60623-568-3

About the Author

Matthew D. Selekman, MSW, is a family therapist and addictions counselor in private practice and the co-director of Partners for Collaborative Solutions (*www.partners4change.net*), an international family therapy training and consulting firm in Evanston, Illinois. He is an Approved Supervisor with the American Association for Marriage and Family Therapy. Mr. Selekman received the Walter S. Rosenberry Award in 1999, 2000, and 2006 from The Children's Hospital in Denver, Colorado, for significant contributions to the fields of psychiatry and the behavioral sciences. He has published numerous family therapy articles and five professional books: *The Adolescent and Young Adult Self-Harming Treatment Manual: A Collaborative Strengths-Based Brief Therapy Approach; Working with Self-Harming Adolescents: A Collaborative, Strengths-Based Therapy Approach; Pathways to Change: Brief Therapy with Difficult Adolescents (Second Edition); Solution-Focused Therapy with Children: Harnessing Family Strengths for Systemic Change;* and *Family Therapy Approaches with Adolescent Substance Abusers* (coeditor with Thomas C. Todd). Mr. Selekman has presented workshops throughout the United States, Canada, Mexico, South America, Europe, Singapore, Indonesia, Hong Kong, and Australia on his collaborative strengths-based brief therapy approach with challenging children and adolescents.

Preface

Prior to 1997, there had not been a book published on brief therapy with children and their families. Seeing this gap in the literature, and with major insurance companies moving in the direction of managed mental health care, I wanted not only to fill this gap, but also to provide a user-friendly, practice-oriented handbook on short-term, goal-oriented therapy for clinicians working with children in a variety of settings. In my earlier book, *Solution-Focused Therapy with Children: Harnessing Family Strengths for Systemic Change*, I stressed the importance of viewing children's difficulties through a strengths-based ecosystemic lens. That book blended together the best elements of traditional child therapy and family systems approaches for children by presenting a wide variety of family play and art therapy techniques and strategies, and demonstrated how to utilize children's and family members' strengths, resources, and resiliencies to empower them to rapidly resolve their difficulties. However, important findings from research in interpersonal neuroscience, psychotherapy outcome, and positive psychology studies were missing.

Fortunately, 13 years later The Guilford Press has afforded me with the opportunity to greatly revise and expand the earlier book. This new volume includes my most current therapeutic ideas for working with children and their families; the latest research from interpersonal neuroscience, psychotherapy outcome, and positive psychology findings that can inform our clinical practices; and four new chapters on parenting skills training, collaborative work with school personnel and pediatricians, and practical suggestions for getting unstuck and creating possibilities with complex and challenging child case situations. Furthermore, three special features in the book are new culturally diverse case examples, six full-length case examples, and the blueprint for change plan. Each of the six full-length case examples is written in such a way that readers will feel as if they are sitting right in the therapy room with the clients and me, experiencing the whole treatment process as it unfolds.

The *blueprint for change* plan invites new clients in first sessions to be completely in charge of deciding what their goals are, and which of their key strengths and resources they will tap into to help them to achieve their goals; selecting from menus of therapeutic modalities and experiments that they wish to try; and determining who attends sessions and the frequency of visits. Since this is a client-driven treatment plan, it is flexible and will evolve over time. The blueprint for change plan optimizes clients' success in treatment and can greatly reduce the likelihood of premature client dropouts, particularly with clients who have extensive treatment histories.

My hope is that my new book will provide graduate students, as well as novice and seasoned therapists, with many useful therapeutic tools and strategies that they can put to immediate use with even the most challenging of child case situations.

Acknowledgments

There are several people I wish to acknowledge for greatly contributing to my professional development and the ideas discussed in this book. First and foremost, I want to thank Michele Weiner-Davis for showing me a variety of shortcuts for empowering clients and rapidly navigating them to "possibility land." I would like to thank the late Steve de Shazer and Insoo Kim Berg for providing me with several exceptional training experiences at the Brief Therapy Center in Milwaukee. From "down under," the late Michael White gets my undying appreciation for introducing me to the creative therapeutic pathway of externalizing problems. Finally, a special thanks to the late Harry Goolishian and to Harlene Anderson for exposing me to important postmodern therapy ideas, particularly, effective ways to collaborate with families who are therapy veterans and all the mental health professionals who are actively involved in those families' lives.

A big thanks to Jim Nageotte, my editor at The Guilford Press, for asking me to write this book.

And, finally, I would like to thank my loving and supportive wife, Åsa, and Hanna, my little angel and other love, who constantly reminds me to make room daily for play and laughter.

Contents

COLLABORATIVE BRIEF THERAPY WITH CHILDREN

1

Expanding the Possibilities

A Collaborative Strengths-Based Brief Therapy Approach with Children

What moves men of genius, or rather what inspires their work, is not
new ideas, but their obsession with the idea that what had already been
said is still not enough.

—EUGÈNE DELACROIX

Introduction: Myths about Children and Therapy

President John F. Kennedy once said: "The greatest enemy of the truth is
not the lie—deliberate, contrived, and dishonest—but the myth—persistent,
pervasive, and unrealistic" (in Dawes, 1994, p. vii). Therapists hold many
sacred cow beliefs about which methods and treatment approaches are best
suited for children. Child therapists argue that family therapy approaches
fail to attend adequately to the developmental concerns and intrapsychic
conflicts of the child client. Family therapists, on the other hand, maintain
that the child's symptoms indicate such family dysfunction as pathological
structures or problem-maintaining interaction patterns. Another widely held
belief among therapists is that treatment with children must be long-term.
In this chapter, I first dispel some commonly held myths about children and
therapy and demonstrate why a collaborative strengths-based brief therapy
approach can be an effective treatment model for clinical work with children and their families. I then present key findings from research on resilient
children and the growing field of positive psychology that provide empirical
support for the major therapeutic tools, strategies, and key elements that
promote change with this therapeutic approach. Finally, I follow with an

1

overview of the major components of the collaborative strengths-based brief therapy approach for children.

"Young Children Should Be Excluded from Family Therapy Sessions"

It is not uncommon for family therapists to instruct parents either to leave their youngest children at home with a babysitter or to place them in a supervised play area in the office waiting room. Some family therapists believe that including young children in family sessions could be "psychologically harmful to them" (which is a concern also raised by some parents) or that they might be "highly disruptive" during the session. Many believe that young children would be unable to participate in session discussions or understand what is talked about, anyway, because of their "developmental limitations."

However, there are several good reasons for including young children in family therapy sessions. Through young children's play and artwork we can gain access to family conflicts less accessible through verbal communications (Bailey, 2000; Zilbach, Bergel, & Gass, 1972). Often children's play and artwork are metaphors for how they view themselves and significant relationships in their families. Eliciting feedback from the parents and older siblings of the young child about his or her play and artwork can open up avenues for challenging outmoded family beliefs and unhelpful parent–child interactions. Keith and Whitaker (1994) maintain that "play is the medium for expanding the family's reality" (p. 194). Young children inject spontaneity and playfulness into family sessions. The young child can serve as a co-therapist in teaching his or her parents how to play again. Finally, young children's presence in family sessions affords the opportunity for the therapist to model positive, nurturing, and playful interactions for the parents.

"Traumatized Children Will Grow Up to Be Emotionally Flawed Adults"

Undoubtedly, some children who have been traumatized by various forms of parental abuse or who have experienced painful losses are subject to emotional scars that could possibly haunt them for the rest of their lives. The trauma literature is filled with examples about the deleterious effects of traumatic events on a child's individual and interpersonal functioning. Yet, over the past few decades there has been surprisingly little discussion about the growing body of resiliency research that has identified children who experienced multiple traumatic events in their lives and yet managed to grow up to be well-functioning adults. As Garmezy (1991) has pointed out, the resilient individual is characterized by "the maintenance of competent functioning despite an interfering emotionality" (p. 416). In commenting on some widely held beliefs in the sex abuse treatment field, Trepper and Barrett (1989) note that "the belief that sexual abuse will lead to severe emotional problems has been the cornerstone of all therapy. Most therapists probably believe this without hesitation, and probably justify some of their most intrusive therapeutic measures on it. The research on the long-term effects of child sexual abuse has been quite mixed, however" (p. 11). Garmezy (1993) also argues that there are not enough empirically based longitudinal studies of long-term outcomes of child abuse cases to support the widely held belief that an abused child will grow up to become an adult abuser.

Here I present two major studies conducted with trauma survivors who "beat the odds" and grew up to be well-functioning adults.

Moskovitz (1983) conducted an exploratory study with a group of Holocaust survivors to determine how they coped with their hellish experiences in the Nazi concentration camps during World War II. None of her subjects succumbed to suicide attempts, alcohol or drug abuse, or psychiatric disorders. She noted that "their hardiness of spirit and their quiet dignity are part of this persistent endurance" (p. 233). Moskovitz further added: "Despite the severest deprivation in early childhood, these people are neither living a greedy, me-first style of life, nor are they seeking gain at the expense of others. None express the idea that the world owes them a living for all they have suffered. On the contrary, most of their lives are marked by a compassion for others" (p. 233).

Festinger (1983) followed 277 children in New York City who were placed in foster care early in childhood until young adulthood. Many of these children were emotionally and physically abused, were abandoned, had a mentally ill or drug-addicted parent, or lost a parent through death. Approximately 69% of her sample had been in three to four foster homes or institutions as young children. When comparing all 277 of these young adults to a sample of subjects from a national survey conducted by the Institute of Social Research at the University of Michigan, she discovered the following: although the foster care subjects showed lower scholastic achievements, their employment rates, health and symptoms status, and personal evaluations of their feelings, future hopes, and current sense of happiness were similar. Festinger noted that her foster care subjects were generous contributors to the study and exhibited a willingness and openness to discuss their lives in the hope that it would help others.

What these two studies did not mention was that each of the subjects possessed a unique set of protective factors that helped insulate each one from the onslaught of multiple stressors and adverse life events throughout his or her childhood. Without these protective factors, such as social competence and nurturing support systems (Garmezy, 1994), the research subjects' adult lives might have turned out differently. Later in this chapter, I discuss further the role of protective factors in the adaptation process as well as how resiliency research can inform our clinical practices.

When working with children who were traumatized, we need to empower them to become masters of their own lives. We can do this by conveying an optimistic attitude, capitalizing on their competency areas, respecting their defenses, and giving them room to tell their painful stories when (or if) they are ready to do so. As therapists, we need to be sensitive to the fact that our theoretical maps and the way we interact with our clients determine what we see. If we operate from a deficit-oriented model, we inevitably see deficits and become expert repairmen and -women. By capitalizing on our young clients' strengths and resources and what is "going right" in their present lives, we can help these children create their own positive self-fulfilling prophecies.

"Children Should Be Seen and Not Heard in the Treatment Planning and Problem-Solving Process"

More often than not, children are not given a voice in their own treatment or school educational planning. Typically, when a family presents for therapy, the parents' goals automatically become the focal point for determining treatment objectives without seriously exploring with the child what his or her goals or expectations might be, such as what specifically the child would like to see changed in the parents' behavior. We see this phenomenon a great deal even in child abuse cases, where the treating therapist, child protective worker, and other involved representatives from larger systems typically determine the treatment goals and treatment plan for the child and family. Often at multidisciplinary school staff meetings, children are altogether excluded when an individualized education plan (IEP) is being developed for them, and, if they are "lucky," they will be invited in at the end of the proceeding to hear what direction their school year will take in terms of special services or placement. Not only do the children have no input in the final individualized education plan, but also they have no opportunity to give any feedback on the school psychologist's case study evaluation results, which are typically discussed in the multidisciplinary staff meeting.

When working with children and their families, I invite the child to share his or her goals and expectations for the therapy. Some children may have a specific goal in mind for their parents (e.g., to "yell" less). I believe it is essential to pay heed to both the parents' *and* the child's goals or objectives. Also, I explore whether the children are having any special problems with siblings or particular teachers with whom they would like me to intervene. To help take the onus off the child client's being labeled by the parents and others as the "bad kid," I recommend to the parents, as an experiment, to carefully observe for 1 week the angelic "good kid's" behavior when he or she is around the client. Frequently, parents discover that their angelic child is a master at pushing their so-called problem child's buttons. This therapeutic experiment helps to show the parents that the problem is essentially *relational* and challenges their belief that the problem is solely confined to the one targeted child. Finally, whenever possible, I try to include the child in any collaborative meetings with school personnel and involved helpers. By hearing their young voices directly in these collaborative meetings, school and other helping professionals learn firsthand what the child's unique needs, attributes, and best hopes are, in addition to revisiting what has and has not been helpful in their interactions to date with him or her.

In an exploratory study with children who had received family therapy, researchers discovered from the children themselves that they expected to be fully included in family sessions and to have an active voice in discussions and participate meaningfully in the problem-solving process. The children also appreciated therapists who displayed warmth and concern toward them (Stith, Rosen, McCollum, Coleman, & Herman, 1996). Research of this kind provides empirical support for the importance of giving children a significant voice in their own treatment.

"Severe and Chronic Child Behavioral Difficulties Will Require Big and Complex Solutions"

In an earlier work (Selekman, 2005), I discussed the evolutionary process through which cases become "difficult." Typically, the so-called difficult case keeps receiving "more of the same" type of treatment (Watzlawick, Weakland, & Fisch, 1974), and the child's and family's problems become further compounded and exacerbated while on the treatment circuit, collecting a variety of labels out of the DSM-IV-TR (the text revision of the fourth edition of the *Diagnostic and Statistical Manual of Mental Disorders*; American Psychiatric Association, 2000). In commenting on the labeling process, Wittgenstein (1963) warned us against prematurely treating as already complete phenomena that are essentially incomplete human activities still in progress: "If you complete it, you falsify it" (p. 257). In other words, once a child is labeled as having a particular problem or disorder, suddenly we find that there is no other way of thinking about this child—past, present, or future!

When working with children and families that have experienced multiple treatment failures, it behooves us to explore with them what they disliked about former therapists and therapies, so as to avoid making the same kinds of mistakes. I like to empower these families by treating them as experts, asking them the following types of questions:

- "You have seen a lot of therapists before me; what did they miss with your situation?"
- "What didn't you like about former therapists?—so I don't make the same mistakes."
- "If I were to work with another family just like yours, what advice would you give me to help that family out?"
- "If you were to work with the perfect therapist, what would he or she do that you would find to be most helpful?"
- (*with clients labeled "noncompliant"*) "On your way to my office, did you think about all of the possible ways I could screw up your case? What are some of those ways?"

It is also helpful with therapy-hardened families to negotiate small but achievable goals, with the family members deciding what they want to work on changing first. With some of these families, past therapists' goals may have driven the treatment: either the therapists had no idea what their clients' goals were, or the clients' goals were too ambitious, such as trying to change too many symptoms simultaneously. When the latter is the case, I find it most useful to break up the family and work with family subsystems or individuals separately (Selekman, 2005).

"The Therapist Is More of an Expert on Parenting Than the Child's Parents"

Many therapists adopt a privileged-expert attitude with the parents and children with whom they work. It is hard not to fall into this trap. The more specialized training and knowledge we secure in a particular therapy approach, the more confidence (verging on overconfidence) we come to have in our therapeutic abilities and therapy models of choice. As Palmarini (1994) cautions us, "We need to be wary of our overconfidence, which tends to be at its greatest in our own area of expertise and where it can do the most damage" (p. 119). There are many popular parenting models that therapists have adopted as their road maps for parent training, such as parent effectiveness training (PET; Gordon, 1970), systematic training for effective parenting (STEP; Dinkmeyer & McKay, 1989), and Active Parenting (Popkin, 2007). Some child therapists believe that they are better equipped than the child's parents to provide their young clients with missing "selfobject functions" (Kohut, 1971) or to help them resolve their intrapsychic conflicts. The same is true with play therapy, as the parents are rarely included in the child's play or art activities.

It is my contention that our main expertise as therapists should be directed toward eliciting the parents' expertise. Any past successes that the parents have had at resolving other behavioral difficulties can be used as models for present and future successes. In all problematic parenting situations, there are times when the parents are managing their children's behaviors well and are enjoying their tough jobs. Like a Columbo or Miss Marple detective, we need to inquire about what specifically parents are doing during those nonproblem times that is working for them. These key parental problem-solving and coping strategies can serve as building blocks in the solution construction process. Similarly, taking the time in the first family session to find out from the parents what their strengths and talents are in their work roles can provide therapists with valuable information that they can utilize in developing potential solution strategies. Finally, why not include parents in the child's in-session play and art therapy activities? Doing so can help reduce family stress, improve family communications, and teach parents and children fun ways to resolve conflicts and problems.

Superkids: How Resiliency Research Can Inform Our Clinical Practices

In speaking out against the "Diseasing of America" (Peele, 1985) trend in the media and in the world of mental health care—which continues into the present, owing to popular talk shows that devote whole programs to the "disorder of the day"—Wolin (Wolin, O'Hanlon, & Hoffman, 1995) has argued that "we need a list of strengths as powerful and as validating as the florid vocabulary of diseases found in DSM-IV to combat our national obsession with pathology" (p. 24). Wolin (Wolin & Wolin, 1993) and a group of psychologists and psychiatrists have been studying high-risk children's psychosocial competencies and resourcefulness over the past three decades. These researchers found that, when faced with adversity and stressful life events, many of the children in their studies consistently "bounced back" quickly and "beat the odds" (Anthony & Cohler, 1987; Haggerty, Sherrod, Garmezy, & Rutter, 1994; Wolin & Wolin, 1993).

Table 1.1 provides an overview of the three categories of key protective factors that are found in these researchers' studies of high-risk children reared in poverty and high-stress family environments characterized by violence, parental alcoholism and substance abuse, divorce, and parental mental illness. Following this overview, the discussion turns to how to develop, enhance, and utilize these key protective factors in our therapeutic work with children and their families.

Effective and Creative Problem Solvers

One of the most frequent findings in all the reviewed studies with high-risk children was that these children had strong problem-solving abilities. These children were described as "resourceful," "creative," and "acting"

TABLE 1.1. Key Protective Factors of Resilient Children

Individual factors	Family factors	Extrafamilial support factors
Optimistic explanatory style	Caring and supportive parents	Nurturing support system (relatives, friends, teachers, neighbors, and inspirational significant others)
Good sense of humor	Strong parent–child relationships	Church involvement
Self-efficacy	Low levels of family conflict	Successful school experiences
Strong social skills	Optimistic parenting explanatory styles	
Cognitive competence		
Good-natured temperament		
Pronounced self-sufficiency		
Robustness		
Sense of coherence		
Perseverance		
Involvement in creative activities		
Intelligence		
Strong problem-solving skills		
Good management of emotions		
Keen sense of self-awareness		

rather than "reacting" to the problems and crises they faced (Anthony, 1987; Garmezy, 1981, 1994; Masten, Best, & Garmezy, 1990; Masten & Garmezy, 1985; Werner, 1987a, 1987b; Werner & Smith, 1982, 1992; Wolin & Wolin, 1993). Many of these children viewed problems as challenges they were confidently prepared to face and master—a finding in studies on children deemed optimistic (Diener & Dweck, 1978; Dweck, 1975; Seligman, Reivich, Jaycox, & Gillham, 1995). As a way of coping with crises and problems, some of these children would seek solace by going to church, spending time with a close friend or an inspirational other, or engaging in sports or other recreational activities (Anthony, 1984, 1987; Masten et al., 1990; Wolin & Wolin, 1993).

Anthony (1987) has identified two types of cognitive competence displayed by resilient children: *constructive competence* and *creative competence*. Constructive competence is characterized by a practical and concrete approach to tasks and problem solving. These children are independent and self-confident when carrying out tasks. Creative competence is demonstrated by the child's ability to move from practical ways of solving problems to more abstract and novel ways of problem solving.

In applying this important protective factor to clinical practice, in the initial family assessment session I explore with the child and his or her parents what the child has done in the past and does presently to resolve problems or better cope with them. I have some children visualize memorable successful problem-solving experiences and utilize these movies of success to empower them to resolve their presenting problems. It is also helpful to find out from the parents what they have done successfully in the past to help the child better cope with life stressors and resolve difficulties. These successful problem-solving strategies can be used in the current problem area. Sometimes I have a child create a *victory box*. He or she records on paper any personal triumphs, achievements, and problem-solving efforts in school, at home, in sports events, or with the creative arts, including the steps he or she took to achieve these wonderful accomplishments, and then places these slips of paper in the box. The victory box serves as a storehouse for blueprints of success and mastery for the child and his or her family.

If a child is presented by his or her parents or the referring person as having "poor problem-solving abilities," I still explore with the child and his or her parents what interests, talents, and skills the child has that I might be able to further activate. For example, if the child has a strong interest in science and performs well academically in this subject area, I have the child identify his or her favorite scientists and inventors and discuss how they solved problems. I then ask the child to adapt some of these well-proven problem-solving strategies to experiment with the problems he or she faces. Role playing the child's problem situation can also be useful as a skill-building technique for teaching the child new problem-solving strategies. However, it is even more effective to include the child's identified "pal" in the role-play activity, as the friend may be able to offer and model more effective problem-solving strategies than the therapist could provide.

Strong Social Skills

Another important protective factor for resilient children is their strong social skills. Many of the researchers who studied these high-risk children were struck by the children's knack for establishing and maintaining relationships with peers, neighbors, clergy, and other adults. Not only were these children naturals at establishing support systems for themselves, but also they could reach out with ease to a friend, parent, or other adult for support in times of crisis (Anthony, 1984, 1987; Garmezy, 1994; Masten et al., 1990; Kauffman, Grunebaum, Cohler, & Gamer, 1979; Wolin & Wolin, 1993). Their solid assertiveness skills were an important strength that helped shield them from becoming clinically depressed (Garmezy, 1981, 1994; Hauser, Allen, & Golden, 2006; Masten et al., 1990; Masten & Garmezy, 1985; Seligman et al., 1995). In his St. Louis Risk Research Project with inner-city African American children, Anthony (1984, 1987) found that many of these children sought out and established a relationship with a charismatic or inspirational person in their community who "turned them on," sustained them, and continued to have long-lasting effects on them throughout their lives.

Most of the researchers observed that the resilient children's social competence served to help build their self-esteem and contributed to their success in school (Garmezy, 1994; Masten et al., 1990; Werner & Smith, 1982, 1992). Most of the emotional needs for some of the resilient children in these studies were met through their social involvement with concerned neighbors, teachers, clergy, and friends' parents.

Clinically speaking, we can capitalize on a child's strong social skills by incorporating his or her close friends, inspirational others, and other concerned adults in the treatment process as consultants. These consultants may offer the therapist, the child, and his or her parents some useful ideas about how to solve the presenting problem and better cope with life stressors. For children who have poor social skills, we can use role playing to teach assertiveness skills. The child's friends can be used as participants in the role-playing exercises and can serve as a natural relapse prevention support team between family sessions (Selekman, 2005, 2009).

Supportive and Responsible Caretakers

Most research on high-risk children challenges the widely held belief among social scientists and mental health professionals that these children lack a caring and responsible adult in their lives. In fact, many of the studies reviewed indicated that these children received considerable attention from responsible caretakers in their early years of development and throughout their childhood. Even children who had a mentally ill, alcoholic, or drug-impaired parent described times when their parent was very loving and supportive and met their needs (Anthony, 1987; Bleuler, 1978; Kauffman et al., 1979; Wolin & Wolin, 1993). In some cases, a relative, an adult friend of the family, or the nonsymptomatic parent assumed the main caretaker role for the child. Kauffman et al. (1979) observed in their study that non-symptomatic parents played a critical role in helping their at-risk children function and cope well with family stressors. Many of the supportive and responsible caretaking adults in the studies maintained optimistic parental explanatory styles (Seligman et al., 1995). These parental figures displayed unconditional positive regard, were flexible, modeled the importance of being optimistic when faced with life's struggles, and taught their children how to separate one isolated failure from other experiences and to challenge their pessimistic views (Murray & Fortinberry, 2006; Anthony, 1987; Bleuler, 1978; Garmezy, 1994; Kauffman et al., 1979; Wolin & Wolin, 1993).

In the clinical arena, this research finding provides empirical support for educating parents about the importance of adopting an optimistic parenting style and demonstrates how such education can greatly influence their children's optimism and behavior when they are faced with stressful life events (Murray & Fortinberry, 2006). In fact, Seligman and his colleagues (1995) found in their Penn Resiliency Research Project that both parental and teachers' optimism serves as a key protective factor in reducing the risk of children's developing difficulties with depression and anxiety. Furthermore, the researchers also found that teaching the children in their study *disputation* skills—that is, specific ways of challenging self-defeating and irrational thoughts triggered by negative and stressful life events—they were better able to develop and maintain an optimistic mindset, to avoid experiencing these emotional difficulties, and to perform better academically than the control group did in the study. Assigning parents observation tasks to keep track of what the child does that is "right" and responsible, asking questions about past successes, and having the parents visualize positive treatment outcomes can help create a therapeutic climate of optimism for the child and his or her family. For families that tend to be overly focused on negative developments, I immediately assign the construction of a *compliment box* (Selekman, 2006, 2009). On a daily basis, family members are responsible for writing on slips of paper one or more compliments for other family members and placing them in an old shoebox with a slit in the top. At dinnertime, family members can take turns blindly reaching into the box and read aloud each other's compliments on the slips of paper. The compliment box system helps to reduce blaming and negativity in the family and creates a more positive atmosphere in the home. Finally, grandparents, other significant extended family members, and close friends from the child's social network can be used as expert consultants in sessions and for added support between visits.

The good news is that children—despite being raised in high-risk family and social environments—can and do survive adverse life experiences. Some children are born naturally resilient, while others are quite skilled at creating nurturing support systems for themselves outside their families. The research on resilient children has uncovered many ways that we, as therapists, can help strengthen family relationships and help children find strength and success beyond their families.

Positive Psychology: Studying What Is *Right* with People and Empowering Them to Flourish in Their Lives

In common with solution-focused brief therapy, "positive psychology" mainly emphasizes what is *right* with people. Martin Seligman, Mihaly Csikszentmihalyi, Christopher Peterson, and Barbara Fredrickson are the major pioneers and leading researchers of this revolutionary new movement focused on wellness in the field of psychology (Fredrickson, 2006, 2008, 2009; Kashdan, 2009; Snyder & Lopez, 2007; Peterson, 2006; Peterson & Seligman, 2004; Keyes & Haidt, 2003; Seligman, 2002). These researchers asked themselves, "Why are we not studying people who are flourishing in the world and learn what their secrets are for having meaningful, productive, and highly satisfying lives?" Peterson and Seligman (2004) took it a step further and identified in their research 24 human strengths and 6 major virtues. As part of their intensive effort to identify and define these strengths and virtues they carefully reviewed the written work of great philosophers, spiritual leaders, and historic figures. Peterson (2006) developed two instruments that can be accessed online (at *www.viastrengths. org*) designed to identify an individual's top-five *signature strengths,* permitting him or her also to print out in order of potency the remaining 19 strengths. The adult version of this questionnaire is called *Values in Action (VIA) Classification of Strengths.* The older child and adolescent version of this questionnaire (which is more streamlined) is called the *Inventory of Strengths for Youth.* In my clinical practice, after building a relationship with new clients, I have both parents and children (age 10 or older) answer the questionnaires online and bring in to our next session their respective printouts identifying not only their top-five signature strengths but also the order of the remaining 19 strengths. The benefit of answering these questionnaires are threefold:

1. We learn about key signature strengths that clients may not have identified at pretreatment or in their first sessions, which can be both illuminating and empowering to them.
2. We learn about latent strengths that clients can begin to develop and use in all areas of their lives.
3. Once clients' top-five signature as well as latent strengths have been identified, these can be used in co-designing, tailor fitting, and implementing therapeutic experiments to help them achieve their goals.

Cszikszentmihalyi (1990, 1997), in studying artists and other professionals immersed in their work and feeling most productive, observed that they all shared the same common feeling, which he called "flow." It was during this segment of their work experience that the professionals lost track of time and were totally oblivious to anything else occurring in their immediate surroundings. Similar to Buddhist monks who have meditated for decades, when these professionals reached their deepest meditative states they experienced a sense of timelessness and nirvana, and they consistently reported that they did their best work while in this flow state. In my work with children, I want to know what their key flow state activities are and have them increase their involvement in them if both their parents and they think this would be a beneficial thing to do, particularly as a strategy to cope with the stressors in their lives. Flow state activities can take many forms, including building models and other constructs, playing an instrument, dancing, or doing artwork.

Fredrickson (2006, 2008, 2009) has developed the *broaden-and-build theory of positive emotions,* having found in her research that positive emotions both broaden people's ideas about positive actions and open their awareness to a wider range of thoughts and actions. Positive emotions open our minds and hearts to be more present with others, to take more positive risks, and to be better and more creative problem solvers. An added bonus of striving to provide ourselves with daily doses of positive emotion is that it also strengthens our immune systems (Fredrickson, 2009). When working with parents, I have them strive to create positive and upbeat home environments and celebrate their children's daily successes, whether at home or at school. I educate parents on the important role that positive emotions play in helping their children flourish and be better problem solvers.

These positive psychologists have helped develop several therapeutic activities designed to reduce negative emotions, trigger positive emotions, raise happiness levels, maintain an optimistic mindset in the face of adversity and stressful life events, and assist individuals in leading more meaningful and fulfilling lives. Two positive psychology activities I use regularly with children are the *you at your best story* and the *plan out your perfect day exercise* (Peterson, 2006; Seligman & Dean, 2003). The first involves having the child write a short story (of three to four paragraphs) about something he or she has accomplished (and of which he or she is proud) either very recently or in the past. In a concrete way, I like to teach children about *agency thinking* and *pathway thinking* (McDermott & Snyder, 1999). By "agency thinking," I mean how the child activates him- or herself to pursue a particular goal or particular objective. Agency thinking can include useful self-talk, visualization, or even inviting one's close friends to help one get fired up—almost like a cheerleading squad. Pathway thinking consists in knowing the right steps to take to accomplish a given goal or objective. After the child writes a you-at-your-best short story of success, I have him or her underline with colored pencils (using two different colors) both their agency and pathway thinking and bring the story to our next session. In reviewing the story together, the therapist helps the child see how he or she could use bits of agency and pathway thinking to perhaps achieve other current goals or to change something else in his or her life.

The "plan out your perfect day" exercise is designed to co-create positive self-fulfilling scenarios with clients. The night before each selected day, the child plans out what his or her most perfect day would look like. This exercise entails deciding what needs to be accomplished, identifying what types of pleasurable and meaningful activities he or she needs to engage in, and whom he or she needs to see or be with that would trigger positive emotions and put him or her in good spirits. The clearer and more concrete the child's road map for success is, the more likely he or she will be able to make most of these things happen, if not all of them. At the end of each day, the child rates the day on a scale from 10 to 1, with 10 being "the best day of my life" and 1 "the worst day of my life" (see Chapter 4 for more details on the rating scale). It is best to have the child engage in this exercise over a 2-week period, thereby providing ample time for both the child and his or her parents to see what patterns emerge (i.e., what activities and people trigger the most positive emotions, resulting in days rated 6 or better; or, conversely, which activities and people need to be steered clear of). On a cautionary note, it is important to let children and their parents know that things happen beyond our control and sometimes despite our best intentions we fall short of our goals or don't accomplish everything we set out to do on any given day. It is important to emphasize that it is the effort that counts and that low-rated days are not a reflection of the child's lack of strengths or willpower. Finally, it is advisable to map out a "Plan B" with the child and the parents. Whenever the child's day begins to take a negative turn, he or she can then spell out the steps that one might take to save the day. By doing so, the child is encouraged to think ahead and will be better equipped to constructively manage the situation and become more resilient in the future.

An Evolving Integrative Solution-Focused Brief Therapy Model for Children and Adolescents: The Collaborative Strengths-Based Brief Therapy Approach

Like all therapy models, the basic solution-focused brief therapy approach has its limitations with certain types of child and adolescent cases, even after exhausting all the therapeutic options within the model. Having worked with the solution-focused brief therapy model since 1986 and experienced great clinical results using it, I was discovering that there were certain child and adolescent case situations where using the model in its pure form was not leading to the kinds of changes the families desired, even after fostering cooperative relationships with them and negotiating achievable treatment goals. Furthermore, I was also finding myself feeling stifled by the base model's being too formulaic, that I was limited to specific categories of questions and therapeutic tasks and not free to bring in ideas from other therapeutic approaches or to contribute my own creative ideas and therapeutic experiments. Before discussing three clinical case situations in which it may be necessary to expand the basic model and integrate and apply therapeutic ideas from individual and other family therapy approaches, I discuss some of the limitations of the solution-focused brief therapy approach with children.

To begin with, the basic solution-focused brief therapy approach is a "talk therapy," which does not mesh well with young children's natural tendencies to express themselves best through nonverbal means (e.g., play and art activities). Berg and Steiner (2003), however, have begun to break new ground in this area by developing art and play activities for children that are informed by the solution-focused brief therapy approach. Young children are not capable of cognitively understanding such abstract concepts as "miracles" and "goals." Some of these children may respond better to the use of *an imaginary wand or crystal ball* (toy ones can be used as well). The solution-focused questions in general may be incomprehensible or too difficult to grasp for some children, even after the therapist simplifies the wording of the questions. Many solution-focused therapists believe that simply altering parental beliefs and interactions with the child will lead to the latter's changing. This assumption is based on the systems concept of *wholism*; that is, if you change one part of the family system, the other members of the family will change as well (de Shazer, 1985). Most solution-focused therapists, and family therapists for that matter, would not consider the idea that children can serve as the catalyst for changing their parents' and family interactions through the use of family play and art activities. de Shazer (1988) has suggested that therapists should draw from the set of "all known tasks" once they have exhausted all the standard therapeutic tasks typically used within the basic solution-focused model. What he does not provide for therapists, however, are recommended therapeutic interventions and strategies from other therapy approaches that may be useful with particular types of children's problems and clinical case situations. I began to ask myself the following question: "Why do I have to stay so loyal to the solution-focused brief therapy approach that I have to wait until I have exhausted all the possibilities within the model before integrating some new ideas or trying a completely different approach?" I started giving myself permission to improvise more and to bring in compatible therapeutic tools and strategies from other therapy approaches. As a result, I began getting better clinical outcomes with some of my toughest child and adolescent clients.

At this point, I present three case situations in which I found it helpful to expand the basic solution-focused model and to be more therapeutically flexible:

1. The parents change their ways of viewing and interacting with the client; however, the child remains symptomatic.
2. The parents' treatment goals are achieved, but the changes in the client are not perceived by them as sufficiently "newsworthy"; thus, their outmoded beliefs about the child and their situation remain intact.
3. Multiple helping professionals are involved with the case, many of whom are highly pessimistic about the client and his or her family's ability to change.

By expanding the basic solution-focused brief therapy model and being therapeutically flexible, the therapist can adequately manage each of these situations. In the first case scenario, mindfulness meditation, visualization, disputation skills training, positive psychology exercises, and family play and art therapy tasks can open the door to a child's inner world and help remove constraints or blocks in affective or cognitive areas of functioning that may be preventing symptom alleviation.

In the second case scenario, there may be family secrets, unresolved traumas and losses, or other family concerns not being talked about, or the therapist may have blocked family members from sharing their long, problem-saturated stories by overemphasizing positive talk in sessions. Two common parental concerns typically voiced in these types of situations reflect either my reluctance to accept and confirm the DSM-IV-TR label to which the parents are committed or my imputed failure to take their child's chronic presenting problems "seriously enough." By asserting that the therapist is not taking their child's presenting problems seriously enough, the parents may be trying to express that they want the therapist to work with their child individually or on a longer-term basis. Open-ended conversational questions (Anderson, 1997; Anderson & Goolishian, 1988a, 1991a, 1991b; Selekman, 2005, 2009) can be used to give family members ample space to share their concerns and the "not yet said," such as disclos-ing a family secret or a painful life event. Another option would be to use a "reflecting team" (Andersen, 1991, 1995) to offer the family a multiplicity of views on their family concerns and difficulties. This alternative could help loosen up fixed family beliefs and open up space for family members to view their situation differently.

In the third case scenario, a therapist hosting a family–multiple helper collaborative meeting or attending a multidisciplinary school meeting may come across as too optimistic or overzealous about reporting the positives in a chronic child case, and group conversations and input from the more pessi-mistic helpers attending these meetings may be shut down. Therefore, when hosting or attending such meetings, therapists, no matter what their theo-retical persuasion, should adopt the Buddhist stance of "don't know mind," which is a true "both/and" perspective (Selekman, 2005). As the hosting therapist, he or she must be able to suspend his or her assumptions about the helpers' and family's concerns to learn to view them as assumptions and not facts, and to hold them in front of the group for all to see (Scharmer, 2007; Selekman, 2005, 2006; Isaacs, 1993). Similar to attending to the concerns of a pessimistic family member, the therapist needs to create a safe space for the pessimistic helpers to voice their concerns about the case. It is important to remember that there are many ways to view a child or family's present-ing problems and that consensus in the family–multiple helper collaborative meetings or among school staff is not required in order to have effective group problem solving and to generate new family narratives. Finally, thera-pists need to view these concerned helping professionals as allies in the treat-ment process who bring to us and the clients a wealth of strengths, expertise, and wisdom from working with similar children and families in the past that we can tap to cogenerate high-quality solutions together.

A final reason for expanding the basic solution-focused brief therapy model and utilizing a more integrative approach is that such expansion increases our repertoire of interpretation schemes and offers us a broader range of therapeutic options when intervening with clients and their families. Research also indicates that there is compelling evidence for the effective-ness of integrative family therapy approaches for children and adolescents with behavioral problems (Henggeler, Schoenwald, Borduin, Rowland, & Cunningham, 2009; Lebow, 2005; Lebow & Gurman, 1996).

Applying the Collaborative Strengths-Based Brief Therapy Approach with Children

What is unique about collaborative strengths-based brief therapy is that it is a flexible family competency-based model that targets interventions at all levels of the child social realm and logically brings together the best elements of change-based and meaning-based postmodern systemic therapy approaches. Although my model continues to evolve, it presently integrates the best elements of MRI (Mental Research Institute) brief problem-focused therapy (Fisch & Schlanger, 1999; Fisch, Weakland, & Segal, 1982; Watzlawick et al., 1974); narrative therapy (White, 1995, 2007; Freeman, Epston, & Lobovits, 1997; Epston, 1998; White & Epston, 1990); collaborative language systems therapy (Anderson, 1996, 1997; Anderson & Goolishian, 1988a, 1988b, 1991a, 1991b); client-directed, outcome-informed therapy (Murphy & Duncan, 2007; Duncan & Miller, 2000; Hubble, Duncan, & Miller, 1999); positive psychology (Fredrickson, 2006, 2008, 2009; Kashdan, 2009; Snyder & Lopez, 2007; Peterson, 2006; Peterson & Seligman, 2004; Seligman & Dean, 2003; Keyes & Haidt, 2003; Seligman, 2002; Csikszentmihalyi & Csikszentmihalyi, 2006; Csikszentmihalyi, 1990, 1997); Buddhist mindfulness practices and teachings (Lantieri & Goleman, 2008; Hanh, 1991, 1997, 1998, 2003, 2007); Navajo First Nation healing and teaching practices (Alvord & Cohen-Van Pelt, 2000); cognitive therapy (Seligman et al., 1995); the stages of change model (Norcross, 2008; Prochaska, Norcross, & DiClemente, 1994); the multiple intelligences framework (Gardner, 1993, 2004); interpersonal neurobiological therapeutic ideas (Siegel & Hartzell, 2003); and art, drama, and creative writing expressive therapy ideas (Selekman, 2005, 2009; Malchiodi, 2003; Bailey, 2000; Wachtel, 1994; Gil, 1994). Clients take the lead in determining their treatment goals, session agendas, who they think should attend sessions, the frequency of visits, and in each session are free to choose from a menu of therapeutic activities that they wish to try between visits.

The collaborative strengths-based brief therapy approach is sensitive to gender power imbalance, cultural, spiritual-wellness, and wider societal social injustice issues that often play a part in the development and continuance of human difficulties. The collaborative strengths-based therapist views the therapeutic encounter as being a political enterprise, particularly with women and clients of color who are marginalized and disempowered in our society. In partnership with clients, the therapist actively collaborates both in and out of sessions with involved and concerned members of their social networks and helping professionals from larger systems. Thus, this ecological family therapy approach targets interventions at the individual, family, social network, larger-systems, and community levels. In this section, I present the major therapeutic components of the collaborative strengths-based brief therapy model as applied to clinical work with children and their families. Case examples are provided.

Honoring Clients' Stories and Concerns

The renowned philosopher and educator John Dewey believed that any problem that is truly well defined is already half-solved (Parnes, 1992). For a number of reasons (e.g., managed health care), there is a strong tendency among therapists to try to find the quick solution for their clients' problems without taking the time to determine collaboratively with the clients what the "real" or "right" problem is. Leading proponents of the basic solution-focused brief therapy model argue that therapists do not need to know a great deal about their clients' problems to solve them and that therapists should avoid at all costs engaging in "problem talk" (Berg & de Shazer, 1991) with their clients. However, going with an ill-defined client problem (or goal, for that matter) will make any constructed or selected solution ineffective in the long run. In this light, zeroing in on the right client problem is equivalent to finding the right solution for resolving it. Problems and solutions are close relatives and do not always need to be separated for effective problem solving (Van Gundy, 1988).

Numerous studies have provided empirical support for the key importance of defining the problem properly and precisely in creative problem solving (Csikszentmihalyi & Getzels, 1970; Getzels & Csikszentmihalyi, 1976a, 1976b; Moore, 1985; Hall, 1995; Isenberg, 2009; Roberto, 2009). Doug Hall (1995), a creativity expert and master marketing consultant, found that deferred judgment, or *incubating,* is one of the most important steps in developing creative ideas and high-quality solutions. Csikszentmihalyi and Getzels (1970) investigated the relationship between problem defining and artistic creativity. The artists in their study were instructed to produce a drawing using a variety of objects that had been placed on a table in front of them; a panel of well-known artists and art critics judged the drawings. The results of the study suggested that the artists who approached the task with no set solution in mind and who avoided using predetermined patterns or formulas produced more original and creative drawings than did those who began with a predetermined approach. Interestingly, the most highly rated artists spent considerably more time than the others manipulating the objects on the table. Two important dicta can be extracted from this study that should inform our clinical practices: (1) take the time to determine with the family what it considers to be the "right" problem to begin addressing first, and (2) avoid using a predetermined formula for problem solving.

Frank Gehry, the great modern architect, when offered a new building project, spends a lot of time during the early stage of the design process playing with ideas about the task at hand, doodling and building models of his most intriguing notions to gain as much knowledge as possible about the problem or task. The more he plays with all of these different ideas about the problem or task at hand with his doodles and models, Gehry increases his knowledge about it, and potential solutions to take form, paving the way for a well-constructed and unique final product (Isenberg, 2009).

Families that have been oppressed by their problems for a long time and have experienced multiple treatment failures may feel invalidated and unheard when a therapist fails to give them ample space to share their long, problem-saturated stories. According to Anderson (1996), "Understanding too quickly cuts a client's story short and risks eliciting the story that a therapist wants to hear, rather than the story a client wants to tell" (p. 202). Throughout my professional career, I have worked with numerous children and adolescents who had extensive treatment histories and yet were given little opportunity to voice their individual concerns, expectations, and what specifically they wanted to work on changing individually or with their family situations. Fraser (1995) argues that, unless we take the time to elicit from clients and families their attempted solutions and views of the problem, we will have no idea when their problems are really solved, and we run the risk of replicating unsuccessful attempted solutions that have not worked in the past. The case below helps illustrate the importance of both taking the time to collaboratively determine with the family the "right" problem to work on first and making room for their story about the problem situation.

> Ellen, a 10-year-old Caucasian girl, was brought in for therapy by her mother for attention-deficit disorder (ADD), "stealing," "lying," "doing poorly" in school, "fighting" with her siblings, and "breaking" her mother's "rules." According to her mother, Ellen had been sexually molested when she was 6 years old by an uncle. Sensing the mother's strong feelings of hopelessness and despair about being able to help her daughter, I gave her plenty of opportunity to share her problem-saturated story. I also gathered detailed information about her attempted solutions, particularly what past therapists had tried to do with Ellen and her mother that the mother did not find helpful. After receiving ample time to ventilate her frustration about former therapists and the problem situation, the mother became much more receptive to clarifying with me what she perceived as the right problem to work on first. She believed that Ellen engaged in all these objectionable behaviors because of "the trauma" of Ellen's being sexually molested at the age of 6. The stealing behavior in particular began at this time, which was the mother's "greatest source of irritation." The mother agreed with me that it would be too daunting a task to try to change all of Ellen's behaviors at once. For both the mother and Ellen, the right problem to work on changing first was the stealing behavior.

After hearing the mother's frustrations with past therapists and Ellen's chronic behavior problems, it was clear to me that the mother would have felt slighted and would have viewed me as being too much like all the over-zealous therapists she had seen in the past if I had moved too quickly to talk about exceptions or prematurely asked the miracle question (which, in essence, is "What would be different if, by a miracle, everything were suddenly okay?"; de Shazer, 1988; see Chapter 2, this volume). By giving the mother ample time and space to share her long, problem-saturated story without interruption, I was in a much better place to define the problem to work on first. Future therapy sessions were focused on systematically stabilizing each of Ellen's behavior problems and collaborating with concerned school personnel.

Finally, although pure solution-focused therapists do spend time consolidating clients' treatment gains throughout the treatment process, they also unfortunately tend to steer clients away from sharing concerns that may be unrelated to the primary treatment goal. From a solution-focused purist perspective, this type of extraneous exploration would be considered "problem talk" to be avoided at all costs. Not addressing these concerns, however, could lead to clients getting derailed and feeling as though they were back at square one. Therefore, it is crucial that therapists conduct sessions in a balanced manner, where we both amplify and consolidate clients' gains and we *cover the back door* by making room for them to share any concerns or new problems as they arise, addressing these difficulties immediately (Selekman, 2009).

Doing What Works: Integrating Key Research Findings into Our Practices

Hubble, Duncan, and Miller's (1999) ground-breaking research and therapeutic ideas have enabled therapists to have better outcomes with a wide variety of treatment populations. These researchers took the four common factors found in successful treatment outcome research and developed streamlined questionnaires to measure their presence in a given session in the process of creating a treatment approach that they called *client-directed, outcome-informed therapy*. The four common factors are *the clients' extratherapeutic factors* (clients' strengths, theories of change, treatment preferences and expectations, self-generated pretreatment changes and effective coping strategies, stages of changes, and random events that had benefited them); *the therapeutic relationship* (such relationship skills as empathy, warmth, and validation and such structuring skills as the therapist's timing in the use of interventions, taking charge in sessions, and structuring of sessions as well as overall competence); *expectancy and hope* (how well the therapist conveys with confidence his or her client's ability to change while instilling hope); and *therapeutic models and techniques* (the ability to create a good fit between the therapeutic model and techniques employed and the client's unique characteristics). Interestingly, the variable category that counts the most in terms of successful treatment outcomes is the client's extratherapeutic factors, while the second most important is the therapeutic relationship or alliance. The most surprising finding in close to 50 years of psychotherapy outcome research is the fact that therapists' beloved treatment models and techniques account for only about 15% of treatment success!

The questionnaires Hubble et al. developed that have been so well validated are called the *Session Rating Scale (SRS)* and *Outcome Rating Scale (ORS)*. The SRS assesses the quality of the therapeutic relationship with the client—that is, whether or not a strong therapeutic alliance has been established—while the ORS solicits feedback from clients throughout the course of treatment on whether they are experiencing change process or not (Miller, Mee-Lee, Plum, & Hubble, 2005). These two important inputs from clients help therapists carefully tailor treatment options to clients' unique needs throughout the course of treatment, which helps prevent premature dropouts from occurring and optimizes the likelihood of positive treatment outcomes. Some therapists and clients feel uncomfortable with or do not like to fill out questionnaires. In those situations, therapists may solicit the same information verbally at each session and make the necessary adjustments based on clients' feedback.

Since the inception of managed health care and owing to reductions in federal and state funding for mental healthcare, there has been a strong push for agencies, mental health clinics, and hospital-based programs for children and adolescents to employ empirically validated individual and family treatment approaches. For a time, solution-focused brief therapy was being highly touted by managed care companies and health maintenance organizations as one of the most strongly endorsed treatment approaches. Many of these companies provided extensive training opportunities in solution-focused brief therapy for both their in-house staff and provider networks. Over time, however, such empirically validated therapy models as cognitive-behavioral therapy (CBT; Weisz, McCarty, & Valeri, 2006; Compton, Burns, Egger, & Robertson, 2002), multisystemic therapy (Henggeler et al., 2009), functional family therapy (Sexton & Alexander, 2005), and brief strategic family therapy (Horigan et al., 2005) came to be more in vogue because they all had strong outcome data to back their efficacy as the treatments of choice for child and adolescent behavioral difficulties. To my knowledge, there have not been any well-controlled experimental research studies with large samples of children that combined both qualitative and quantitative methods with the solution-focused brief therapy model. There are, however, numerous qualitative studies conducted with both the solution-focused brief therapy and, more recently, the collaborative strengths-based brief therapy models where clients rated their treatment experiences very highly (Selekman, 2009; Selekman & Shulem, 2007; Macdonald, 2007; Gingerich & Eisengart, 2000).

The just cited empirically validated family therapy approaches have clearly demonstrated the importance of being integrative, working with subsystems (i.e., allowing separate session time for parents and children), being sensitive to child developmental and family life cycle issues, and intervening in the clients' social ecologies (collaborating with involved helping professionals from larger systems and concerned others in their social networks). However, some of the limitations posed to mental health professionals by having to use these empirically validated approaches *exclusively* are (1) having to stay rigidly true to the model with only minimal integration of other insights, (2) having one's own creativity needlessly stifled, and (3) with certain approaches having to be available 24/7, which is highly unrealistic for many therapists. Ethically it is my contention that, as practitioners, we should never permit research considerations to outweigh the unique needs of our clients. Furthermore, one-size-fits-all clinical thinking clearly does not work with every child and family. We need to allow our preferred therapy models to evolve, be flexible and integrative therapists, and look for logical ways to combine the best elements of empirically validated treatment approaches with our own clinical experience and wisdom regarding what works with particular types of child behavioral and family difficulties.

Applying the Multiple Intelligences Model to Family Therapy with Children

I have written in earlier works about the many benefits of utilizing Howard Gardner's *multiple intelligences model* in psychotherapy (Selekman, 2005, 2006, 2009). Gardner (1993, 2004) has identified 10 distinct human intelligences, as follows: *linguistic* (likes to write poetry and creative stories and read), *logical-mathematical* (strong analytical and mathematical skills; likes puzzles, science, computers), *musical* (likes to play an instrument and/or sing), *bodily-kinesthetic* (expresses self best through movement; may like to dance or play sports; likes acting and drama), *visual-spatial* (likes art and photography; strong visualization skills; inventive and has strong sense of imagination), *interpersonal* (strong social skills, natural leadership abilities; likes group projects), *intrapersonal* (introspective; likes journaling about thoughts and feelings), *naturalist* (loves learning about and being out in nature; loves animals, has pets; likes camping), *existential* (searches for the meaning of events and things; curious and reflective), and *spiritual* (may be very religious and believes in a higher power; has learned to believe in him- or herself and have faith during tough times).

The beauty (and special utility) of the multiple intelligences model is that it can aid therapists in matching what they do with clients' particular learning styles and main channels for expressing themselves, thereby capitalizing on their key strength areas and helping to guide the therapeutic experiment construction process. As a nice complement to solution-focused ideas, the multiple intelligences model takes capitalizing on children's and other family members' strengths *to the next level*. The case below illustrates how, by capitalizing on a child's key intelligence area, the therapist was able to custom-tailor a therapeutic experiment more precisely to the client.

Antonio, a 9-year-old from Spain, was having grave difficulty coping with his parents' recent divorce. Since the divorce, he had not seen his father for 8 months. He had been picking on his 7-year-old sister Cecilia, not following his mother's rules, talking to her in a disrespectful way, and engaging in disruptive behaviors in his classroom at school. Lucinda, the mother, openly admitted that she had been yelling at and punishing Antonio quite a bit lately. The family was struggling financially as well. Lucinda had recently lost her job working in a restaurant. She was now cleaning houses in her community to earn some money. One area Antonio excelled at was playing soccer. According to the mother, he was the top scorer in his local community league for children. I really captured Antonio's undivided attention when I invited him to talk about his favorite professional soccer star, the Spanish team, and his best game. The whole room lit up at that point, and he was "all smiles." I learned that his best game of the whole season was when his six goals had won the league championship for his team. He also shared with me that the professional soccer team he really disliked was Barcelona because they seemed to be the champions every year. Learning that Antonio's key intelligence area was *bodily-kinesthetic* and that soccer was his life's passion, I proposed a family soccer ritual for them to experiment with over the next week. The major objective over the next week was for Antonio to see how many "goals" he could score with his mother in 1 week's time. When asked what he would call his team, he said, "My Mother's Team." Lucinda smiled, obviously touched by Antonio's coming up with this team name. The team he was trying to beat and was pitted against was his arch enemy, "Barcelona." Lucinda came up with the scoring criteria. He would score a goal with her by doing any of the following: no phone calls from his teacher about getting in trouble at school; not picking on his sister; and not breaking her house rules and talking to her in a nicer and more respectful way. Whenever he engaged in formerly troublesome behaviors, the Barcelona team would get goal points placed in their column on the chart keeping track of both teams' scores. Antonio did not like the idea of Barcelona beating his team and appeared fired up to lead his team to victory. With the help of Lucinda's supportive coaching and patience, Antonio successfully led "My Mother's Team" to victory over Barcelona. In fact, he set a personal best scoring record—20 goals in 1 week's time! Lucinda was very proud of him and also wanted to let me know that Antonio's sister had also had a few positive "assists" with some of his goals. Lucinda was very proud of Antonio for working really hard to turn his behavior around. She also discovered that they needed to play more together as a family. Finally, now Lucinda had a system she could put in place if Antonio began to have difficulties again in the future.

Using Family Art and Play Therapy Techniques

For decades, child and family therapists have vigorously debated which treatment modalities are best suited to children. Child therapists would argue that the child's behavioral and emotional difficulties are caused by faulty parenting, which results in intrapsychic conflicts, developmental arrest, and/or possible psychic deficits. By employing art and play therapy methods, the therapist provides a safe climate for children to play out their conflicts and uses his or her relationship with the child to try to heal the psychic deficits (Kohut, 1971). The parents are typically seen separately or by another therapist. Family therapists would argue that the child's problems should be viewed through a broader lens. The "problem" child's symptoms or dramatic behavioral difficulties may serve a particular function in the family (Haley, 1987; Madanes, 1981) and may be attributable to structural problems in the family (Minuchin, 1974), perpetuated by problem-maintaining parental attempted solutions (Watzlawick et al., 1974), and maintained by constraining beliefs and dominant oppressive stories (White, 2007; Epston, 1998; White & Epston, 1990). Most family therapists would actively involve the parents in the treatment process. Depending on the model being used, the family therapist focuses most of his or her attention on changing parental outmoded beliefs about the child and altering family patterns of interaction that may be maintaining the problems. Some family therapists focus most of their therapeutic attention on changing the parents and spend very little time interacting with the child alone.

It is my contention that both the individual child therapy and the family therapy perspectives offer therapeutic tools and strategies that complement one another—as long as what the therapist chooses to do therapeutically is purposive and accords with both the child's and family's goals. In general, children (and particularly young children) like to play and rarely respond well to talk therapies alone. Sometimes the parents' ways of viewing and interacting with the child change but yet the child remains symptomatic. One therapeutic option in such cases is to use art and play therapy techniques. However, rather than seeing children alone to perform these experiments, I have found it most advantageous to include the parents as both participants and observers in these activities.

Wachtel (1994) and Gil (1994) use a similar format in their clinical work with children and their families. With some cases, it might be a novel experience for both the child and the parents to play with one another or to create a family mural or collage together. Family play and art therapy experiments can take the sting out of presenting problems, reduce stress levels, loosen up fixed beliefs about the problem, and alter the family dance in which the problem is embedded. The therapist also gains access to destructive problem interactions and family conflicts which he or she can address directly in a relaxed context in which anything is possible. Sometimes children's art creations can serve as the catalyst for changing and healing their parents. The following case example illustrates this point.

> Sandra, a 6-year-old Caucasian girl, was brought for therapy by her parents, Bill and Evelyn, who were separated after their second marriage to each other. The couple separated after Bill began slapping and pushing Evelyn around when they got into an argument. Both parents were quick to point out their long history of arguing and getting physical with each other.
>
> Sandra lived with her mother and 10-month-old brother, Evan. Despite the parents' difficulties, they were both concerned about Sandra's passivity and wondered whether she was "depressed." Sandra appeared to be very timid and shy. Efforts to engage her went nowhere until I asked her to draw a picture of her family. The parents were quite shocked and even cried when they saw Sandra's drawing. Sandra drew a picture of her family floating in air around the interior of the house; she placed herself outside the front door. She drew very thick lines around the house and had the front door closed.
>
> Seeing this drawing proved to be an eye-opening and emotional experience for the parents. Sandra was also able to talk about how she did not feel "safe" when her parents were together. The child protection and local police departments had a history of involvement with this case and were still involved as a result of domestic disputes. Despite all the chaos in the home, the children were never physically harmed. By the end of the session, the parents were open to working on their problems with anger management, conflict resolution, and violent behavior. We established a no-violence contract as well. I also secured signed consent forms to collaborate with the child protection worker and a local police officer involved with their case.
>
> Through the use of the family portrait drawing, the parents in this case were confronted in a powerful way and began to take responsibility for their problematic behaviors. Sandra's drawing successfully reached a place in the parents' minds that served as the impetus for committing to changing their destructive behaviors. Interestingly enough, the parents disclosed in our session that no therapeutic intervention had ever had more of an "emotional impact" on them than Sandra's family portrait drawing.

Integrating Narrative Therapy Ideas

Michael White and David Epston's narrative therapy approach is quite compatible theoretically with the solution-focused brief therapy model in several ways. Both approaches share strong Batesonian theoretical influences, are family empowerment models, and capitalize on family members' strengths and resources. The leading proponents of these models believe strongly that children should be advisers when the subject is their own lives (de Shazer & White, 1996). However, since some important elements of narrative therapy are unique to it, I have found it beneficial to integrate them into the basic solution-focused brief therapy model.

Narrative therapists approach cases with a political lens; that is, they bring gender, cultural, and social justice issues into the therapy room. The narrative therapy approach tends to be more meaning-based and historical and makes more room for the family's problem story than does the basic solution-focused brief therapy approach (White, 2007; Epston, 1998; Chang & Phillips, 1993; de Shazer & White, 1996; Jenkins, 1994). By taking the time to elicit the family's story about the problem, narrative therapists can learn a great deal about family beliefs and the various ways family members influence and are influenced by the oppressive problem. With this important information, the narrative therapist can engage in externalizing conversations (White, 1995, 2007; Epston, 1998; White & Epston, 1990) with the family to tease out story lines of competency that can help liberate them from their dominant problem-saturated situation. Externalizing the problem in this way is an effective therapeutic pathway to pursue with families that do not respond well to the basic solution-focused brief therapy approach, have been oppressed by the problem for a long time, have experienced multiple treatment failures, and describe the problem as having a life of its own. Often families that are therapy veterans such as these do not notice times when they are not pushed around by the problem because such events do not fit with their dominant problem-saturated stories. Some therapy veterans may also experience a solution-focused therapist's over-emphasis on positive talk as not taking their problem story seriously, being sarcastic, and/or minimizing their plight.

The following case example demonstrates the effectiveness of externalization (White & Epston, 1990) with a 9-year-old African American boy (Jimmy) and his parents, for whom Jimmy's chronic stealing habit of 3 years had become oppressive. I was the fifth therapist the parents had taken Jimmy to see for his stealing problem.

> Jimmy had been stealing money from his parents since he was 6 years of age. According to his father, he also had a long history of using his "slick fingers" to take things from his teachers' desks. Throughout

the initial family interview, the father called Jimmy's stealing problem "slick fingers." The mother referred to Jimmy as being a "slick thief," able to find their money hidden in shoe boxes and other inconspicuous places around the house.

The use of the miracle question (de Shazer, 1988), coping, and pessimistic sequence questions (Selekman, 2005; Berg & Miller, 1992) proved to be unproductive in the interviewing process; so, I decided to capitalize on the father's externalizing of the problem into "slick fingers." The "slick fingers" construction of the stealing problem was also much more treatable than the parents' other explanations, such as "He must have a character flaw," "We must have spoiled him," and "He is never happy with what he has."

The parents and Jimmy both shared feelings of frustration and hopelessness about ever being able to conquer this problem, with Jimmy readily disclosing that he had "no control" over his stealing problem. By consciously externalizing the problem in our conversation, the parents began to see how they and Jimmy were being victimized by "slick fingers." As a way to help empower the family to win back control of their lives over "slick fingers," I offered them an "honesty test ritual" (Durrant & Coles, 1991; Epston, 1989) to experiment with.

The parents were instructed to leave money out in various locations around the house. After securing a signed consent form from the parents, I contacted Jimmy's teacher to let her know what we were doing to help defeat "slick fingers." The teacher placed previously stolen items on top of her desk for 1 week to test Jimmy's ability to stand up to "slick fingers" and not allow that urge to push him around. I emphasized to the parents, Jimmy, and the teacher the importance of this being a team effort. I also pointed out that stealing habits do not die easily.

One week later, the family came back in good spirits, reporting a perfect week. Jimmy openly admitted that on two occasions he almost succumbed to "slick fingers'" attempts to brainwash him to steal, but he fought back with useful self-talk. The parents also admitted that they had some moments of distrust with Jimmy but avoided the temptation to confront him. The teacher had reported to the parents that there were no signs that "slick fingers" had gotten the best of Jimmy in 1 week's time.

Since the honesty test strategy proved to be so successful, I continued to use it throughout the course of family therapy. I ended up seeing the family four more times. In our final session together, I threw a party for Jimmy and his parents to celebrate their victory over "slick fingers." The teacher joined the festivities as well.

One of the most compelling features of White and Epston's (1990) narrative approach is the use of an "audience" of friends, relatives, and significant others in the identified child client's life to bear witness to his or her competencies and to pioneer a new direction within the family and in other social contexts. The telling and retelling of the child's new evolving story of competency is empowering and can create possibilities (White, 1995, 2007; Epston, 1998; de Shazer & White, 1996). The therapist also is decentralizing him- or herself within the life of the family by having key members of the clients' social network serve as their main support structure for staying on track and accentuating their progress.

White and his colleagues have developed several effective therapeutic rituals that can empower families to gain their freedom from the problem's reign over them (White, 2007; Epston, 1989, 1998; Durrant & Coles, 1991; White & Epston, 1990). One quite effective ritual with children's behavioral problems is the *habit control ritual*. Using this therapeutic ritual, family members keep track of their victories over the problem and the problem's victories over them on a daily basis. The therapist can raise dilemmas with family members around their need to be a unified team rather than caving in to having arguments about the best course of action for defeating the problem or continuing to blame the identified child client for their difficulties. I typically instruct families to work out together in order to be as fit as possible to do battle with the tyrannical problem. Once the family has defeated the problem, we can celebrate the change process by giving the family a party, certificates, ribbons, or trophies (Epston, 1989, 1998; Durrant & Coles, 1991; White & Epston, 1990). Celebrating change with families in this manner nicely complements the positive-oriented basic solution-focused brief therapy approach and is an effective way to further amplify "news of a difference" for them.

Quieting the Mind: Teaching Children How to Achieve Inner Peace with Mindfulness Meditation and Related Practices

One valuable life skill and coping strategy we can teach children as young as 6 years old is *mindfulness meditation* (Selekman, 2005, 2009; Lantieri & Goleman, 2008; Thomas, 2003; Hanh, 2003, 2007). Growing up in a world of extremes and high levels of stress, children can greatly benefit from learning how to wind down from all of the media and high-tech stimulation they are bombarded with daily by quieting their minds and deliberately focusing on their internal core and well-being. Thomas (2003) calls this quiet time "heart and soul time" and believes that parents should establish as a daily ritual a specific time for children to meditate.

When introducing mindfulness meditation to children, I present it in a very concrete way by having them experiment with such simple activities as carefully watching how they breathe by focusing their attention on their chests expanding and contracting, paying close attention to every step they take while walking, or listening carefully with their eyes closed to sounds they hear around themselves, simply labeling each sound they hear to themselves. Another mindfulness practice I have children do is *cloud-shape watching* (Selekman, 2009). This activity entails going outside and while looking up at the clouds trying to identify familiar-looking shapes of animals, human heads, and other recognizable objects. Not only is this a fun activity to do, but also it can become like a game for children in that each time they go out and cloud-watch they can try to identify new recognizable animals, human heads, and other familiar objects. I have them bring in their written-down cloud-shape discoveries to talk about. Parents can encourage their children to go outside and cloud-watch when they are being pushed around by negative thoughts and feelings, which can help disrupt the inner turmoil they are experiencing in their heads.

Many psychological and physical health benefits accrue to children who engage in daily mindfulness meditation. Psychologically such practices help them to temper their wild stallion thoughts and feelings and also to enhance their concentration and problem-solving abilities. Physically, we know that mindfulness meditation lowers our breathing and heart rates and strengthens our immune system (Selekman, 2009; Lantieri & Goleman, 2008).

Integrating Contributions from Winnicott, Siegel, and Other Developmental Theorists

In reviewing the solution-focused brief therapy literature, we see little mention of the importance of developmental theory in informing what we do clinically with children and their families. Having a good grasp of developmental theory can aid us in determining how best to communicate with the child and in designing and selecting therapeutic experiments that he or she is capable of understanding and performing. According to the brilliant child psychiatrist D. W. Winnicott, "One must have in one's bones a theory of the emotional development of the child and the relationship of the child to the environmental factors" (1971b, p. 3). For the remainder of this section, I discuss important contributions from Winnicott, as well as from other interpersonal neurobiological or related developmental theorists that therapists should consider in their clinical work with children and their families. Winnicott (1971b) always took into account the strengths and resources of the child as well as the parents' availability and capability to facilitate the child's maturational process. He believed that clients want to be co-collaborators and inevitably guide therapists toward what they really need. When stuck with a case, Winnicott knew how to tolerate and make clinical use of the "not knowing." He had "the capacity to tolerate feeling ignorant or incompetent and a willingness to wait until something genuinely relevant and meaningful emerged" (Casement, 1985, p. 9).

Winnicott (1971b) attempted to create what he called a "holding environment" in which children believe they will get help for their difficulties. He would try to create a natural and free-flowing human relationship in which clients surprise themselves by sharing important thoughts and feelings (Casement, 1985). Winnicott (1985) believed that some clients' difficulties arise simply because no one has ever "intelligently listened" to their story. Finally, Winnicott practiced somewhat like a brief therapist by increasing the time intervals between sessions once progress occurred. One of Winnicott's (1971a) most famous play therapy techniques was the Squiggle Game. He would say to the child:

> "Let's play something. I know what I would like to play and I'll show you. This game that I like playing has no rules. I just take my pencil and go like that … (do squiggle blind). You show me if that looks like anything to you or if you can make it into anything, and afterwards you do the same for me and I will see if I can make something of yours." (pp. 62–63)

Not only does the Squiggle Game help build rapport with the child, but also it furnishes the therapist with valuable information about the child's inner world and provides opportunities to indirectly offer children new ideas or solutions to their difficulties. Winnicott believed strongly that therapists working with children had to be able to play and could enjoy playing.

In expanding on Winnicott's Squiggle Game technique, I like to include the parents in the process. I may have the parents draw a squiggle and have the child construct a picture out of the squiggle and tell a story about their picture. The child then draws a squiggle, and the parents follow the same procedure (see Chapter 5). Gil (1994) has developed another version of the Winnicott Squiggle Game in her clinical work with abused children.

Dan Siegel (Siegel, 2007; Siegel & Hartzell, 2003), one of the leading pioneers in the growing field of *interpersonal neurobiology*, has demonstrated in his research that our brains are socially oriented organs and the kinds of mental interactions that children have with their parents shape their capacity for developing empathy for others. He believes that when children consistently sense being "emotionally felt" by their parents and have strong connections with them, they develop *mindsight*. Mindsight is the capacity to perceive our own thoughts, feelings, perceptions, sensations, memories, beliefs, attitudes, and intentions—*and those of others*. Children master this ability through their parents regularly sharing their own thoughts, feelings, and memories with them. Through these kinds of meaningful interactions with their parents, children gain self-understanding and build social skills (Siegel & Hartzell, 2003).

Another important concept that has grown out of both Siegel's and attachment theorists' research (Ainsworth, 1978; Bowlby, 1979, 1988) is *narrative coherence,* which is one's ability to access and make sense of one's personal life story. Narrative coherence paves the way for an individual's ability to establish and maintain solid interpersonal connections with others. In my clinical practice with children, I regularly invite parents to share their personal stories of growing up—their struggles and the high points, what their relationships were like with their parents, and what their grandparents were like as people, including valuable words of wisdom and life experiences they shared with them. Parental storytelling strengthens their relationships with their children and helps them to trace and make sense of their roots and heritage.

Historically, there has been a heated debate across all mental health disciplines whether "nature" or "nurture" is responsible for childhood problems and personality development. Greenspan (1995) argues that we should instead look at how nature and nurture work in tandem. Using the metaphor of a lock and key to describe the unique and continuous interplay between nature and nurture, Greenspan says:

> The child brings his "nature" and the parents bring warmth and love wrapped up in a particular pattern of caring. This interplay operates like a lock and key. Finding the right key creates new patterns of interactions. Each stage of child development has its own goals, which are in turn associated with new ways for nature and nurture to work together. For each stage of development, there is a special "key." With the right knowledge about how to find the "keys," parents can learn how to greatly influence this interplay of nature and nurture in their children. (p. 7)

Therapists who treat children need to be knowledgeable about child development. By educating parents on what to expect developmentally of their children and helping them find the right "keys," or courses of action, for supporting their children's mastery of developmental tasks, we can have a much more meaningful impact on families. Through the use of education and normalization, therapists can dispel parental concerns about what they and referring persons may be identifying as "pathological" behaviors. In reality, such behaviors often turn out to be the child's struggle with particular developmental tasks. As Achenbach (1990) stated:

> Many behavioral/emotional problems for which professional help is sought are not qualitatively different from those most individuals display to some degree at some time in their lives. Instead, many problems for which help is sought are quantitative variations and characteristics that

may normally be evident at other developmental periods, in less intense degree, in fewer situations or in ways that do not impair developmental progress. (p. 4)

From a Piagetian cognitive-developmental perspective, Cowan (1978) contends that children's problems, struggles, and conflicts are necessary and inevitable for their growth. At each developmental stage, children have to confront and negotiate personal and environmental mismatches (i.e., the complex interactions between their psychological functioning at a given stage with situational demands and the values of their families, peers, schools, and communities) in order to minimize the extent of the mismatch. This can lead to *disequilibrations* and new problems. In our clinical work with children and their families, we need to encourage parents to be supportive of their child's attempts to cope with these disequilibration periods during their development.

Another important developmental area that therapists should be sensitive to are children's *temperaments*. Each child brings into the world this unique innate part of him- or herself (Kagan, 1994). Often when parents do not match up their responses well with their children's unique temperaments, such as becoming inflexible and too emotionally reactive, they end up clashing with and frustrating one another or feeling misunderstood. Taffel (2009) recommends that parents first try to identify their children's unique temperaments and determine what types of responses from them seem to fit best when the children are emotionally distressed. For example, a "clingy child" may need more one-on-one time with a parent prior to each transition (say, at bedtime) or a strong-willed child may need to be offered two options instead of one (both acceptable to the parents).

For numerous reasons, most family therapists do not use developmental theory to guide their assessment observations and to design appropriate therapeutic experiments. When training and consulting with family therapists, I frequently hear the criticism that one's thinking in developmental terms about a particular family member or the identified child client is "too linear" or "not systemic." The child client is not some innocent victim in his or her family drama but, instead, plays an active part in contributing to family stress and difficulties. The child's role in the family drama can be determined by directly observing family interactions in therapy sessions and may be graphically depicted in the child's art and play activities. We need to be sensitive to the effects of the child's own adaptation to his or her developmental struggles on other family members and how family members, in turn, respond to the child. For example, if parents provide a great deal of assistance to help their child master toilet training, they may enable the child to achieve competence quickly; however, such a "solution" may fail in the long run because the child may lack the self-confidence to use the potty alone. The rewards of independence and confidence go to the child who is allowed to try and fail, struggle, and then finally succeed. Lastly, we also need to examine and explore how family life cycle issues affect the child's functioning (Carter & McGoldrick, 1988; Haley, 1986).

Flying Out of the Center: The Art of Therapeutic Improvisation

Jazz critic Robert Levin (1987), in describing the creative, even brilliant, improvisational abilities of the late saxophonist and reedman Eric Dolphy and other pioneers of the avant-garde jazz movement, rhapsodized that "the new jazz is about learning to fly, to fly out of the center. ... To fly means to end the pursuit of the original, the given, the order, to break that circle, and to pursue instead the rediscovery of surprise—which is to say the rediscovery of reality and the vital."

Levin's sentiment captures the essence of how we as therapists can help liberate the families with which we work from their oppressive problem-saturated life stories. Through the use of humor—even to the point of absurdity now and then—and surprises in the therapeutic process, we can move our clients out of the center, bring back lost spontaneity and playfulness, and alter fixed beliefs and entrenched family interactive patterns that keep them stuck. Similar to what chaos theorists refer to as *fractals*—that is, unique patterns left behind by unpredictable movements (Briggs, 1992) that occur in nature—I want to inject humor and surprises into each family session to help introduce novel ways for family members to look at their original problem-saturated situations. To fly out of the center and be effective improvisors, we have to feel free to step out of our comfort zones and allow our creativity to run wild! When flying out of the center with a family, a therapist can tell jokes, explicate or exaggerate a family pattern in a humorous way, share anecdotes and stories, use metaphors, and be as unpredictable as possible. The therapeutic experience with children and their families should be a fun, surprising, and at times wacky adventure. Two case examples of flying out of the center offer possibilities.

Alison, a 6-year-old Caucasian girl, was brought into therapy for "low self-esteem," "isolating herself from the rest of the family," and looking "depressed." Alison came to the session with her parents. Her 13- and 16-year-old sisters were involved in school-related sporting events, so they did not attend our first family session. No precipitant was identified for Alison's symptoms. Earlier in the session, I felt that I had joined well with the parents but failed to connect with Alison. Alison would not say a word to me, even after I asked the imaginary magic wand question, which is not unlike the miracle question, except with a wand and tried to engage her in a board game on the floor. It appeared that my approach with Alison was too straightforward, and what I really needed to do was something funny and unpredictable. I decided to fake crying and say in a sad childlike way, "I'm telling my mommy that Alison won't play with me" (I put a super sad look on my face). Suddenly, Alison began to smile and laugh at me. She then got on the floor and asked me to play a board game with *her*! By the end of the session, Alison opened up about what was making her so sad. Apparently, she had recently stopped getting the kind of attention she was used to getting from her dad because of his new involvement in coaching her sisters' softball teams. Hearing Alison's concerns proved to be a newsworthy experience for the parents, and the father promised that he would set aside more individual quality time to spend with Alison.

There are many popular children's stories written both in this country and abroad whose main characters, themes, and story lines parallel our young clients' stories. As another way of engaging a child, improvising, and introducing new angles on the child's story, I sometimes share with the child and his or her family a story that seems to fit their situation.

Walter, an 8-year-old Caucasian boy, was brought for therapy shortly after his father, Curtis, had gotten custody of him. Walter and his mother, Michele, had a strained relationship, and she no longer wanted custody. Following the parents' divorce, it had been decided in court that Walter would go live with Michele. According to Curtis, while Walter lived with his mother, she would "yell at him a lot," "neglect his needs," and "favor Monica," his 10-year-old sister, who also lived with Michele. It was Curtis's hope that Walter would use counseling to get out all of his "bad feelings" about his "awful experiences" living with Michele. Walter looked sad when I first saw him in the waiting room.

When I greeted the family in the waiting room, I observed that Walter was reading Dr. Seuss's *The Cat in the Hat Comes Back*. Thus, in thinking about the pervasive theme in Walter's story of being an "invisible" child when living with his mother, I decided to share the book *Moomin's Invisible Friend* (Jansson, 1962) with Walter and Curtis. The story in many ways paralleled Walter's. Moomin, the main character, and a friend, Too Ticky, one day brought home a new friend, Ninny, for Moomin's parents and friends to meet. However, nobody could see Ninny because she was invisible. Ninny was being raised by her nasty aunt, who was so horrible to Ninny that Ninny became invisible. Moomin's parents and friends were the nicest people in the Moomin Valley. On a daily basis, Moomin, her parents, and the former's friends would treat Ninny very nicely and compliment her. With almost every act of kindness and compliment, a different part of Ninny's body would appear. After some time had passed, most of Ninny's body could be seen except for her head. Moomin's family decided one day to take Ninny to the sea to relax and swim. Moomin's mama was standing on the edge of a rock hesitant to jump in, for the water was very cold. Moomin's papa decided to push his wife into the water. As he snuck up behind her, Ninny thought this was wrong and bit his tail to stop him. While Moomin's papa was screaming in pain, Ninny's head suddenly appeared. Everyone jumped for joy! Finally they could see all of her! Ninny was really happy too because she was no longer invisible. Moomin urged Ninny never to make herself invisible again. Ninny promised, "Never! Oh, never!"

After hearing this story, Curtis vowed that he would not allow his son ever to become invisible while living with him. Walter liked the story a great deal and said he could identify with Ninny. We used this story as a vehicle for discussing his thoughts and feelings about when he lived with his mother. Over time, Walter's view of himself changed as well as his pessimistic outlook on the future. His father was highly invested in building a nurturing relationship with Walter.

To conclude this discussion on flying out of the center—outside the comfort zone—with children and their families, let me share this thought from the pioneer humanistic psychologist James Bugental: "The seasoned therapist is able to 'work on the edge of awareness' and is a true artist rather than a technician. True art is only to be found on the edge of what is known—a dangerous place to be, an exciting place to work, a continually unsettling place to live subjectively" (Bugental, 1987, p. 95).

Using Postmodern Therapy Ideas

According to Fruggeri (1992), therapists who consider themselves to be postmodern practitioners should acknowledge their premises, points of view, and biases with their clients. She argues: "It is through this acknowledgment that they [therapists] can observe their own way of constructing the phenomena they are observing and their relationship to them" (p. 50). Postmodern therapists avoid adopting a privileged expert position with their clients by trying not to present them with some "higher truths" or final explanations about their problem situations. Alternative constructions of the client's problem situation and therapeutic tasks are presented in a tentative way: "I wonder if ... " "Could it be ... ?" "This task may be useful as an experiment. ... " Postmodern therapists recognize that there are a multiplicity of views for any given client problem situation, with all views constantly in flux (Hoffman, 1990, 2002).

Family problems are viewed as being an "ecology of ideas" (Bogdan,

1984). Often parents get the idea that their child may have a *problem* from people outside their immediate and extended families, such as an adult friend, the pediatrician, a school principal or teacher, or even a popular talk show host. Operating from this postmodern perspective, the main role of the therapist is to facilitate the renegotiation of the meaning system within which "the problem" exists. Thus, the therapist actively enters into dialogue with those individuals who maintain the problem definition and becomes a collaborator in the construction of new client narratives (Anderson, 1997; Anderson & Goolishian, 1988b; Spence, 1982; Schafer, 1994). The family can be invited to share with the therapist which involved helping professionals are part of the problem system and with whom the therapist should collaborate. I view these helping professionals as potential allies that can serve as key members of the *solution-determined system*—that is, offering us creative input in the solution construction process (Selekman, 2009).

In a fascinating postmodern study of expert practitioners from a variety of professional disciplines, including therapists, Schon (1983) discovered that these practitioners utilized two processes when managing work tasks: *reflection-in-action* and *reflection-on-action*. He found that the critical reflective thinking that the practitioners employed in their work was an artistic process, not purely a cognitive process of analysis and speculation. For Schon, reflection-in-action is the capacity to keep alert, listen intently, and improvise in the midst of action that does not require the practitioner to stop and think. Reflection-on-action consists of asking oneself questions about action already undertaken from a critical perspective.

In a therapy context, reflection-on-action entails thinking about one's motivations for behaving in a particular way in a session (questions asked and/or interventions tried) and what aspects of the client's story one has taken most seriously (problem-saturated beliefs or solution talk). With reflection-on-action, a therapist seeks new ways of approaching a client's problem situation in a future therapy session, accepts the possibility that it may not fit into any pattern of understanding in the therapist's present repertoire, or accepts that he or she has tried to make it conform to a particular theoretical orientation. When we find techniques that are unusually effective with particular clients, in similar cases the memory of that response jumps to the forefront of our minds and we try out the same techniques again to see if they will work. If they do, the initial registration or "logging" of their success in our memory is reaffirmed, and the same set of techniques may well become a tried and trusted response to situations characterized by similar patterns. In other words, it becomes a theory in use (Brookfield, 1987; Schon, 1983).

One famous reflective practitioner was the great physicist Niels Bohr. Bohr was never fond of axiomatic systems and declared repeatedly, "Everything I say must be understood not as an affirmation but as a question" (in Capra, 1988, p. 18). In a similar vein, psychology researcher and critic Robin M. Dawes (1994) argues, "Responsible practitioners should practice with a cautious, open and questioning attitude" (p. 31). Through the use of reflection-in-action and reflection-on-action, we can become better improvisers, be more critical of our therapeutic assumptions and interventions, and be more therapeutically flexible.

2

The Collaborative Strengths-Based Family Assessment Session

There are always flowers for those who want to see them.
—HENRI MATISSE

Child psychotherapists and many family therapists have traditionally viewed the diagnostic evaluation or assessment process as a separate stage of therapy that needs to be completed before the *real* treatment can begin. It is still common clinical practice among child psychotherapists to evaluate and treat the child separately from the parents. Moreover, many therapists maintain the need for a few sessions to arrive at an accurate diagnosis for the child. Some family therapists operating from the "functionalist" school of thought (Bogdan, 1986) may need a session or two to determine the "function of the symptom" (Haley, 1987) and structural family pathology, such as "enmeshment" and "disengagement" (Minuchin, 1974). Yet, in today's managed care world, most therapists have only one assessment session authorized to arrive at a DSM-IV-TR diagnosis and to construct with the client an appropriate treatment plan. Therefore, therapists not only need to learn how to conduct assessment sessions in an efficient manner but also need to be able to negotiate solvable client problems and goals and design realistic treatment plans with children and their families in their first family session.

In this chapter, I present a collaborative strengths-based family assessment session format that not only is comprehensive and efficient but also designed to create possibilities with clients in their very first family session. I discuss how to secure sufficient information about the referral process, presenting problems and concerns, developmental and background factors, cultural and gender issues, and family members' resiliencies. This discussion is followed by another about how to collaboratively construct treatment

39

plans with families consisting of well-defined treatment goals and a clear and straightforward therapeutic action plan. I conclude this chapter with a discussion of postassessment session critical reflection.

Eliciting Client Expertise through Their Self-Generated Pretreatment Changes

Prior to first meeting the parents in the initial family assessment session, I like to give them this precounseling assignment or experiment by phone, saying something like this:

> "My colleagues and I have been so amazed over our many years of working with children and their families how creative, resourceful, and resilient our clients are in preventing their difficulties from getting much worse—and even beginning to resolve their problems well before we see them for the first time. In order for me to learn what your special strengths, resources, and resiliencies are, I would like you between now and our first appointment to carefully observe daily for any encouraging steps you see your child take or any other signs of improvement that you would like to see continue. In addition, I want you to keep track of what you are doing during those times that is contributing to or promoting his [or her] positive behavior. Please write down all of your important observations between now and our first appointment."

As a result of this experiment, parents occasionally cancel their appointments after discovering that the child's positive behaviors greatly outweigh the negative ones or because their problem views change about the original complaint. In some cases, parents come in with lists of 5–10 significant pretreatment changes that occurred between the time of first calling our office and their first appointment. After amplifying on and consolidating all of the child's and family's improvements at the initial assessment, the parents may decide that one session is enough, or they may want to keep the door open and schedule a checkup session a few weeks later. During the amplification and consolidation process, we learn a lot about the family members' key strengths, resources, and resiliencies that can be utilized in behalf of the client. Once we learn about what clients are doing that works, we want to encourage them to increase these solution-building or -maintaining patterns of behavior. Assigning this precounseling experiment enables the first session to become more like the second session, potentially reducing clients' length of stay in treatment. This precounseling experiment also helps empower families that have to be placed on waiting lists owing to an inability to see them right away. Talmon (1990) and Weiner-Davis and her colleagues (1987) were the first brief therapy practitioners to write extensively about the benefits of capitalizing on clients' pretreatment changes. Finally, Allgood and his colleagues (1995) found in their study that clients' pretreatment changes continued to persist years after the conclusion of their therapy experiences.

Overview of the Family Assessment Session

After taking time to connect closely with each family member about his or her personal strengths and talents, I explain the assessment session format, sharing with them the following general description:

> "There are two parts to this assessment session. In the first part we will talk about what difficulties and concerns led you to come in at this time, and in the second part of the session we will talk about solutions and change—where you want to be when we have a successful outcome here."

By structuring the assessment session in this way, the therapist empowers the family by confidently conveying to them that there are solutions to their difficulties and that he or she believes that the family has the strengths and resources to change. Research supports this approach in that therapists' expectations and beliefs in their clients' abilities to change have been found to have a great impact on treatment outcomes (Selekman, 2009; Selekman & Shulem, 2007; Hubble et al., 1999; Campbell, 1996; Gingerich, de Shazer, & Weiner-Davis, 1988; Leake & King, 1977; Thomas, Polansky, & Kounin, 1955). Families that have already experienced multiple treatment failures are pleasantly surprised to encounter a confident, optimistic therapist who is ready to discuss their concerns and yet also interested in their areas of competency and in rapidly steering them toward change.

This format also enables the clinician to get enough information to complete the forms required by many managed care companies directly following the session. Whenever possible, it's also in the assessor's best interest to call the case manager on the same day of the assessment session to discuss the case and provide a good estimate of the number of visits needed to complete treatment with the clients. Thus, future appointments can be scheduled without delay. With practice, therapists will discover that it is possible to use the first half of the assessment session time to gather sufficient information about the presenting problems, the child and family background, past treatment experiences, and school functioning to fill out the managed care company's assessment summary forms and, in the same hour-long session, open up the door for change and possibilities for the clients.

The collaborative strengths-based family assessment format consists of five major areas of therapeutic inquiry and collaboration:

1. Defining and clarifying the problem
2. Meaning making, or eliciting the family story
3. Determining the real customer(s) for change
4. Coauthoring a new family story
5. Co-constructing the "blueprint for change" plan

To a great extent, these areas of inquiry and collaboration blend together, complementing one another to provide the therapist with a broad understanding of the family's problems, beliefs, and goals. For example, when collaborating with families about problem definitions and explanations, we are also engaged in the meaning-making process. However, the meaning-making process goes well beyond problem defining and clarification; it also includes the referral process and treatment history, including major illnesses and medications; inquiring about family members' attempted solutions and resiliencies; assessing child and family developmental issues; assessing gender and cultural issues and how they may affect the presenting problems; and assessing who is most motivated to do something about the presenting problems in the client system.

In the second half of the family assessment session, the therapist can inquire with family members about pretreatment changes and solutions to help them begin to coauthor a new problem-free family story. As part of the collaborative treatment planning process, treatment goals are negotiated into achievable terms, treatment modalities and an action plan are agreed upon, and a DSM-IV-TR diagnosis is selected with the family's input. Like the four Buddhist mind-training principles discussed in the next section, the self-reflection part of the postassessment session serves as a useful exercise to prevent us from becoming too wedded to any one way of thinking about the family, to remain both curious and flexible, and to be self-critical of what we chose to do, avoided doing, or forgot to do with the family during the assessment session. By listening to our clients with a "beginner's mind," therapists can avoid the common mental error of assuming we understand our clients' problem stories and family situations before we really do.

Assuming the Buddhist Perspective, with a Twist

When conducting collaborative strengths-based family assessment sessions with children, therapists need to operate from the Buddhist perspective of "don't know mind" (Barrett, 1993; Mitchell, 1988), which is eternally fresh, open, and fertile with possibilities (Selekman, 2005, 2009). *The bottom line is that our clients are much better experts on their lives than we are.* We need to give them plenty of slack and space to share their problem stories to help us better understand their world views, mindsets, and difficulties. However, research indicates that many therapists have a tendency to crystallize their diagnostic impressions within the first 30–60 seconds after meeting their clients in assessment interviews (Gauron & Dickson, 1969; Yager, 1977). Explaining how therapists arrive so quickly at diagnostic impressions and labels for their clients, Dawes (1994) argues, "The heuristics that we use for assessing our clients, *availability* (searching in one's memory for cases similar to the one in front of us) and *representativeness* (matching cues or characteristics with a stereotype or a set of other characteristics associated with a category), most commonly lead to inaccurate case formulations." (p. 130).

The following four Buddhist mind-training principles serve as helpful guidelines for therapists when conducting collaborative strengths-based family assessment interviews with children and their families. Therapists will find that all four of the principles can help us to be better listeners and to maintain an open and curious mind when gathering information from family members and trying to understand their clients' problem stories.

Pull Out the Rug

There once was a wise teacher in India named Saraha, who counseled his students thusly:

> Those who believe that everything is solid and real are stupid, like cattle, but those who believe that everything is empty are even more stupid. Everything is changing all of the time, and we keep wanting to pin it down, to fix it. So whenever you come up with a solid conclusion, let the rug be pulled out. (in Chodron, 1994, p. 19)

This good advice captures the essence of the mental traps that therapists too easily fall into when assessing their clients. Chodron (1994) suggests that whenever our thoughts become solidly entrenched we should "self-liberate even the antidote" and consciously label our thoughts as mere "thinking." By upbraiding ourselves, we begin to see the insubstantiality of our thoughts, their illusory aspects, and "acknowledge that you just made them all up with this conversation you are having with yourself" (Chodron, 1994, p. 20). We need to let go of small-mindedness and the tendency to fixate on any particular explanation for the child or family's difficulties by pulling the rug out from under our belief systems.

Cultivate Patience

One therapeutic skill not typically taught in postgraduate family therapy training programs and in workshops is the gentle art of being patient with our clients. We need to learn how to become better observers and listeners. Tao-Wu, once said: "If you want to see it, see into it directly; but when you stop to think about it, it is altogether missed" (the Buddhist sage, in Barrett, 1993, p. 51). Whenever Milton H. Erickson would make an observation in a therapy session, he would write it down on a piece of paper, put it in an envelope, and stick it in his desk drawer. Later, he would pull it out and compare it to other observations he had made to see whether there was any consistency to what he was observing with his clients (Erickson & Havens, 1985).

> My colleagues and I once worked with a Caucasian family in which the mother, a pediatric nurse, was convinced that her 11-year-old son, Bill, was clinically depressed. Bill had been "isolating himself" from the family, appeared to have "low self-esteem," and became "increasingly more noncommunicative." At the intersession break, all three of my colleagues were convinced that Bill was depressed because he was so "soft spoken," "slouched low" in the corner of the couch, and kept his "head down" for the first half of the session. As the interviewer, I had similar observations. Yet, I remained open to the possibility that Bill's nonverbal attitude and soft-spoken voice could indicate any of the following: normative preadolescent behavior, his upset about his parents making him go for counseling (after all, he was not even a window shopper for counseling; the parents were the real customers), and the possibility that Bill's demeanor had always been this way. It was not until our second session with this family 4 weeks later that my colleagues began to view Bill differently, particularly when both his parents had very positive reports about his behavioral changes between sessions. Interestingly enough, Bill's nonverbal attitude and soft-spoken voice had not changed at all!

This case helps demonstrate the common therapist mental trap of, "What you will see is what you will get." By being patient with my observations and impressions with Bill's case, I left the door open for many possibilities in viewing his situation.

When listening to our clients share their problem stories, we need to try to suspend our own therapeutic agendas, forget about what questions we might want to ask next, and concentrate deeply on the language, themes, and beliefs the clients use to describe their situations. Nichols (1995) maintains that "a good listener is a witness, not a filter for your experience" (p. 17). We have to be careful not to allow our personal and therapy model assumptions to totally predetermine what we truly "see" about and "hear from" our clients. By listening intently to our clients' descriptions of their problem situations, we can get to know the problem's nature and let it teach us what it will.

Take a Bigger Perspective

There is a sacredness to our clients' wisdom about their problem stories. For them, the map *is* the territory (Hoffman, 1990). Some families may come to the assessment session armed with a DSM-IV-TR label to which they are closely attached and for which they are seeking confirmation. Rather than trying to talk them out of this DSM-IV-TR label or reframing the problem, therapists need to respect their unique understanding of their problem situation (Selekman, 1996). As therapists, we need to be curious about the second and third possible explanations for a client's presenting problem. The client's responses to our questions should be followed up with more curiosity and questions, to enlarge the meaning of their problem story. We will never find the final explanation for the client's story because knowledge is "always on the way." Frank Howell, the famous Native American painter, put it best when he said, "We need to create 'windows' which other people can't make for themselves—windows that provide the way to a greater awareness" (in Wood & Howell, 1993, p. 7). What prevents our clients from adopting a larger perspective and creating "windows" for themselves are the emotions and outmoded beliefs that keep them stuck.

Another technique in family assessment sessions that can help families adopt a larger perspective on their problem situations is to ask problem-tracking questions (Selekman, 2005, 2009; O'Hanlon & Weiner-Davis, 1989; Palazzoli, Boscolo, Cecchin, & Prata, 1980). Asking a family member to provide a very detailed, videotape-like description of what every family member does when the child client is symptomatic or acting up and how family members interact recursively with one another can help operationalize the problem and challenge outmoded family beliefs that the problem lies solely in the child being treated. Problem-tracking questions also help to assess how family members interact with involved helpers representing larger systems, such as school personnel concerned about the child client. In some cases, the same interactive dance occurring between the parents and the child at home gets played out between the child and his or her teachers and other involved school personnel.

The Tao That Can Be Spoken Is Not the Ultimate Tao

Applied to the world of therapy, the principle "The Tao that can be spoken is not the ultimate Tao" means that when the therapist becomes wedded to one way of looking at the client's presenting problem, he or she cannot see or hear anything else. Our favorite therapy models are not a panacea for every presenting problem. Lao-tzu used to teach his students that "the more you know, the less you understand" (in Mitchell, 1988, p. 47). As mentioned earlier, by being both actively curious and duly patient with our clients, we can avoid inadvertently substituting tunnel vision for accurate perceptions.

One of my favorite Dr. Seuss short stories is the tale of *The Sneetches,* which is a nice metaphor for this Buddhist principle. On the beaches there were two types of Sneetches, star-bellied ones and Sneetches without stars. The star-bellied Sneetches held their heads up high and viewed themselves as being superior to the Sneetches without stars on their bellies. The latter were always excluded from the star-bellied Sneetches' hot dog roasts and marshmallow-toasting parties. The plain-bellied Sneetches spent most of their days "moping and doping" on the beaches until one day a man drove up to them in a strange-looking car. His name was Sylvester McMonkey McBean, and he called himself the "Fix-It-Up-Chappie." He pushed some levers and buttons on his car, and it turned into a "star-on" machine. For $3 apiece, all the plain-bellied Sneetches went through his machine to get the highly prized stars put on their bellies. The Sneetches were so happy with their star bellies that they rushed over to the original star-bellied Sneetches to show off their beautiful new bellies. The original star-bellied Sneetches were defensive and made it clear to the other Sneetches that they would always be the first star-bellied Sneetches. Amid the heated anger and consternation, McBean appeared with yet another machine that he called the "star-off" machine. For $10 per Sneetch, he convinced the original star-bellied Sneetches that stars were out of style and that having a plain belly was presently "in" and more contemporary. After having their stars removed, they approached the other Sneetches to show off their new look and make it clear to them that they were the superior ones. This greatly angered the original plain-bellied Sneetches, who then approached McBean. In a very clever and cunning way, McBean convinced the original plain-bellied Sneetches to have their stars removed. Finally, both groups of Sneetches ended up exhausting all their finances having the stars removed and put back on again and so on. After McBean drove off, now a rich man, both groups of Sneetches decided together that "Sneetches are Sneetches, and no kind of Sneetch is the best on the beaches" (Seuss, 1961a, p. 24).

Defining and Clarifying the Problem

Most experts on solving problems would argue that properly defining the problem at the outset is equally as important as finding, or divining, its solution (Berns, 2008; Csikszentmihalyi & Getzels, 1970; Dillon, 1992; Getzels, 1992; Hall, 1995; Hurson, 2008; Isenberg, 2009; Mackworth, 1965; Roberto, 2009; Van Gundy, 1988). Many therapists in this age of managed health care have a tendency to be too solution-minded rather than problem-minded. Finding the "quick" solution becomes our primary goal, when, in fact, accurately pinpointing the client's real problems—and the "right" one to tackle first—should be the initial priority.

Taking insufficient time to explore family members' views of the real problem and editing their problem-saturated story too quickly generates "solutions" unlikely to work in the long run. Problems are not static or fixed but are in a constant state of evolution. The better we clarify with clients the different problem states and further build on our perceptions of their problems, the more likely we properly define what the clients view as the "right" problem.

Sometimes asking productive questions about presenting problems is more challenging than generating solutions. Swedish family therapists Salamon and Grevelius (1996) have found in their innovative clinical work with families that eliciting from the families their "key questions" about their problem situations provides important clues for solution finding. Two examples of key parents' questions might be:

- "Do you think he [or she] has anger inside about the divorce?"
- "What should we do as parents [to try to solve the problem]"?

Some examples of productive problem-finding questions are:

- "If there was one question that you were dying to ask me about your problem situation, what would that question be?"
- "In what ways can I be most helpful to you?"
- "What's your theory about why this problem exists?"
- "If there was one question that you were hoping I would ask you while we are working together, what would that question be?"
- "How will you know when you won't have to go for counseling anymore?"

Meaning Making and Eliciting the Family Story

Therapists never approach a new family with a *tabula rasa*. Based on the referral information and past experiences, treating similar types of family problems inevitably triggers in the therapist preconceptions about what to explore or observe in the first family interview. Thus, the meaning-making process begins with the referral context. Since, early on, the therapist needs to know how the family came to pursue therapy (Andersen, 1991), family members should be invited to share their thoughts about how they ended up at the office by asking them the following questions:

- "Who was the first person who got the idea that you should seek help?"
- "What idea do you think [referral person from larger system] had that made him [or her] decide that you need counseling now?"
- "Who else thought counseling would be helpful now?"
- "Whom did he [or she] consult with first?"
- "How long did it take from the time you first had the idea to seek counseling to eventually pursue it?"
- "Do you have any idea about what [referral person from larger system] needs to see happen in counseling that would convince him [or her] that you wouldn't have to come here any more?"

By securing detailed information about the history of the idea of pursuing therapy, we can learn a great deal about family members' beliefs, who is the most or least concerned about problems, and which helping professionals from larger systems we will need to collaborate with. If there is some discrepancy between what family members tell me about the referral process or their presenting problems and the information I have on my intake form, I explore with them how they think the intake worker got his or her ideas about their situation and whether there is something else important that we have not yet talked about. Finally, we need to be sensitive to the constraints of the referral treatment process in terms of what realistically can be treated, the time factors, and the clinic or agency's treatment philosophy, policies, and procedures that can influence our therapeutic work.

The late family therapy pioneer Harry Goolishian once observed, "I learned to listen, understand and converse in the language of my clients, as opposed to the language of my theory" (1990, p. 179). What made Goolishian a masterful meaning maker and storyteller was his uncanny ability to balance listening, curiosity, and using the client's own language in the therapeutic conversation. Goolishian would "move with the family as they present themselves, with total respect for their rightness" (Phillips, 1986, p. 6). Just like Goolishian, when eliciting the family's problem story, we need to listen carefully to the words family members use to describe it, their beliefs, and important themes in their stories. We must avoid being narrative editors and instead serve as consulting coauthors speaking the client's language and being curious about family members' understanding of their family drama, how it has evolved, and where it is going. Through this meaning-making process, shared understandings can develop that did not exist before the family assessment interview.

What is important is that there are multiple meanings to the words family members use to describe their problem situation and that their problem stories are stories about stories. As Wittgenstein (1963) has pointed out: "Words are not maps of reality. The significance of our words remains open, vague, ambiguous, until they are used in different particular ways in different particular circumstances" (p. 154). For example, the word "run" has 142 different meanings, depending on how it is used (Erickson & Havens, 1985, p. 14). Thus, it is important to have family members clarify the meaning of the words they use with others in the therapy room or when describing their problem situation. The whole therapeutic enterprise is an ambiguous process. We may think we really understand a family's situation and are being helpful to the family when, in reality, they believe we are "totally" missing the boat. "Real understanding of families is but an illusion or delusion that we carry with us" in our clinical work (Newfield, Kuehl, Joanning, & Quinn, 1991, p. 306).

Assessing Family Members' Attempted Solutions

As an integral part of the meaning-making process, therapists need to explore in great detail with the family what their attempted solutions have been and what their resiliencies (successful individual and family coping and problem-solving strategies) are. It is most helpful to explore with the parents everything they have tried to do on their own to resolve their child's difficulties. I like to ask parents some of the following questions when inquiring about their attempted solutions:

- "Has anything you tried in the past to resolve other difficulties with your child worked that we might want to test out with this new problem?"
- "Has there been anything that you thought about trying—maybe something off the wall—but you held back because you didn't think it would work?"
- "When your child misbehaves, what do the two of you typically do to manage his [or her] behavior?"

The answers can furnish the therapist with important information regarding areas for parental intervention and potential building blocks for solution construction. It is also important to find out from child clients what their attempted solutions have been when they were pushed around by the problem.

Another area to explore with families that have been in treatment before is what they liked and disliked about former therapists. I like to empower families by placing them in the expert position in designing the kind of treatment experience they would like to have with me. Such questions as the following can be asked:

- "You have seen a lot of therapists before me; what did they *miss* with your situation?"
- "What kinds of things should a counselor do with a family like yours?"
- "If you could describe what the perfect counselor would be like for you and your family, what would he or she be like?"
- "If I were to work with another family just like yours, what advice would you give me to help that family out?"

For families that have not had counseling before, I like to plant the idea that they are "more ripe for change" than families that have had lots of previous counseling.

Assessing Family Members' Resiliency

The therapist should also inquire about family members' resiliency and family group resiliency. I share with families that I am very interested in their strengths, particularly in learning about the various ways as individuals and as a group that they have successfully managed past and present stressful life events. I ask the following questions:

- "Can you think of any past life events or crisis situations that were pushing your family around—and yet you weathered the storm?"
- "What did you do as a family to pull that off?"
- "What else did you do as a family that seemed to help?"
- "Mom and Dad, can you think of a time in the past when your child was struggling to cope with a painful life event/transition? What did you do to help him or her better cope and get back on track?"
- (*to parents*) "Have you noticed anything your child does that seems to help him or her be less stressed out?"
- "Can you think of anything that your mom and dad could do to help you better deal with your grandpa's death?"
- "What do you do that seems to work in helping you deal with your parents splitting up?"
- "When you were your child's age, what did you do to bounce back when you were teased and bullied at school?"

The answers to these questions can provide the therapist with a wealth of information about key family members' resiliency and family group resiliency that can be harnessed and channeled into the presenting problem area.

It has been my clinical experience that family members take pride and joy in sharing past triumphs in successfully managing a painful or stressful life event.

Assessing the Client's Key Intelligence Areas and Flow State Activities

Two important areas to assess in the initial family assessment session are the subject child's key intelligence areas and flow state activities (Gardner, 1993, 2004; Csikszentmihalyi, 1990, 1997). By learning about the children's unique strength areas, avenues of expression, and learning styles, we can design and tailor-fit therapeutic tasks or experiments to their key intelligence areas. Children are more likely to cooperate with and try out therapeutic experiments that tap into their expertise and what they are passionate about doing. Their favorite flow state activities often overlap with their key intelligence areas, such as visual-spatial intelligence and doing artwork or logical-mathematical intelligence and mastering tough puzzles.

One way we can reduce the likelihood of acting-out behavior and other difficulties with children during after-school and early evening hours and after they have had a snack and some playtime is to increase their involvement in their favorite flow state activities. Not only does this provide them with structure, but also they are engaging in meaningful activities that bring them great pleasure, such as playing an instrument, dancing, doing artwork, playing their favorite sport, building models, spending extra time taking care of their pets, and so on. Once I know what children's key intelligences and flow state activities are, I use the language and metaphors of these strength and talent areas in our conversations in sessions and in devising rationales for trying out carefully designed therapeutic experiments that tap their skills in these areas. The change process thereby becomes a playful and fun endeavor for them.

At times, I also will use the parents' key intelligence areas and flow state activities to help foster a cooperative relationship with them and for related therapeutic experiment design and implementation as well. Not surprisingly, parents find it empowering to employ what they do best to help resolve their child's difficulties.

Assessing Child and Family Developmental Issues

When inquiring with parents about their child's developmental issues, past illnesses, prescribed medications, and psychosocial functioning, it is important to remember that the child developmental theories we use as frameworks for assessing the child are not etched in stone. Each child we interview is unique and does not typically experience a smooth transition from one developmental stage to the next. Observed behavior may not tell the full story about the child's underlying capacities. It is also important when assessing a child's development to be self-critical about our conclusions and try to consider how things might look and feel *to the child*. Besides asking parents about their child's mastery of major developmental milestones, I like to gather information about the child's functioning in the following eight areas: temperament, self-awareness, mood management, problem-solving capacity, self-motivation, empathy for others, social competence, and school functioning. When discussing with the parents their child's functioning in these areas, I also want to find out how well the parents are coping with their child's developmental struggles, particularly how they typically respond to the child. Where the child is at developmentally dictates the level of skill development in each of these areas. I look for certain things in each of the skill areas, and I ask the parents certain kinds of questions when gathering information about their child's mastery level in these areas.

TEMPERAMENT

The child appears to have a balanced temperament and does not respond in extreme ways when experiencing frustration, emotional distress, stressful life events, separation from the parents, and having to manage transitions. He or she is flexible and adapts well to changes in both the family and school environments.

Questions: How does your child respond to frustration and emotional distress? How well does your child handle separations from you and other transitions like getting out of bed in the morning, going to school, and at his or her bedtime? How well does your child cope with new situations, like trying new activities and meeting new people?

SELF-AWARENESS

The child appears to know what he or she is feeling. He or she is congruent with his or her thoughts and feelings. When upset, the child can readily express him- or herself to the parents. The child displays a good understanding of changes that occur around him or her in the home environment and in other social contexts.

Questions: When your child is sad/mad/happy, can she express herself? Does he appear to be aware of his feelings when he looks sad or angry? Can your daughter express to you when she is having difficulties coping with changes/stressors/crises at home? Do his words seem to match how he looks when expressing himself?

MOOD MANAGEMENT

Mood management is the child's capacity to self-soothe when anxious, feeling bad, or under a great deal of stress. The child also has the capacity to bounce back quickly from setbacks.

Questions: Does your child appear to have the ability to comfort herself when upset (sad/mad)? How well does your child manage disappointments? How long does it typically take for your child to rebound from feeling frustrated/sad/angry? Does he rebound quickly or slowly? Do your child's moods fluctuate a lot, or are they pretty balanced? What does your son typically do when he is frustrated/mad/sad?

PROBLEM-SOLVING CAPACITY

The child is skilled at managing tasks through to completion. He or she has no difficulty staying focused and concentrating on the task at hand. The child acts rather than reacts to daily and life challenges.

Questions: When faced with a challenging or upsetting situation, what does your son typically do? Does he tend to think things through before taking action, or does he react impulsively? When you and your daughter are at odds, how does she typically respond?

SELF-MOTIVATION

The child approaches tasks and challenges with desire and enthusiasm. Parents and other significant adults do not have to be the motivating force for the child. The child takes responsibility for completing assigned tasks, such as chores or putting toys away when finished playing with them.

Questions: Does your child take the initiative to get chores/homework done, or do you have to be the motivating force to get the job done? When involved with a new sports activity or task, does he commit to it through completion, or does he lose interest quickly and want to give up?

CAPACITY FOR EMPATHY

Although children by nature show signs of empathy for others before becoming toddlers, the capacity for adultlike empathy does not occur until they are 5–7 years of age (Greenspan, 1995). At this time, they can begin to see the world through others' eyes and try to comfort others in distress.

Questions: Does your child show concern for or try to provide support for others when they are in distress? Is your child sensitive to your needs and expectations? What about with his or her brothers' and sisters' needs and feelings?

SOCIAL COMPETENCE

Between the ages of 7 and 8, the child seeks peer group affiliation (Greenspan, 1995). The child has to master the ability to negotiate multiple relationships, learn how to assess group dynamics, and perform well in group activities. The child has the ability to make and sustain friendships.

Questions: Does your child have any difficulties making and sustaining friendships? Does your child have a close friend? In group situations, does your child tend to withdraw or socialize freely with confidence?

SCHOOL FUNCTIONING

The child has no difficulties with auditory and visual memory or perceptual processes, with staying on task, and with completing assignments and tasks. He or she is able to follow directions and respect the classroom rules and the teacher's authority; he or she has no behavioral problems or difficulties with other students. The child displays the ability to delay gratification, ask for help when necessary, and express opinions or needs.

Questions: Does your child have any difficulties academically or with the learning process? Has the teacher voiced any concerns with your child's ability to stay on task, complete assignments, or get along with peers in the classroom? Are there any reported problems with following the rules or testing the teacher's limits? Are there any problems with your child doing, completing, or turning in her homework assignments?

By gathering this important developmental information from the parents and the child, we can collaboratively identify target areas for intervention, elicit valuable information about the child's strengths and competency areas, negotiate treatment goals, and have the family assist us with therapeutic task selection and construction.

Family developmental life cycle issues are also important to consider as part of the meaning-making process. For example, symptoms may develop in a child going to school for the first time or following the birth of the second child in the family. One way to look at the firstborn child's symptomatic behavior is as a normative protest to being "dethroned" by the newborn. He or she will now have to share or relinquish center stage in the family, which is a major adjustment for most children.

Gender and Cultural Issues

Two final areas to assess in the meaning-making process are gender and cultural issues. It is helpful to assess in what ways power imbalances among family members and patriarchal assumptions contribute to the maintenance of the presenting problems. Recently, I treated a family in which the 6-year-old identified child client was "depressed" and "diagnosed by the school as exhibiting ADD." In the family assessment session, the mother proceeded to blame herself for her son's problems and cited a multitude of reasons why her husband could not participate in family therapy. At the same time, she disclosed how she felt "all alone" with her son's "problems" and wished she could "go out with girlfriends more." I gently challenged the mother's patriarchal-based beliefs that it was up to her to resolve her son's problems alone and that she should sacrifice her social life for the sake of motherhood. In reflecting on her own mother, she disclosed how her mother too was oppressed by traditional values and expectations about how women should be. We agreed that it was necessary for her husband to participate in future family therapy sessions and that she should have a life outside the family. She confronted her husband a few hours after our session about the need for him to come to the next session. She also made plans with some longtime friends to go away for a weekend. The husband's involvement in subsequent family therapy sessions helped us to quickly resolve their son's difficulties, probably because the son had reported that his father's absence from the home, due to several business trips, was why he was feeling "sad" and having problems in school.

Feminist family therapists have argued that most family therapy and brief therapy models fail to address power imbalances between family members, do not challenge traditional patriarchal assumptions about women's role behaviors, and emphasize the importance of establishing a nonhierarchical therapeutic relationship with women and their families (Almeida, Del-Vecchio, & Parker, 2008; Bograd, 1990; Goodrich, 1991; Luepnitz, 1988; Walsh & Scheinkman, 1989; Whipple, 1996). In discussing the myth of therapeutic neutrality, Avis (1986) contends that "therapists who adhere to this myth inadvertently adopt political positions by what they choose to focus on, respond to, challenge, or ignore, which may reinforce traditional values oppressive to women" (p. 217).

The last important assessment area to explore in the meaning-making process with families is cultural and spiritual wellness issues that are interwoven with their problem stories and are played out in the context of the therapeutic relationship. When working with families from different ethnic, cultural, and religious backgrounds, it is helpful to ask ourselves and our clients the following questions:

- [If you are a white therapist] "Have I examined my own white identity in terms of what it means to be white in our society?"
- "How do I feel about being white and my own ethnic and/or cultural background?"

- "How does being white and/or being from a different ethnic or cultural background affect what I can see, hear, and think about this family?"
- "In what ways does being white in our society grant me a privileged status?"
- "How does this privileged status (and the implied power imbalance) affect my relationships with the African American families I am working with?"
- "If you were African American, Asian, or Latino, how comfortable would you feel working with a white therapist?"
- "What would your concerns be with a white therapist?"
- "How did you choose your spiritual orientation?"
- "What is your relationship with God?"
- "Do you see God as an adviser or a bystander?"
- "How did you become the author or the owner of your spiritual values?"

According to Pinderhughes (1990), therapists must learn how to monitor and manage "feelings, perceptions and attitudes mobilized as a result of one's clinical and cultural group status role" (p. 133) in order to have effectual culturally sensitive clinical practices. Therapists should actively employ curiosity as a respectful way to try to better understand the client's cultural background.

Other important areas to explore with families from different ethnic and cultural backgrounds are the various ways they may feel oppressed or marginalized by particular groups in our society or by negative discriminatory interactions with larger systems representatives; how they feel about working with a therapist of another ethnic and/or cultural background; and whether or not they would like a referral to a therapist with the same ethnic and/or cultural background as themselves (Almeida et al., 2008). I also like to explore with families of color the role that spirituality plays in their lives and whether or not we should include a mentor or spiritual adviser in our family work together. Finally, with families that are recent immigrants, one should assess how well family members are adjusting to such transitional stressors as language barriers and significant differences in religion, education, family values, and lifestyles (Landau-Stanton, 1990; Sluzki, 1979). When there is transitional conflict occurring with immigrant families, we may observe such difficulties as social isolation, extremes in family boundaries (either being too loose or too rigid) and parent–child conflicts related to cultural differences, such as the child's struggles to cope with traditional family values while also adopting mainstream societal values (Landau-Stanton, 1990).

Determining the *Real* Customer(s) for Change

de Shazer (1988) has developed a highly practical and useful therapeutic guide for determining who in the client system is truly motivated to work with the therapist in resolving the presenting problem. In some cases, the *real* customer(s) for change may be the referring person or other involved helping professionals from larger systems. de Shazer (1988) has identified three observable therapist–family relationship patterns, distinguished by their true sense of involvement: *visitors, complainants,* and *customers.* These patterns are not fixed but change as the therapist develops *fit* (de Shazer, 1985, 1988) and cooperative working relationships with family members. It is important to remember that each family member has a unique cooperative response pattern and may be at a different stage of change (Norcross, 2008; Prochaska et al., 1994). Therefore, therapists need to match their questions and therapeutic tasks carefully with the stage of change and response pattern of each family member.

Visitors

Most children brought for therapy are initially visitors: it is typically their parents or an outside social control agent who is most concerned about their behavior. When asked about the particular behaviors that parents or the referring person is most concerned about, the visiting child often shrugs and says, "I don't know," or doesn't respond at all. Older latency-age children may deny that they have a problem or blame their parents, teachers, or other external forces for their difficulties. Prochaska et al. (1994) maintain that visitors are in the "precontemplation" stage of the change cycle. Precontemplators/visitors want their parents and social control agents to stay "off their backs."

In some cases, the whole family could be considered visitors. I like to refer to these families as "no-problem problem" families (Eastwood, Sweeney, & Piercy, 1987) in that not even the parents are alarmed that their child got into trouble at school or in the community. With no-problem problem families, the identified child client is typically a "good student," has never had any major behavioral problems warranting the need for treatment in the past, and is described by the parents as being basically "a good kid."

When working with visitors, we need to be warm and caring hosts and hostesses. We can empathize with the visiting child or parents' dilemma about having to see us for court-ordered or school-referred family therapy and accept whatever goal they may have for themselves. Some children may want help with dealing with their annoying siblings, a problematic peer, one of the parents, or teachers who are always on their back. With a highly oppositional child, it can be helpful to set up a split so that together the therapist and the child can prove the pessimistic referring person wrong: for example, the therapist can have the child pretend to engage in positive prosocial behavior as an experiment in a class in which the child was having difficulties, to "blow the teacher's mind!"

The "Columbo" approach (see Selekman, 1995, 2005) is particularly useful when a child or parent is making the therapist feel highly incompetent as a therapist. The celebrated TV detective Columbo was a master at seemingly using his confused and bungling presentational style to throw potential murder suspects off guard, who (by politely submitting to his copious questions) inevitably led him to important clues for solving the crime. Similarly, when confronted by our simulated feelings of incompetence and confusion, the child and parents may well want to be more helpful to us, will be more inclined to clarify the referral process and presenting concerns, and possibly will be more receptive to exploring problem-solving strategies.

If the foregoing therapeutic strategies fail to foster a cooperative therapist–family relationship or produce a treatment goal, I simply compliment family members on whatever they report doing for themselves that has been good for them, such as showing up for our first scheduled appointment, and I do not offer them therapeutic tasks. The following case example illustrates the utility of the Columbo approach with a no-problem problem family.

> Melissa, a Caucasian precocious 8-year-old, was school-referred by her teacher because of her "aggressive behavior" in the classroom. This was the third time Melissa had been reprimanded for "kicking and punching" the same male student in her class. The teacher also requested that the school social worker evaluate Melissa for her "violent tendencies." According to Jane, the mother, she was surprised to receive phone calls from both the teacher and the school social worker, for Melissa was an A student and "not violent or aggressive at home." Although Melissa was quite talkative in the session, she denied any family problems or worries early in our session. When asked if she would have ever considered taking Melissa for counseling if the school crisis situation had not occurred, Jane responded with, "Why ... there were no problems." Feeling stuck, I decided to put on my imaginary wrinkled trenchcoat and utilize the Columbo approach.

> THERAPIST: (looking puzzled) I'm really confused ... help me out with this. Both the teacher and school social worker called you about Melissa's punching and kicking this boy in the class. Do we know if he might have "pushed her buttons" or was bothering her in some way?

MOTHER: Well ... I don't know. (*looking at Melissa*) Was that boy annoying you?

MELISSA: Yeah! Jason is always calling me names and bothering me. So I punched him, and he kept up, so I kicked him. He never quits—I mean, I tell him to stop, but he keeps it up.

THERAPIST: How long has he been bothering you?

MELISSA: Since the beginning of the school year.

JANE: You're kidding! Why didn't you tell me, sweetheart?

THERAPIST: Where is the teacher when Jason is pushing your buttons? Do you ever ask for her help?

MELISSA: She doesn't do anything. I mean, sometimes she will talk to him, but it doesn't do any good. It felt good to punch him!

THERAPIST: Sounds like you are frustrated and mad about the Jason situation. So, if Jason has been bothering you since September, what has stopped you from asking your mother for help with this?

MELISSA: Well, since Miss Brown [the teacher] can't do anything about it ... what could my mom do?

THERAPIST: (*turning to mother*) I wonder how your daughter got the idea that she could not call upon you for support when the going gets rough for her?

JANE: I don't know ... I mean, I have always been there for her in the past. I have been pretty stressed out a lot lately because of some changes at my job, and my husband has been out of town on business quite a bit. (*looking at Melissa*) I'm surprised that you didn't come to me for help way back in September ... I would have tried to meet with your teacher.

THERAPIST: (*looking at mother*) Do you have any idea what the teacher and school social worker need to see happen in counseling that would convince them that you wouldn't have to come here anymore?

JANE: Well, I guess Melissa would not be punching and kicking Jason—or any other students, for that matter. (*turning to Melissa*) What do you think, Melissa?

MELISSA: It's going to be hard, Mommy. Jason never quits ... I mean ... I will try.

THERAPIST: What do you guys think about the idea of my setting up a meeting at school for the three of us with Miss Brown and the social worker to see if we can together resolve the difficulties between Melissa and Jason?

JANE: That sounds like a great idea! What do you think, Melissa?

MELISSA: Yeah, that sounds fine if it works.

I ended up seeing the family twice in my office and twice in collaborative meetings at the school with the teacher and social worker. In therapy sessions, Melissa and her mother came up with several good ideas for avoiding the temptation to swear at, kick, or punch Jason. In the school meetings, the teacher agreed to refocus her attention on Jason's behavior, which led her to discover that he was instigating fights daily and causing problems with other students. By the time of our first school meeting, the teacher began to notice that Melissa was displaying "good self-control" and "no aggressive behavior."

Complainants

Complainants can be parents, school personnel, or other social control agents. They are typically very concerned or worried about a child's behaviors and want the "expert" therapist to "fix" the child. Often complainants do not include themselves initially when describing the family's problem-maintaining interaction patterns, nor do they view themselves as co-collaborators in the solution construction process. Prochaska et al. (1994) would argue that the complainant is in the "contemplative stage" of the change cycle: he or she recognizes that there is a problem but is not yet ready to take action. Many complainants expect therapists to see their children alone and "figure out why" they "act out" and have "low self-esteem" or "attitude" problems. These parents often claim that their hectic work schedules prevent them from being able to attend their children's therapy sessions regularly.

Because complainants are excellent supersleuths by nature, it makes a great deal of sense for therapists to capitalize on their excellent observational skills by giving them an observation task (de Shazer, 1988; Selekman, 2005). The parent is given the following directive:

> "I am struck by your tremendous insight into your child's behavior, but in order to give me a more complete picture of what we are looking at, I would like you to do a little experiment for me over the next week. I would like you to pull out your imaginary magnifying glass and notice all of the encouraging steps [child's name] will be taking on a daily basis. Please write those encouraging steps down and bring that information to our next appointment."

The following case example demonstrates how to engage a complainant who has been involved in multiple treatment experiences for her own alcoholism as well as for her son's stealing, lying, and ADD. At the beginning of the first interview, I considered William a visitor due to his lack of desire to be in another counseling situation again.

William, an African American 10-year-old boy, was school-referred for counseling due to his "disruptive, clowning behavior" in class. His grades were slipping because he failed to complete homework assignments or to turn them in when he did complete them. He also had a tendency to "mouth off" to his teacher when she reprimanded him. On the homefront, Renee, the mother, described William as "always getting under her skin" by "stealing money" from her and "bullying his two younger sisters." According to Renee, William had been stealing from her "since he was a toddler." She also reported that whenever William came back from a weekend visitation with his father, George, he was "totally wired" and "difficult to manage." Renee's two final complaints concerned William's lack of closeness with his stepfather, Steve, and his worsening "ADD condition," despite the fact that his pediatrician had placed him on Ritalin. After getting absolutely nowhere with the miracle question (de Shazer, 1988; see also below), I shifted gears and asked Renee how she managed to cope with all the problems to better cooperate with her pessimism. I decided to meet alone with Renee.

THERAPIST: I am curious how you have managed to cope with all of these difficulties. I mean, some parents would have thrown in the towel already.

RENEE: Well ... as much as William is a pain in the butt sometimes, I still love him. Who knows ... maybe it is a self-esteem problem.

THERAPIST: What steps have you taken to prevent this situation from getting worse?

RENEE: Well, I am in regular contact with his teacher and counselor at school. I mean, I keep taking him for counseling ... but it doesn't seem to work. Part of the problem is his father, George. He is also in recovery, but from drugs. We really can't stand each other. I mean, I think he sabotages what Steve and I try to do at home with William.

THERAPIST: With all of your past counseling experiences with William, do you remember if any of the therapists incorporated George into the treatment process?

RENEE: No. None of them did.

THERAPIST: Do you think that could be helpful for me to try and engage his father to work with us to help William?

RENEE: Good luck! He is one of most hard-headed men I have ever met … but I guess it is worth a shot.

THERAPIST: Do you think it would also be a good idea for me to collaborate with William's teacher, school counselor, and the pediatrician?

RENEE: Definitely. The school people are totally fed up with William and have discussed the possibility of putting him in a therapeutic day school. I would really like to avoid that at all costs.

By shifting gears and better matching my questions with Renee's pessimistic stance, we did a complete U-turn from my fielding complaints to eliciting her strong desire to help William out and explore potential avenues for solution construction. I also gave Renee an observational task of keeping track, on a daily basis, of the various things she was doing to prevent William's behavior from getting worse, particularly those strategies that seemed to work in eliciting positive responses from him.

In future sessions, I successfully engaged the father around the school's threat of placing William in a therapeutic day school, an outcome he wanted to avoid as well. I was also able to unify the adults around the importance of parental consistency with limit setting and working together as a team when William would try to split them. The teacher and school counselor were very cooperative, and I was successful in building a bridge between the school and the home around problem-solving efforts. William's stealing behavior stopped once he was more receptive to learning positive ways to "steal his mother's attention." In collaboration with the pediatrician, we mutually agreed to revisit the Ritalin issue. It turned out that an adjustment in the Ritalin dosage was necessary, and the adjustment helped William to be less hyper and more focused with his school assignments. I ended up seeing the family for 10 sessions over 1 year's time.

Customers

The customer is a parent, extended family member, the referring person, or another involved helping professional from a larger system who is genuinely concerned about the child client's problematic behaviors and wants to work closely with the therapist in generating solutions. Theoretically, having just one real customer in the family sessions is all it takes to resolve the presenting problem. The same is true at school. If the teacher is the customer, getting him or her to look at the child's behavior differently, abandon unsuccessful attempted solutions, and try new behaviors in response to the child's problematic behaviors can promote changes with the child. The following questions are useful in sessions when the therapist is trying to determine the true customer(s) in the client system:

- "Who in your family is most concerned about this problem?"
- "Who else?"
- (*to the identified client*) "On a scale of 1 to 10, 10 being most concerned about you, what number would you give everybody in your family?"
- "What difference will it make to each person in the family when the problem is solved?"
- "If things get worse with this problem, who will suffer the most?"
- "Who next?"
- "Who at school is most concerned about this problem?"
- "Who else?"

Coauthoring a New Family Story

Once the therapist has gathered sufficient family and child background information and clarified with family members what they view as the key problem they want to work on changing *first,* the second half of the family assessment session is devoted to eliciting from each family member what his or her initial treatment goals and desired outcome pictures will look like. By moving the interview discussion in this positive direction, we are helping family members coauthor a more preferred solution-determined story in which they are the lead authors. As a lead-in to this discussion, I share with the family the following: "Now we can talk about solutions and change—where you want to be when we have a successful outcome here." Sometimes the family and I go into a completely different room when beginning this part of the family assessment session so that we can turn the light switch off on "problem talk" (Gingerich et al., 1988), thus heightening the family's awareness and expectation that something positive and surprising is about to happen. There are four parts to this portion of the family assessment session: goal setting, co-constructing the "blueprint for change" plan, the editorial reflection, and the postassessment session self-reflection.

Goal Setting

To begin the goal-setting process with the family, I may use the miracle question (Selekman, 2005, 2009; de Shazer et al., 2007; de Shazer, 1988; de Shazer & White, 1996; Miller & Berg, 1995) or other presuppositional questions (Selekman, 2005, 2009; O'Hanlon & Weiner-Davis, 1989) to elicit from each family member what the ideal treatment outcome would look like when all their problems are solved. With both of these categories of questions, it is most advantageous to expand the possibilities with each family member—that is, have them all spell out in great detail the changes they envision in all their familial and extrafamilial relationships and in every social context in which they interact, such as the peer group and the school. Family members absent from the assessment session can be introduced into the miracle question inquiry as well, for example, by asking the client the following: "If your father were sitting here, what would he be most surprised about that changed with you after the miracle happened?"

THE MIRACLE QUESTION

When asking the miracle question, it is important that the therapist be patient and give family members plenty of time to think and respond. If they appear to be having difficulty answering the question, I ask them to pretend or play around with the idea that all their problems are magically solved. Typically, this helps open up the imagination doors for family members who are initially having difficulty answering the miracle question. The therapist should avoid asking leading questions, allowing family members to introduce their own unique solutions and envisioned changes in the miracle picture spontaneously. Once family members have shared their miracle pictures, the therapist can naturally use curiosity to explore with them other changes they wondered about that might be happening and to ask whether any of their miracles are occurring a little bit already. The miracle question sequence is as follows:

- "Suppose you go home tonight and go to bed, and while you are sound asleep a miracle happens and all of your problems are solved. When you wake up the next day, how will each of you be able to tell that this miracle really happened?"
- "What will be different?"
- "What else will have changed with your situation?"
- "What difference will that make in your relationship with your [mother, father, brother, sister, son, or daughter]?"
- "What else will be better?"
- (to client) "Who will be the most surprised—your [mother, father, brother, sister]?—when you do that?"
- "What effect will that have on your relationship with your mother when you do that more often?"
- "How will your mom and dad have changed?"
- "When they are yelling less, how will the three of you be getting along better?"

- "What else will you be doing instead with your parents?"
- (*to parents*) "When he [or she] does that, how will you treat him [her] differently?"
- "How will you get that to happen?"
- (*to client*) "What about at school? What will your teacher notice first that changed with you?"
- "What else will you be doing differently in class that will help you and your teacher get along better?"
- "I'm curious ... have there been any times lately when you have seen pieces of this miracle happening already?"
- "When was the most recent piece of the miracle?"

With younger children who are cognitively unable to grasp the concept of a miracle, I may hand the child an imaginary magic wand (any toy wand will do) and have him or her wave it in the air and "zap" each family member with it—as well as explore what changes he or she would make happen with the teacher, friends, or any peers with whom he or she is having trouble at school or in the neighborhood. After the child client is finished, I hand the imaginary magic wand to the parents and siblings present in the family assessment session. The following case example demonstrates the usefulness of the imaginary magic wand with a child and his parents.

Charlie, a 6-year-old Caucasian boy, was brought for counseling because of his severe temper tantrums and for not responding to his mother's limit setting, particularly when his father was not around.

THERAPIST: If I gave you [Charlie] an imaginary magic wand—careful, don't drop it (*reaching over to hand Charlie the wand*)—and asked you to wave it in the air to warm it up first and then zap your family with it, how would you make your family better? What would you change first?

CHARLIE: They would be happy ...

THERAPIST: What would make everyone happy?

CHARLIE: We will play together a lot. Dad will be home more ...

THERAPIST: What will you play together?

CHARLIE: We don't make puzzles no more ... I like to make puzzles with Daddy ... but he's at work a lot.

THERAPIST: When Dad's home more, will you make puzzles again?

CHARLIE: Yeah! Daddy ... Daddy ... I want to make the airplane puzzle ... Can we?!

MARILYN [mother]: I wonder if this is why Charlie is so upset these days

... because he misses not playing with you? (*looking at George, her husband*) Matthew [therapist], do you think this is why he is having such bad temper tantrums—because he is angry about this?

THERAPIST: I don't know. What do you think about this, George?

GEORGE: Marilyn might be right. I've had to be out of town a lot on business, and I can understand why Charlie is so upset. We used to play a lot together in the past. Charlie, what do you think? ... Have you been mad because I've been away a lot?

CHARLIE: (*hugging his father*) I miss you ... I want to play more with you. Can we make the airplane puzzle when we get home?

MARILYN: I miss Daddy too, honey. (*looking at Charlie*)

THERAPIST: (*looking at George*) Will your business trip situation be changing soon, or will this be a regular part of your job responsibilities?

GEORGE: Yeah, it should be slowing down in a few weeks for a while. (*looking at Marilyn and Charlie*) I miss you guys a lot when I'm away.

THERAPIST: Charlie, you did a nice job with the magic wand. Are there any other wishes you would like to make come true with it, or should we let Mom and Dad try it out?

CHARLIE: Here, Daddy, (*handing the wand to his father*) you try! What do you wish?

GEORGE: Not as many business trips. Charlie is happy and not mad anymore. We go on a nice family trip together.

THERAPIST: Where do you want to take your family?

GEORGE: Out west ... maybe the Rockies or the Grand Canyon.

MARILYN: That sounds great. When are we going?

The remainder of the interview was upbeat. When it was Marilyn's turn to use the magic wand, she wished for Charlie to be "happier" and for her husband to be "around more," and she also thought it was "time for a family trip." Earlier in the family assessment session, Marilyn thought Charlie's "temper tantrum" problem was related to his having "low self-esteem," "looking depressed," and having "anger management" problems. With the help of the imaginary magic wand, we were able to open up space for possibilities and operationalize the concept. All the family members, including the father, "missed" each other because of George's mandatory business trips. As a devoted husband and father, George was eventually able to negotiate with his boss a reduction in business trips. Once George started spending more time with Charlie, the child's behavior improved a great deal. We terminated after three sessions of therapy, including the family assessment session.

PRESUPPOSITIONAL QUESTIONS

Presuppositional questions (Selekman, 2005, 2009; O'Hanlon & Weiner-Davis, 1989) can be used to amplify pretreatment changes and exceptions, to convey with confidence the certainty of change to families, to elicit the family's treatment outcome goals, and to help co-create a context for change with the family. Presuppositional questions can also produce significant changes in family members' outmoded beliefs and behaviors. In the interviewing process, we should listen carefully to individual family members' own presuppositional language and try to match our presuppositional language to theirs. For example, if the mother in a family uses past-tense presuppositional words such as "fixed" and "resolved," it makes sense for the therapist to ask questions laced with such words as "accomplished" or "did." Like the miracle question, presuppositional questions are a powerful therapeutic tool for eliciting from family members the "who," "what," "when," "where," and "how" of goal attainment. Some examples of presuppositional questions are:

- "Let's say that all of you were driving home from today's session, and it proved to be highly successful; what will have changed with your situation?"
- "If we were to look at a videotape of this family when all of your problems are solved, what will we see happening on that video that will convince you things are better?"
- "What else do we see that changed?"
- "How will you know when you don't have to come here anymore?"
- "I'm curious ... what have you noticed that is better since you first called here to make an appointment?"
- "Let's say I were to hand you my imaginary crystal ball, and I asked each of you to look into the crystal ball and tell me what you see that changed over the next week with your situation? What would that be?"
- "How surprised will you be when that happens?" (*to identified child client*) "Which one of your parents will faint first when you do that?"
- "What will be a small sign of progress over the next week that will tell you that you are really making headway?"
- "In what ways can you see yourself succeeding over the next week?"
- "How will you know that the problem is really solved?"

The following case example illustrates the therapeutic value of presuppositional questions in co-creating a context for change with families.

> Lisa, a bright 11-year-old, was school-referred for "underachieving," "not turning in her school assignments," and "talking back to her teacher." In past school years, Lisa had always received A's and B's on tests and assignments. Present in the family assessment session were Lisa; her mother, Jane; and Chester, her relatively new stepfather.
>
> THERAPIST: Let's say I handed you my imaginary crystal ball and I asked each of you to look into the crystal ball (*all family members are staring at my hands holding the crystal ball*) and tell me what each of you see that changed over the next week with your situation. What would you say?
>
> CHESTER: Well, Lisa will be completing all of her school assignments and turning them in daily.
>
> THERAPIST: When she does that next week, how will the two of you be getting along better?
>
> CHESTER: Well ... I will be yelling at her less ... I know she is capable of doing better. She is a bright girl.
>
> THERAPIST: Lisa, when Chester is yelling at you less, what will he be doing instead with you that will help you guys get along better?
>
> LISA: I would be very surprised if he would be nicer to me. I mean he is always pushing me with the schoolwork. I'm sick of it! Mom, why do you let him do that?
>
> JANE: You know school is very important to us. Chester and I just want you to do better in school. We know you can do well if you just try. Do you really feel like we are putting too much pressure on you to do well in school?
>
> LISA: Yes! Just leave me alone. Miss Smith [Lisa's teacher] is just like you guys. "You can do better, Lisa—I know you can." That is how she sounds. That makes me mad!
>
> THERAPIST: Lisa, please look into the imaginary crystal ball and tell me what Miss Smith is doing differently that will help the two of you get along better.
>
> LISA: Well ... she is not trying to be my mom.
>
> THERAPIST: What else?
>
> LISA: She is not always asking to see my homework as soon as I walk in the door.
>
> THERAPIST: Let's say that now I am gazing into the imaginary crystal

ball, what do I see you doing differently at school that is helping you get along better with Miss Smith?

LISA: I will turn in my homework first thing. Treat her nicer. I mean not be mean to her.

THERAPIST: What about at home? What do I see you doing differently in the crystal ball with your parents?

LISA: Getting my homework done. Making sure they see I am taking it to school with me. I know what can help a lot!

THERAPIST: What?

LISA: If Mom and Chester would not push me.

THERAPIST: How so?

LISA: I will want to do my schoolwork if they leave me alone about it.

With the help of my trusty imaginary crystal ball, we were able to identify specific behaviors that maintained Lisa's difficulties with her parents, her teacher, and completing and turning in her school assignments. At the same time, by capitalizing on her own expertise, Lisa was able to identify clearly what the parents and teacher could do to resolve the difficulties. In a school meeting with the teacher, Jane, and Lisa, Lisa was able to share with her teacher that she felt as if her teacher was trying to "mother" her, which led to Lisa's "mouthing off" to Miss Smith and not doing the schoolwork. Once the parents and the teacher began to experiment with "backing off" of Lisa, particularly regarding her school assignments, Lisa's behavior improved dramatically. I ended up seeing the family three more times after the family assessment session.

SCALING QUESTIONS

Scaling questions (Selekman, 2005, 2009; Berg & de Shazer, 1993; de Shazer, 1991, 1994) are very useful for securing a quantitative measurement of the family's presenting problem prior to treatment and presently and of where they would like to be on a scale of 1 to 10 in 1 week's time. Frequently, family members report that they have already taken constructive steps to resolve their problem situation when comparing where they were on the scale 4 weeks prior to the assessment session and where they are presently. Like Sherlock Holmes and Miss Marple detectives, we need to elicit in great detail from each family member the useful coping and problem-solving strategies he or she has employed to advance higher on the scale. Having family members talk about their unique creative strategies for trying to resolve the presenting problems and other difficulties empowers them and helps make it newsworthy that they are on the path to a solution. Cheerleading, handshakes, and high-fives are also useful for highlighting important pretreatment changes (Selekman, 2005, 2009; de Shazer, 1988, 1991).

Once the family rates where they are on the scale presently, I ask the following question: "Let's say we get together in one week's time and you proceed to tell me that you took some steps and got to a 7 [the family was at a 6] ... what will you tell me that you did?" The answer to this question becomes the family's initial treatment goal, particularly if these steps are what they want to accomplish first in treatment. The therapist's job is to collaborate with the family in negotiating an achievable initial treatment goal, especially if the family's suggestions sound too grandiose or unrealistic. Well-conceived treatment goals are small, concrete, realistic, and behavioral. The therapist can ask the following kinds of questions:

- "Do you really think it is possible for your son to have a whole week without even *one* temper tantrum, given that he has been having one or two daily for the past year?"
- "What will be a small sign of progress over the next week that will tell you [the parents] that we are heading in the right direction?"
- "What has to change first that will indicate that we are really succeeding here?"
- "How else will you be able to tell that we made it up to a 7 [the parents' baseline rating for their son's temper tantrum problem was a 6]?"
- "How many days out of seven will he have to go without a temper tantrum that would make you [the parents] feel like we are making good headway?"
- "On a scale from 1 to 10, with 10 being 'I am totally satisfied with my situation,' what number would you use to rate your situation today?"

In some cases, the therapist can establish separate goals for the child and his or her parents. This is particularly useful when the child is quite outspoken about a specific parental behavior that he or she contends is contributing to the maintenance of the difficulties. For example, if the parents' "yelling" is a major concern to the child, I may have the child rate the parents' yelling on a scale from 1 to 10, both 4 weeks prior to treatment and presently. The next step would be to identify as clearly as possible what the parents would need to do in a week's time (in the child's view) to cut back on their yelling behavior.

Scaling questions can be used to measure family members' confidence levels regarding their ability to resolve the presenting problem. I may ask the parents to rate their confidence levels regarding their ability to resolve their son's temper tantrum problem by asking: "How confident are you today on a scale of 1 to 10 that we will resolve your son's temper tantrum problem, 10 being most confident?" With children who experience difficulty grasping the number rating process, I may use a feeling face scale, with a happy face at the top of the scale and a sad face at the bottom of the scale, and draw this out on a flip chart or pad of paper. The child can make a dot or "X" mark in our first family assessment meeting on the scale to provide us with a baseline where he or she sees him- or herself presently. Throughout the course of treatment, the child can change his or her marks as he or she moves closer to the happy face.

Finally, with more chronic child cases, highly pessimistic parents, or families that have had multiple treatment experiences, I may offer a subzero scale to more accurately reflect their pessimism, with –10 being the worst and –1 being the best possible rating of the presenting problem situation (Selekman, 2005, 2009). Often, the subzero scale instills hope for highly pessimistic clients who have had lots of treatment by increasing their awareness levels that they are already taking constructive steps to cope and resolve their problems.

The following case example illustrates how scaling questions not only can pave the way for eliciting news of a difference from family members but also can assist the therapist and the family in establishing a clear focus for the treatment process.

Juan, a Puerto Rican 10-year-old, was brought for therapy by his mother, Maria, because he did not follow her rules, had temper tantrums, and fought with his 8-year-old sister, Isabella. Out of respect for cultural differences, I explored with the family how they felt about working with a non-Latino therapist; this was not a problem for them. After expanding the possibilities with the miracle question, I then asked the family scaling questions.

THERAPIST: Maria, on a scale from 1 to 10, how would you have rated Juan's behavior 4 weeks ago?

MARIA: A 2! He never listened to me. Juan used to break anything he could get his hands on when having one of his temper tantrums.

THERAPIST: What about today? How would you rate him on that scale now?

MARIA: Well ... I think he is doing better ... maybe he is at a 5.

THERAPIST: A 5! That's quite a leap? (*Juan is smiling in response to my reaction.*) What steps have you seen him take to get from a 2 to a 5?

MARIA: Well, we are not having any more battles about making his bed and putting his toys away. When he does have his temper fits, he is not destroying things anymore.

THERAPIST: How did you help make all of those good things happen? What are you doing differently?

MARIA: Well, I am more patient. I am not yelling as much. You know what really works?

THERAPIST: What?

MARIA: Avoiding the power struggles.

THERAPIST: How did you come up with that great idea?

MARIA: Well, before ... I used to try and win the battles by screaming and taking away everything ... but that only made the situation worse.

THERAPIST: Are there other things that you are doing that helps?

MARIA: When Juan has had a good week, I reward him by taking him out for pizza and a movie.

THERAPIST: Wow! You are really creative as a parent. What is your consultation fee? I want to use you as an expert consultant with some of my other single-parent family cases. (*laughing*)

MARIA: It's been hard raising these two kids, but I keep telling myself, "You're going to make it ... "

THERAPIST: (*looking at Juan*) What is your mom doing now that helps the most, so that you don't get into trouble?

JUAN: She is not yelling. Pizza and movies! (*smiling and hugging his mother*)

THERAPIST: What do you like on your pizza?

JUAN: Lots of sausage and cheese!

THERAPIST: Maria, let's say we were to get together in a week and you proceed to tell me that Juan took some further steps to get up to a 6! What will you tell me he did to get to a 6?

MARIA: He won't be fighting as much with his sister.

THERAPIST: What will be a small sign of progress over the next week that will tell you we are making headway with the fighting situation?

MARIA: Rather than punching his sister when she teases him or makes him mad, he will come to me instead.

THERAPIST: Do you think it is realistic that he will be able to do that every day?

MARIA: No, probably not.

THERAPIST: How many days over the next week would you be happy with?

MARIA: If he could do this twice I would be thrilled!

THERAPIST: (*looking at Juan*) Do you think you can pull that off?

JUAN: Yeah. I want pizza!

I ended up seeing Juan and his family three times. Juan had a great week, in that he fought with his sister only once and had no temper tantrums. The added bonus in this case was working with a mother who was so committed, creative, and resourceful as a parent that it made my job easy. There also were many client self-generated pretreatment changes to amplify and consolidate.

Co-Constructing the Blueprint for Change Plan

Once the family's initial treatment goals have been negotiated, the therapist can introduce the *blueprint for change plan* (Selekman, 2009). The blueprint for change plan empowers clients to be the lead authors or architects of their road maps for change. It consists of six parts: (1) My/Our Identified Pretreatment Changes, (2) Target Behaviors and/or Relationship Changes Desired Now, (3) My/Our Identified and Key Strengths Tapped for Goal Attainment, (4) Identification of Solution-Determined System Membership and Whom to Include in Future Sessions, (5) the Treatment Modality and Adjunct Services Selection Menu, and (6) the Therapeutic Experiment Menu (see Figure 2.1). I discuss each one of these sections in turn below.

My/Our Identified Pretreatment Changes

In this section we revisit with clients the self-generated pretreatment changes that they think will help them to achieve the initial treatment goals. These may include past successful parenting strategies that they just reinstated or even experimenting with suggestions from a parenting self-help book that seemed to help in reducing the frequency of their child's objectionable behavior. Children can be asked about what they think the parents should increase doing with them that can help them get along better. In addition, we should inquire with them whether they think increased participation in certain flow state activities, hobbies, or social involvements will help them be in a better mood and less likely to get into trouble.

Target Behaviors and/or Relationship Changes Desired Now

Clients take the lead in determining what problems they want to change first. Our job is to negotiate with them well-formulated incremental behav-

FIGURE 2.1. The blueprint for change plan.

My/Our Identified Key Pretreatment Changes:

1.

2.

3.

4.

5.

Target Behaviors and/or Relationship Changes Desired Now:

1. Parents' Goals:

    a.

    b.

    c.

2. Child's Goals:

    a.

    b.

    c.

My/Our Identified and Key Strengths Tapped for Goal Attainment:

1.

2.

3.

4.

5.

6.

(cont.)

FIGURE 2.1. (*cont.*)

Identification of Solution-Determined System Membership and Whom to Include in Future Sessions:

1.

2.

3.

4.

5.

6.

Treatment Modality and Adjunct Services Selection Menu:

_____ Individual Therapy

_____ Couple Therapy

_____ Family Therapy

_____ Solution-Oriented Parenting Group

_____ Collaboration and Advocacy with Larger Systems Professionals

_____ Mindfulness Meditation Training

_____ Art Therapy

Therapeutic Experiment Menu:

_____ Therapeutic Experiment #1

_____ Therapeutic Experiment #2

_____ Therapeutic Experiment #3

Parents:

Name _____ Date _____

Name _____ Date _____

Children:

Name _____ Date _____

Name _____ .Date _____

Name _____ Date _____

Therapist:

Name _____ Date _____

ioral goals that the clients wish to pursue. It is important to emphasize to families that even attained goals represent the start of something new, not ends in themselves. Moreover, they must recognize that the journey to goal attainment requires hard work and good teamwork and that there will be bumps in the road along the way. Both parents and children are invited to establish both joint and individual goals.

My/Our Identified and Key Strengths Tapped for Goal Attainment

Clients determine which of their key individual and family strengths they will use to achieve their initial treatment goals. The strengths may include successful use of self-talk, increasing positive family interactions, such as spending more high-quality family time together or expressing more appreciation toward one another, using one's key intelligence skill areas to achieve the goal, and the like. The whole process of having clients identify and articulate the details about how specifically *they* will use their key strengths boosts their self-confidence and raises their expectations that they will achieve their goals and it is only a matter of *when*.

Identification of Solution-Determined System Membership and Whom to Include in Future Sessions

In this section of the change plan, clients are asked who is actively involved and most concerned about their difficulties other than the referring person(s). The resulting list can include teachers and other school personnel, the pediatrician or psychiatrist, spiritual mentors or advisers, child protective workers, older siblings out of the home, grandparents, and other extended family members. With children, I want to include any adult sources of inspiration as well as concerned peers whom they may wish to include in future family sessions. I like to view concerned helping professionals from larger systems and key members from the clients' social networks as resourceful allies who should be actively involved in the solution construction process. The parents and their children take the lead in determining which of these individuals should participate in future sessions and at what stage of the treatment process they should be physically present in our sessions. Finally, I have children who are old enough to print their names and their parents sign consent forms so I can begin the collaboration process with the involved helpers.

Treatment Modality and Adjunct Services Selection Menu

To help honor clients' treatment preferences and theories of change, I invite them to choose from a menu of treatment modality options and adjunct services what they think will best meet their unique needs. For the treatment modality options, they can choose among individual, couple, and family therapies and a modified *solution-oriented parenting group* adapted for parents with latency-aged children (6–11 years old; for more details about conducting solution-oriented parenting groups, see Selekman, 2005, 2009). Some parents, while filling out the blueprint for change plan, will voice a desire to have separate couples sessions in addition to family therapy. When parents voice a strong desire for individual therapy for their child, I will share my own preference for family therapy or, as another option, the possibility of seeing them concurrently but separately to address the child's relationships with them and offer parenting tools and strategies. Additional adjunct services offered include collaboration and advocacy with larger-systems professionals, mindfulness meditation training, and art therapy. Although all of these adjunct services will to some extent be integrated into their family treatment experiences anyway, if the family seeks additional involvement in these activities, it can be provided by either me or a trained colleague.

Therapeutic Experiment Menu

Once I know what my clients' theories of change, stages of readiness for change, pretreatment changes and key strengths, and treatment goals are, during the intersession break I come up with two to three therapeutic experiments for them to choose from as options to try out over the next week. I find that letting clients take the lead in choosing what they think will work best for them gives them ownership of the change process, helps strengthen the therapeutic alliance, and prevents premature client dropouts from occurring. Finally, I write out each therapeutic experiment for the clients, describing the concrete steps for implementing it.

On the last page of the blueprint for change plan, the parents, child, and therapist can sign their names and note the date it was signed. (I like to have younger children print their names so they feel empowered as part of the family change effort and to make the contract official.) The family receives a copy of it to refer to throughout the course of treatment. We will revisit the blueprint for change plan periodically to see how family members are doing with goal attainment or if there are new goals they would like to work on or if they would like to add or drop any of the treatment modalities or adjunctive services they had selected during the initial family assessment session. The blueprint for change plan is totally fluid and flexible, and clients appreciate having the freedom to customize their treatment experiences.

Although there is no special section on diagnosis or for a Global Assessment of Functioning rating, this can be added to the last page of the blueprint for change plan after the therapeutic experiment menu section. When selecting a DSM-IV-TR Axis I diagnosis for the identified child client for insurance purposes, I like to involve the family in the decision-making process. If the child's diagnosis could be one of three possibilities, I show the family the DSM-IV-TR descriptions for each of the diagnostic categories and have them pick the one they think best fits their situation. Many children's problems are some form of an adjustment disorder; so, I often give the family a grand tour of this section of the DSM-IV-TR volume. When in doubt, we may go with the "adjustment disorder, not otherwise specified" label. Because many insurance companies do not accept V codes, we are often forced to select an Axis I diagnosis for the identified client even though the truth of the matter is that we are usually dealing with a family problem. When families are precommitted to a particular Axis I DSM-IV-TR diagnostic label, I go with their label initially and work with it in the treatment process, often by externalizing the problem (Selekman, 1996; White, 2007; Epston, 1998; White & Epston, 1990). In a similar collaborative fashion, I invite the family to be coauthors in writing any treatment updates and summaries and letters for involved helpers from larger systems, the court, schools, and managed care companies. By doing this, we as therapists empower families to be in charge of their destinies.

The Editorial Reflection

Approximately 45 minutes into the hour, I take an intersession break to compose my editorial reflection for the family. The editorial consists of positively relabeled problem behaviors, normalizing concerns, compliments for each family member on their pretreatment changes, various problem-solving and coping strategies they reported engaging in that were helpful to them, questions to think about regarding their situation, and therapeutic experiments to test that fit with the unique cooperative response patterns of each family member.

When complimenting family members, carefully gauge where each member is in terms of optimism, pessimism, and customership. For instance, if the therapist showers highly pessimistic complainant-type parents and their child with too many positively toned compliments, the parents may think the therapist is being sarcastic or not taking their situation serious enough. The same is true with too much positive relabeling: more pessimistic family members may think the therapist is trying to talk them out of their problems.

While composing the editorial reflection, if there are certain elements of the family's story about which I am curious, I share with the family my questions as part of the reflection process. I begin my questions with such qualifiers as "I wonder if … " or "Could it be … ?" Sometimes I leave the family with some questions to think about when concluding the session and do not offer them experiments. The case of Lisa and her family (see pp. 68–69) can provide an illustration of using questions in the editorial reflection portion of the session. I asked Lisa and Chester the following questions I was pondering:

- "I wondered ... how was it decided that Chester be in charge of monitoring Lisa's schoolwork?"
- "Could it be that this is a tough spot for a new stepparent to be in?"
- "I wondered ... wouldn't Lisa and Chester get along a lot better if he did not have this responsibility?"

By asking such questions, therapists convey to the families that the therapist is not a privileged expert on their problem situation and that the therapeutic process is truly collaborative. The input can also open up space for new possibilities.

When engaging in the editorial reflection, it is most important to utilize the family members' language and speak to their beliefs about themselves and their problem story. By doing this, any new ideas offered or tasks prescribed are more likely to be acceptable to the family. There are two advantages to taking an intersession break 10–15 minutes prior to the end of the hour: (1) the therapist has time to compose a thoughtful editorial reflection as well as select or construct therapeutic tasks that fit with the unique cooperative response patterns of family members, and (2) family members are more than likely sitting at the edge of their seats wondering what the therapist has to say about them. Families that have had past negative experiences with therapists are usually surprised to be complimented on their strengths and resources and to be working with a therapist who appears to be trying very hard to understand their problem story and to help navigate them in the direction of change.

Finally, after the family chooses the therapeutic experiments they wish to try out over the next week, I solicit family members' perceptions of their experience in the session. This practice offers excellent feedback on the new relationships we are beginning to forge and addresses any concerns family members may have. During this concluding phase of the session, I ask the following types of questions:

- "What was today's meeting like for all of you?"
- "What ideas did you find to be most helpful?"
- "How specifically was that idea most useful to you?"
- "Did you learn anything new about yourselves or your situation?"
- "Was there anything that you were surprised I did not ask you about your situation?"

- "Do you think we need to address that issue in the next session?"
- "Was there anything I said or did that was upsetting to any of you that you would like me to stop doing?"

The Postassessment Session Self-Reflection

Following the family assessment session, I like to set aside a little time to reflect on my therapeutic actions in a given session and my clinical impressions and formulations of the case. As questions and ideas pop into my mind, I write them down as a checklist for future thinking and pathways to pursue with the case. I divide my self-reflection process into two different areas: (1) reflections on actions taken during the session and areas to explore with the family and (2) alternative therapeutic actions to pursue in the next family session. With reflection-on-action taken, I may ask myself the following questions:

- "If I were to conduct this session all over again with this same family, what would I do differently?"
- "What should I ask them more about?"
- "Should I use less or more humor with this family?"
- "What family member strengths and resources did I fail to capitalize on?"
- "Who responded the best to being complimented?"
- "Who responded the least to the compliments?"
- "What family members do I need to spend more time engaging in the next session?"
- "What other therapeutic experiments could I have offered family members that might have better fit with their unique cooperative response patterns?"

When thinking about my clinical impressions and formulation of the case, I may ask myself the following questions:

- "Do we have a customer here?"
- "If not, who should I try to engage for future sessions?"
- "Which involved school personnel should I begin collaborating with first?"
- "What else am I curious about with this case?"
- "I wonder if the parents' goal is still too ambitious?"
- "If we renegotiated their goal into more achievable terms, what would that look like?"
- "What are the key solution-building patterns?"

- "What are the patterns that connect?"
- "Have I been sensitive to cultural issues?"
- "Are there power imbalances related to gender in this family?"

With the second and subsequent sessions, the same critical self-reflective process can be used to monitor our clinical thinking and therapeutic actions closely with each family with which we work. By viewing ourselves in relationship to our clients through a critical lens, we can remain therapeutically flexible, maintain a kaleidoscopic view of families, and carefully tailor what we say or do to the uniqueness of each family.

3

Interviewing for Change

Co-Creating Compelling Future Realities with Children and Their Families

If we learn to see, then there is no end to the new worlds of our vision.
—CARLOS CASTANEDA

Inviting families to talk about their past successes, their strengths, and where they want to be when they have an ideal outcome empowers them to create their own positive self-fulfilling prophecies. Questions can be used as therapeutic tools for promoting self-healing, challenging outmoded family beliefs, and sparking curiosity, which can lead to possibilities for stuck families. The quality of the learning process for families depends on the quality of the questions we ask. Bold and intriguing questions that elicit a full range of responses are more likely to open up space for new learning and the emergence of creative solutions with families (Brown & Isaacs, 1997, 2005).

In this chapter, I present five types of therapeutic questions that can be utilized at any stage of family treatment. Family members' unique cooperative response patterns, the age of the child, and the nature of the family's presenting problem dictate which types of questions are used to best effect in the interviewing process. Unlike the conversational (Anderson, 1997; Anderson & Goolishian, 1988b) and goal-setting questions discussed in Chapter 2, the five types of questions described in this chapter are particularly useful in challenging rigid family beliefs and moving the treatment system (therapist, family, involved professionals from larger systems, and key members of the client's social network) away from any impasses. Children also tend to respond well to questions that draw upon their creativity and expertise, such as the imagination and reversal questions presented later in this chapter.

Interviewing for Change

The collaborative strengths-based therapist asks questions in a purposeful manner, by carefully assessing family members' unique cooperative response patterns and matching questions with those patterns (Selekman, 2005, 2009; de Shazer et al., 2007; de Shazer, 1988, 1991, 1994; Lipchik, 1988; O'Hanlon & Weiner-Davis, 1989). The purposeful interview is a circular process in which family members' verbal and nonverbal feedback guides the therapist in his or her choice of subsequent questions. For example, if I ask the miracle question (de Shazer, 1988) and, in the middle of the miracle inquiry, a family member has a concern he or she wishes to address, has a troubled look on his or her face, or is tearing up, I shift into more open-ended conversational questions (Anderson, 1997; Anderson & Goolishian, 1988a, 1988b; Andersen, 1991) to address his or her concerns and make room for storytelling. Once the family member's concerns have been adequately addressed, the therapist can move back to the miracle question inquiry and invite other family members to share their ideal miracle pictures. Collaborative strengths-based therapists must, like ballet dancers, be flexible and on their toes, ready to move in any direction family members wish to take them. If the therapist finds a particular category of questions that appears verbally and nonverbally to be creating possibilities with family members, it is most advantageous to do more of what's working with the family. Finally, when interviewing children, it is especially important for the therapist to concretize his or her language and to use words that the child can readily grasp.

Five types of therapeutic questions—imagination, resiliency, reversal, future-oriented, and externalizing-the-problem questions—are demonstrably useful in the interviewing process. I discuss each type in turn, supplementing each discussion with guidelines for use and a case illustration.

Imagination Questions

Developmentally, children begin displaying signs of imaginative play and pretending after 1 year of age. Parents can help cultivate their children's abilities to engage in imaginative play by modeling make-believe play. Research indicates that very imaginative children tend to be better at concentrating, developing creative solutions to problems, and displaying good self-control (Bodrova & Leong, 2006; Schaefer & DiGeronimo, 1995). The child's current stage of development dictates the level of sophistication that the therapist's imagination questions and scenarios can assume. For example, we know that 3- to 6-year-olds have vivid fantasy lives and are at the peak of their ability to pretend and use their imagination abilities (Schaefer & DiGeronimo, 1995). Bodrova and Leong (2006), authors of the *Tools of the Mind* early childhood curriculum, which is heavily based on the theoretical ideas of Russian psychologist Lev Vygotsky, contend that imaginative dramatic play is the training ground for how children can best develop their self-regulation capacities. Imagination questions fit nicely with children's developmental need to dramatize their social worlds through play and pretending.

Before selecting the type of imagination questions I want to use with a particular child and his or her family, I first assess the following: Who or what are the child's favorite TV, movie, and book characters? What are the child's favorite pastimes, hobbies, and talents? Who are the child's favorite music stars? If the child could be someone famous in history, in the music world, on TV, or a movie or book character for a day, who would the child want to be and why? If the child could choose one TV show or movie in which he or she could star, which TV show or movie would it be? What role could she play and why? If the child created his or her own TV show or movie about his or her family, what would the show or movie be about? Such questions can help spark creativity in both the therapist and the child when collaborating for solutions in the interviewing process. Children typically respond enthusiastically when therapists can tap into their natural creative abilities. Through the use of imagination questions, therapy sessions become more fun and adventurous for both children and their families.

> Marci, a Caucasian 4-year-old, was brought for therapy by her mother for "power struggles" around bedtime and for "night terrors," which were diagnosed by their pediatrician. Except for this time of the day, Marci reportedly was highly "cooperative," "friendly," not anxious, and "a pleasure to be around." According to the mother, Melinda, Marci's preschool teacher consistently found Marci to be a "real joy" in class. Marci was an only child, but her mother described her as being very sociable and having friends in the neighborhood. In exploring with Marci what her favorite TV shows were, she shared with me that she liked "Barney" a lot. I noticed that Marci brought with her a purse with Baby Bop illustrations on it. Because Marci appeared to be a Barney fan club member, I decided to capitalize on her fondness for Barney in the interviewing process.

> THERAPIST: Marci, let's say your mother turned on the Barney show for you tomorrow and we saw Marci on the show. We saw you as a friend visiting Barney and Baby Bop. You came to see Barney and Baby Bop to find out if they could help you go to sleep when you have to go to bed. What would Barney say to help you on TV?

MARCI: Barney would hug me; tell me, "Don't be scared."

THERAPIST: Would Barney say anything else to you?

MARCI: I don't know ...

THERAPIST: Do you think Barney might say, "Most girls and boys get scared when they go to sleep, but it will go away"?

MARCI: Yeah.

THERAPIST: What do you think, Melinda? Do you think Barney would say that to Marci?

MELINDA: Yes! And I think Barney would tell her this "will go away." "Don't be scared."

THERAPIST: Marci, what do you think Baby Bop would tell you?

MARCI: She would be nice to me; hug me; tell me, "It's okay ... I'm your friend."

THERAPIST: What would Barney and Baby Bop do with you on TV to help you?

MARCI: Sing me songs. Watch me when I sleep so I'm not scared.

THERAPIST: So, on TV we would see Barney and Baby Bop in your bedroom standing over you to help you sleep? Does that help?

MARCI: Yeah. I'm sleeping. Barney will say, "Remember, I love you!"

Based on the success of these questions in eliciting images of Marci's receiving support from Barney and Baby Bop with the sleeping problem, the mother and I designed a nighttime ritual in which she and her daughter would carry her stuffed Barney and Baby Bop dolls from the playroom into her bedroom prior to going to bed. Marci would then hug each one of the stuffed dolls and place them in toddler-sized chairs that she would position around her bed. Not only did this ritual eliminate the power struggle problem, it had a profound impact on the night terror difficulty as well.

Resiliency Questions

Family members' resiliencies are our main allies in the solution construction process. Having family members talk about their past successes, how they triumphed over crisis and adversity, can offer therapists important clues about potential problem-solving and coping strategies to capitalize on and channel into the presenting problem area. Families are often surprised when they are asked about their strengths. Families that have experienced failure in previous treatment can be empowered by a therapeutic focus on their competency areas and what is "right" about them.

At times, I have family members describe themselves in detail as a group successfully mastering a past crisis situation as if they were watching a videotape. I use this videotape of mastery as a guide to help them resolve the current presenting problem. Similarly, I may have athletic children use a hypothetical videotape of themselves in the past performing with excellence in a sporting event and have them visualize the video to cope with current stressors. It is also quite helpful to have parents share with the identified child client what they did as children to cope with or to resolve similar difficulties.

George, an African American 10-year-old, was brought for therapy by his mother, Elizabeth, for somatic complaints, such as "headaches" and a "nervous stomach," and some decline in school performance. Elizabeth also thought that George might be "depressed." George was an only child. His parents had been separated for more than 1 year because of his father's severe alcoholism problem. George had been having a hard time for the past 3 years coping with his father's "arguing" with his mother and "passing out on the floor in his vomit" after being highly intoxicated and all the "forgotten promises." George had been receiving some supportive counseling at his school. George had infrequent contacts with his father, who had moved out of state. The father, Bill, had been through four inpatient treatment experiences for alcoholism, all unsuccessful. Inevitably, he would start drinking again a few weeks after being discharged. Because this family had experienced so much emotional pain and suffering, I was curious about their resiliencies—what was keeping them going? How did they bounce back after a crisis with the father? I invited the family to share with me what they viewed as their strengths.

THERAPIST: I am amazed how resilient you guys are, in terms of what you have been through together and how you keep pushing ahead. What's your secret? I mean, I've worked with a lot of families that have been oppressed by alcoholism problems for years, just like yours, and their situations were a lot worse. What are your family strengths, so I can teach other families the tools that work?

ELIZABETH: Well, George and I have really pulled closer together. I really try to be there for him. He knows (*looking at George*) that I really love him and will always be there for him.

THERAPIST: Besides being there for support, what other strengths do the two of you have?

ELIZABETH: He is a big help in the kitchen.

THERAPIST: George, what are your house specialties? I mean, what do you like to cook? (*Both laugh.*)

GEORGE: Well, I can make eggs, macaroni and cheese ... peanut butter and jelly sandwiches.

THERAPIST: Wow! How did you learn how to make all of those dishes?

ELIZABETH: He's really a good cook. We also bake chocolate chip cookies together.

THERAPIST: Elizabeth, I want to go back in time for a few minutes. Can you think of other things you used to do when Bill was in the home to help George weather the storm after a crisis situation, like Bill's passing out or after witnessing you guys arguing?

ELIZABETH: I would take him into his bedroom and tell him, "It's not your fault"; "We love you"; "Only Daddy can decide to stop drinking, we can't stop his drinking."

THERAPIST: Does that seem to help?

ELIZABETH: I think, sometimes. George loves his father and really misses him.

THERAPIST: George, when Mom used to do those things, were they helpful?

GEORGE: Yeah, I guess ...

THERAPIST: Anything she did or is still doing that helps you deal with your dad's drinking?

GEORGE: Well, telling me that I can't stop my dad's drinking. I like when she hugs me when I'm upset.

THERAPIST: Anything else?

GEORGE: No. Mom, can I go get a pop? (*Elizabeth gives him money to buy a soft drink.*)

THERAPIST: Elizabeth, if somebody stopped you on the street and asked you, "What are your strengths as a family?", what would you say?

ELIZABETH: We are loving, very close, and we manage to do fun things— despite all of the problems.

THERAPIST: How about three adjectives to describe your family?

ELIZABETH: Courageous, strong, and bright. What should I do about George's headaches and stomachaches?

THERAPIST: Have they been medically checked?

ELIZABETH: Yes, the pediatrician could not find anything. He thinks it's stress. (*George returns with his Coke.*) What do you think?

THERAPIST: It sounds like, George, you have had to stomach a lot with your dad's passing out, being drunk, and when your parents used to argue. George, this is going to sound like a strange question but, if your stomach could talk to us about what's been going on with you and your family, what would it say? (*George smiles and laughs.*)

GEORGE: (*looking at his mother, smiling*) You're right ... that's a weird question.

THERAPIST: Just play around with it ... pretend your stomach could talk to us.

GEORGE: Well ... it hurts, I guess ... "Stop making me hurt."

THERAPIST: Would it say anything else?

GEORGE: I don't know what else ...

THERAPIST: "Stop making me hurt." Do you think your stomach is trying to tell you and your mom something?

GEORGE: I'm not sure.

ELIZABETH: Maybe the stomach is trying to tell us that we are hurting, both of us, because of all of the problems—you know, the drinking situation.

THERAPIST: What do you think, George?

GEORGE: I don't know ... maybe.

By inviting family members to talk about their resiliencies and past successes, we can learn about what coping strategies we need to mobilize and increase in frequency to help this family resolve their current difficulties. Elizabeth's resiliencies of parental optimism, emotional support, and good problem-solving abilities were instrumental in helping George through some rough times. George's key protective factors for coping were his intelligence, good problem-solving abilities, and seeking his mother's emotional support in times of trouble. I also had the family construct a victory box to serve as a constant reminder of their resilience and creative problem-solving abilities.

When clients are oppressed by somatic problems, I have found it most advantageous to invite the client to put a voice to the affected body part. Not only does it externalize the problem (White, 1995), but it helps challenge outmoded beliefs about the somatic complaint because family members begin to see it as a metaphor for the family drama. I used a similar strategy with George's headache problem. We were quickly able to stabilize the presenting problems by using this therapeutic strategy and capitalizing on family members' resiliencies.

Reversal Questions

In my clinical work with children and their families, I like to use the children as expert consultants in the interviewing process. For some therapists, it may seem illogical to invite children to give their parents advice on parenting and problem solving. However, I have been consistently impressed with how bright, insightful, and creative children are when it comes to solving family problems. When asked, children clearly spell out what specific parental behaviors contribute to the maintenance of the presenting problems and are eager to share with their parents what they can do that can lead to the problem's resolution. While at their friends' houses, children often learn through observation and carefully listening to what their friends' parents do that seems to work in their relationships. Children care about their parents' well-being and often have some good ideas about what their parents can do to help reduce some of the stress in their lives.

By utilizing children as expert consultants in the treatment process, therapists can strengthen their therapeutic alliance with the child, give the child a "voice" in the problem-solving effort, and challenge the parents' unhelpful beliefs about the identified child client. Reversal questions can help interactionalize the problem. Finally, actively involving the child in the solution construction process can greatly reduce lengths of stay in treatment.

> Nadia, a Brazilian American 10-year-old, was brought for therapy by her parents for "emotional problems" related to her chronic difficulties with asthma. The parents came from Brazil, but Nadia was born in the United States. The father was a successful pilot. Sylvia, the mother, "did not work," had only "one friend," and spent most of her leisure time "taking care of" and entertaining Nadia. Nadia was their "special child," for Sylvia lost three babies through miscarriages. Fernando was away a lot on international flights. The parents reported that they almost lost Nadia twice to severe asthma attacks. Sylvia, sitting right next to Nadia, got very emotional when reminiscing about how they almost lost their daughter. The presenting problems with Nadia were temper tantrums, not putting her belongings away, and limit testing with the mother. Because Nadia was an extremely bright and precocious child, I decided to use her as a co-therapist and find out whether she had any advice for the parents that could help improve things at home.

> THERAPIST: We have been talking a lot about your [the parents'] concern with Nadia. It sounds like, Sylvia, that you're with Nadia the most, is that right?
>
> SYLVIA: Yes. Fernando does not have to deal with Nadia during the week because he is away most of the time.

THERAPIST: Since we have not heard much from Nadia and she is such a bright girl, I would like to (*turning to Nadia*) borrow your brain for a few minutes. Nadia, do you have any advice for your mother that can help you get along better?

NADIA: She worries too much. Mom is always asking me, "Did you take your medicine?" "Where is your inhaler?" It makes me mad. She doesn't trust me.

FERNANDO: Nadia, are there not times that you have forgotten to take your medicine and the inhaler to school?

NADIA: Yes, but not a lot.

THERAPIST: Nadia, do you have any advice for your mother that can help her worry less about you?

NADIA: Go out with Yolanda [mother's friend] more. Mom sits around the house too much.

THERAPIST: What else do you think your mother should be doing instead of sitting around the house?

NADIA: Go to the mall. Maybe work again ... remember, Mom, you used to work at that clothing store?

SYLVIA: You're right, honey. I should get out more. I just worry a lot about you ...

THERAPIST: It is obvious to me that you [Sylvia] have a big heart and that you and Fernando have done a super job with Nadia. Thanks a lot, Nadia, for all your good advice. Listen, if I have any problem with my 3-year-old daughter, can I consult with you? (*Everyone laughs.*)

Nadia's expert advice proved to be instrumental in helping create more breathing room in her relationship with her mother. Sylvia, in particular, had not heard Nadia's concerns before, so this was a newsworthy experience for her. Sylvia eventually secured a part-time job and made a few friends at work. Once Sylvia was less vigilant around Nadia, Nadia's behavior greatly improved, especially in taking her medication and carrying the inhaler around with her. In a later therapy session, I helped Sylvia mourn the losses of her three babies. These painful losses and nearly losing Nadia twice to asthma attacks had kept Sylvia stuck in terms of taking care of her own needs outside of motherhood.

Future-Oriented Questions

When the treatment system is stuck or we are working with "past-bound," chronic, or entrenched families, future-oriented questions can be employed to help create possibilities (Selekman, 2005, 2009; Tomm, 1987). The great psychoanalyst Harry Stack Sullivan's core belief was that "the basic direction of the human organism is forward." Always approaching his patients with an optimistic attitude, Sullivan observed at one point, "Thirty years of work has taught me that, whenever one could be aided to foresee the reasonable probability of a better future, everyone will show a sufficient tendency to collaborate in the achievement of more adequate and appropriate ways of living" (in Cottrell & Foote, 1995, p. 203).

Having families envision a future place in time in which they have realized their desired outcomes can be a liberating experience for them, particularly when they are feeling so paralyzed by their presenting problems. The future becomes "the now" for the family. According to cognitive researcher Massimo Piattelli-Palmarini (1994), "The easier it is to imagine an event or a situation, and the more the occurrence impresses us emotionally, the more likely we are to think of it as also objectively frequent" (p. 128). With the help of future-oriented questions, we can co-create with families positive self-fulfilling prophecies.

Cody, a Caucasian 9-year-old, was reluctantly brought for therapy (by his parents) for "stealing," "beating on" his 8-year-old sister, engaging in power struggles, and "not following the rules." Cody was having behavioral "problems in school" as well. The parents were very pessimistic and frustrated by Cody's chronic behavioral problems. After three previous treatment failures with psychologists, the parents were not very hopeful that our treatment experience together would be any different. It was quite clear in the session that there was a lot of conflict between Cody and his father, Dan. Dan reprimanded Cody twice in our session for antagonizing his sister, Tiffany. When I asked the miracle question (de Shazer, 1988), the parents and the children responded with more pessimism. The more I tried to cooperate with the family's pessimism, the more pessimistic they became. At this point in the session I shifted gears and decided to ask future-oriented questions to try to move the family and myself in a different direction. Present in the family interview were Cody, Tiffany, Dan, and Rachel, the mother.

THERAPIST: Let's say that I ran into you guys at a 7-Eleven 6 months down the road, long after we successfully completed counseling together, and I asked all of you what steps you took to get out of counseling—what will you tell me you did?

RACHEL: I would tell you that Cody is cooperative, we are no longer fighting about everything, and he is playing in a nicer way with Tiffany.

THERAPIST: What effect had all of those changes had on your relationship with Cody?

RACHEL: We're getting along better. I am taking him out more to the mall—you know, doing things that he likes to do.

THERAPIST: What else will you tell me that you are doing differently as parents that is now helping you and Cody get along better?

DAN: Avoiding power struggles. Not being so reactive to little things that Cody does.

THERAPIST: What difference has that made when you are doing that?

DAN: Less battles. Less stress.

RACHEL: I like him more when he is not being so difficult.

THERAPIST: What about you, Cody? What will you tell me that is better with your parents when I see you guys at 7-Eleven?

CODY: They are not yelling at me. We are not fighting. Daddy's playing video games with me.

THERAPIST: Cody, if your teacher popped into 7-Eleven right now, what will she tell me you are doing good in her class?

CODY: I'm paying attention, not getting into fights ... doing my work.

THERAPIST: Will she tell me that she is not missing things from her desktop anymore?

CODY: Yeah ... I don't take things anymore.

By using future-oriented questions, we were able to open up the door for possibilities. For the first time in the family interview, family members began sharing creative problem-solving strategies that they believed could work in improving their situation. While sharing their unique solutions, they spoke about the changes in the past tense, as if they had already happened. The future became the now, which liberated the family from feeling stuck in the present. The added bonus for myself was that I no longer felt stuck therapeutically, thanks to the family's guiding me in the direction of change.

Externalizing-the-Problem Questions

Families that have experienced multiple treatment failures and have been oppressed by their problems for a long time tend to be very demoralized and stuck by the time of our initial contact with them. Some of these families will be hard-pressed to identify any newsworthy pretreatment changes or past successes that we can capitalize on to empower them. Therefore, externalizing their oppressive presenting problem (White, 1995, 2007; Epston,

1998; Freeman et al., 1997; White & Epston, 1990; Tomm & White, 1987) through appropriate questions may be a viable therapeutic option to pursue when other means of eliciting information from family members has not made a difference in altering their outmoded beliefs. When externalizing the problem, it is crucial for the therapist to co-construct a new description of the problem that is based on the family's beliefs about their difficulty and the language they use to describe it. Therapists can be as creative as they wish with what they externalize the problem into, whether it be ADD and other DSM-IV-TR labels (particularly with parents who are wedded to the labels with which they come in the door); lying, fears, and other problematic behaviors; the "attitude"; habits; the "temper"; "arguing"; "blaming"; problem patterns; or whatever.

Externalizing the problem is a two-step process:

1. Map the influence the problem has on the identified client, family members, and significant others (peers, relatives, and involved helping professionals).
2. Map the influence the identified client, family members, and significant others have over the problem.

The first step of the process is to explore the effects the problem has had on family members' self-perceptions and relationships with one another and others (White, 1995). A family pushed around by the identified client's "attitude" problem can be asked: "How long has the 'attitude' been pushing all of you around?" "What does the 'attitude' brainwash Billy to do?" Such questions help deconstruct fixed family beliefs about the identified client's behavior and convey the idea to the family that they are all—including the identified client—being victimized by the presenting problem.

Similar questions are critical for the restorying process, as the questions pave the way for creating an alternative family story. Story lines of competency or unique outcomes (White, 1995) are elicited from family members to create a double description of the family's original problem-saturated story. Unique outcome questions (White, 1988) elicit from family members specific instances when they have stood up to or successfully fought back against the oppressive problem rather than succumbing to its powerful influence on them. Some examples of unique-account questions are as follows: "I'm curious, Steve; have there been any times lately when you tricked 'lying' and you didn't allow it to get you into trouble with your parents?" "Can you think of a time lately when the 'temper' was lurking about but you guys [the parents] stood your ground and didn't allow it to divide you?" As part of the restorying process, White (1995) stresses the importance of incorporating an "audience" of involved and concerned others in the lives of the identified client and the family to contribute to the newly developing alternative family story and to help "authenticate" it.

> Johnny, a Caucasian 10-year-old, was school-referred for ADD, being highly "disruptive" in class, and "not following the rules" at home. Johnny's mother, Barbara, was remarried and had three other children from her second marriage. His biological parents had divorced when Johnny was 6. Johnny had regular weekly contact with his natural father. According to Barbara, Johnny had always been in special education programs because of his behavioral difficulties. The parents had also taken Johnny to a "special ADD clinic" where he received several "batteries of tests" that "proved he had ADD." They had seen four other therapists before me. Barbara, Warren (the stepfather), and Johnny described the ADD problem as being oppressive and chronic. I decided to externalize the problem (White, 1995; White & Epston, 1990) because the mother, stepfather, and Johnny were so pessimistic and paralyzed by the wrath of ADD. Present in the first family interview were Barbara, Warren, and Johnny.

THERAPIST: How long has ADD been pushing all of you around?

BARBARA: Three years.

THERAPIST: When ADD is getting the best of Johnny, what sort of things does it make him do?

BARBARA: Well, he is aggravating Ann [7 years old], he doesn't listen to me ... I tell him to put his things away, and he tells me to "shut up." Boy, has he got a mouth on him!

THERAPIST: Does ADD make him swear at you?

BARBARA: Yeah ... and it's sort of strange but I can tell that he's getting an ADD attack when he gets all wound up, swears, and doesn't listen.

THERAPIST: What about you, Warren? Does ADD coach Johnny to push your buttons as well?

WARREN: Yes! I always have to scream at him a few times before he does what I want him to do.

BARBARA: Yeah, sometimes it is like talking to the wall. The child gets taken over by this ADD thing ...

THERAPIST: So, ADD brainwashes him to get out of control—or does it invade his body like an evil spirit?

BARBARA: Warren, wouldn't you say it was like an evil spirit?

WARREN: Yes. He gets mad and mouthy and very difficult to manage.

THERAPIST: When ADD is getting the best of you parents, what does it make the two of you do?

WARREN: We argue a lot about how to manage him. I think she is too lenient. I'm more the screamer.

BARBARA: I don't like when Warren screams so much. So, to try to keep things calm, I let Johnny off the hook ... I know it's wrong ... but I don't know ... I feel frustrated.

THERAPIST: So, ADD divides the two of you? Do both of you feel frustrated by what ADD is doing to this family?

WARREN: Yes, I feel frustrated too. This ADD thing has made our life hell! We can't leave Johnny alone with Ann.

THERAPIST: Johnny, what does ADD coach you to do in class?

JOHNNY: I fight. I don't listen to the teacher. I get mad a lot.

THERAPIST: Does ADD ever make you feel dumb?

JOHNNY: Yeah (*looking sad*).

THERAPIST: What else does ADD try to teach you about yourself?

JOHNNY: I'm not a good boy. I can't do the work.

After mapping the oppressive effects ADD had on individual family members and family relationships, I shifted gears to begin the restorying process by mapping the influence that Johnny, his parents, and the teacher had over ADD. I attempted to elicit story lines of competency and examples of the family protesting against ADD's reigning over them.

THERAPIST: Warren and Barbara, can you think of anything that you guys have done in the past to stand up to ADD and not allow it to get the best of Johnny?

BARBARA: Not yelling a lot. He seems to calm down faster when we don't scream at him.

WARREN: I agree, but it also helps if we work together. You've got to stop giving in to him. You know that makes me mad.

THERAPIST: So, if you guys cut back on the yelling and don't let ADD divide you, it seems to help?

WARREN: Yes, definitely.

BARBARA: He's right ... I need to be tougher with him.

THERAPIST: Can you think of other things you have done to not allow ADD to back Johnny into a corner?

BARBARA: No ... not that I can think of.

THERAPIST: How about you, Johnny? When ADD is trying to get you into trouble with your parents, can you think of anything they do that helps you out?

JOHNNY: Not yelling. Not fighting. When we are happy.

THERAPIST: What do you do as a family that makes you happy?

JOHNNY: We play video games. Warren takes us to the baseball game.

THERAPIST: What about at school? Does Miss Johnson [the teacher] do anything to stop ADD from pushing you around?

JOHNNY: She is not always yelling at me. She's nicer. She sees that I'm trying to do my work.

By the end of the session, the parents and Johnny were viewing ADD as the real villain. The parents began to interact with Johnny in a more positive manner. Once the parents and the teacher stopped their "yelling" and became more of a unified "team," Johnny's behavior improved dramatically. Johnny's view of himself as being an incompetent "bad boy" changed as well. After six sessions over a 6-month period, the label "ADD" was no longer being used to describe Johnny's behavior, and he was mainstreamed back to a regular classroom setting by the end of the school year. Although the school was being cautious about mainstreaming Johnny too quickly, he displayed a great deal of patience, and he continued to prove the skeptics wrong by embarking on a new direction in his school career.

Conclusion

In this chapter, I have presented a variety of pathways that therapists can pursue in the interviewing process with families. Through their responses to at least five types of interventive questions, family members offer therapists valuable feedback about how to better cooperate with them and important clues about what and how they want to change. Interviewing for change also informs the design and selection of appropriate therapeutic experiments.

4

Finding Fit

Guidelines for Therapeutic Experiment Design, Selection, and Implementation

Yes, therapy should always be designed to fit the patient and not the patient to fit the therapy.
—Milton H. Erickson

When designing and selecting therapeutic experiments for children and their families, the therapist should consider four important elements: (1) the family's definition of the problem; (2) key family members' characteristics, that is, language, beliefs, strengths, and theories of change; (3) the unique cooperative response patterns and the stage of readiness to change of each family member; and (4) the family's treatment goals. Unless we make careful use of these important elements, any therapeutic experiment we select or design may fail to fit (Selekman, 2005, 2009; de Shazer, 1985) for family members and may lead to their feeling misunderstood, lacking confidence in our ability to help, and possibly dropping out of treatment.

After a brief discussion of each of the key elements in the therapeutic experiment selection and construction process, I present seven idea-generating strategies that can aid therapists in designing creative therapeutic experiments. The final section of this chapter elaborates on some specific solution-focused brief therapy and positive psychology therapeutic experiments that can be quite effectual in generating change.

The Key Elements for Optimizing Fit
with Therapeutic Experiment Design and Selection

According to problem-solving specialist Arthur Van Gundy, "We must know where we are before we can begin the journey to where we want to be" (1988, p. 19). Therefore, we need to make sure with our clients not only that we have selected the "right" problem to work on but that it is well defined. We can determine the "right" problem with our clients by having them prioritize and clarify which aspect or part of the presenting problem they would like to resolve first. A well-defined and negotiated problem is specific, behavioral, and solvable. For example, a mother brought in her 6-year-old boy for treatment because she felt he had a "low self-esteem" problem. Upon further questioning and in an effort to recast low self-esteem into concrete operational terms, the mother reported that it was her son's "temper tantrum" problem that was the real problem she wanted help with. Because temper tantrum problems are behavioral and much more readily treatable than low self-esteem problems, we were better able to resolve this problem.

The true master and creator of the utilization strategy in psychotherapy was Milton H. Erickson. Erickson would utilize whatever his clients brought to therapy, which included key words and beliefs, life themes, metaphors, nonverbals and subtle verbal communication habits, talents, interests, and hobbies (Havens, 2003; Erickson & Rossi, 1983; Gordon & Meyers-Anderson, 1981). As part of the engagement process, I like to spend ample time finding out from each family member what his or her strengths, talents, and hobbies are. With children, I like to carefully observe what toys, books, and art medium attract their attention the most and the nature of their play style so that I can use these things in both the engagement process and the therapeutic task selection and design. When inquiring about the family's presenting problems, I listen carefully to the words family members use to describe their problems, their beliefs about why the problems are occurring, and any key family themes or metaphors. Asking "why" questions serves as a direct pipeline into family members' beliefs about the causation of the presenting problems and provides important clues for determining the real problem with the family. Parents may be asked, "What's your theory about why this difficulty is happening?" Once we gain access to what the family believes is the real problem, we can use their key words, beliefs, family themes, metaphors, and strengths when constructing and offering them a therapeutic intervention as an experiment. The following case example illustrates the utilization strategy with therapeutic experiment design.

Catherine, a Caucasian mother, brought her 10-year-old son, Dylan, and 11-year-old son, Jaime, for therapy for constantly "mouthing off" to her and "refusing to do their chores" and comply with her "rules." Catherine had divorced their father shortly after Dylan was born, and they had not had any contact with him since then. Early in our first session together I discovered that both boys were not only avid Chicago Blackhawk fans but, according to Catherine, "outstanding hockey players." I spent a lot of time finding out about the positions they played, what techniques and strategies they used to help them score goals, and who their favorite Blackhawk players were. Both Dylan's and Jaime's favorite all-time Blackhawk was Bobby Hull. The brothers had future aspirations of becoming pro hockey players. It was clear that I had engaged the boys around their interest and active involvement in the world of hockey. During my intersession break, I included hockey language in both the rationale for and the description of the therapeutic task. I shared with the family that it sounded like they were losing the game because the boys' *slap shots* were being directed at the wrong target and the *pucks* were missing the real *goal*. I also shared my concerns with the boys that they would continue to lose games (receive their mother's groundings, lose privileges, not be allowed to play in games) unless they started *scoring goals* with their mother by letting her be their cheerleader at home and at games. As an experiment, I left it up to each boy to pick one thing he could do over the next week to *score a goal* with his mother. Once a *goal* was *scored*, Catherine was to give the *hockey player* a high-five and a privilege of her choice. One week later, the mother reported that each boy had "scored two goals apiece" with her.

The last two important elements to consider when selecting and designing therapeutic experiments are family members' unique cooperative response patterns and the family's treatment goals. Once we determine in our relationship with each family member how he or she wants to cooperate in the change effort, we can carefully match our therapeutic experiments with where the family member is in the cycle of change (de Shazer, 1985, 1988; Norcross, 2008; Prochaska et al., 1994). Family members invariably provide us with clues to how they want to cooperate with us. Our job as Sherlock Holmes-type detectives is to listen for and observe carefully clues from family members as to how they want to cooperate and change, particularly in how they respond to our questions, relate to us, and manage in-session family play or art therapy experiments. Finally, whatever therapeutic tasks we select or design have to be in line with the family's treatment goals. Once we have clearly elicited from family members what their ideal treatment outcome pictures look like, therapeutic experiments selected should provide the *how* of empowering them to get there in the most concrete, manageable, and efficient way.

Idea-Generating Strategies for Creative Problem Solving

As therapists, we can be as creative as we allow ourselves to be with any given client problem situation. The more ideas we generate, the greater the odds we will stumble upon a high-quality solution (Van Gundy, 1992). We need to be careful not to get locked into habitual ways of viewing particular types of client problems and rigid therapy model formulas for trying to resolve them. The danger in being too wedded to one particular therapy model for problem solving is that it will rob us of the opportunity to test our own creative powers in coming up with a second, third, or fourth potential solution, which may be much more beneficial than a particular therapy model's first-choice intervention. The seven idea-generating strategies that follow can tap our creative abilities and aid us in achieving high-quality solutions for challenging presenting problems.

Using Mind Mapping for Solutions

Mind mapping was originally developed by educator and creativity expert Tony Buzan (1984, 1989), based on his years of research on note-taking skill development, learning, memory, and creative thinking with college students. In his research, Buzan found that the best note takers shared two major characteristics: (1) they recorded key words used by the lecturer or the authors of the books the students were required to read, and (2) they kept their notes clear and easy to read. Writing down key words stimulates creative association and recall, making the gathered information rich in context (Margulies, 2002; Buzan, 1984, 1989; Gelb, 1995). In a clinical situation, we want to listen carefully for the key words that family members use in describing the presenting problem and write them down as part of the mind map. For example, if a mother uses the words "bad attitude" to describe the cause of her son's behavior, we would want to write that down. Mind mapping works because it creates a positive feedback loop between our brain and our notes. As an idea-generating tool, it trains us to organize our thoughts in a way that makes it easier to see both the bigger picture and the details and to integrate logic and imagination. By capturing a tremendous amount of information on paper, mind mapping can help us to perceive the relationships, connections, and patterns among our ideas (Margulies, 2002; Gelb, 1995).

The four steps of the mind-mapping procedure are:

1. Draw a symbol or a picture in the center of the sheet of paper to represent the family's presenting problem.
2. Print family members' key words used to describe the problem.

3. Connect the family members' key words with lines radiating out from the symbol or the picture.
4. Use color coding or pictures to help produce greater associations; yellow can be used to highlight the most significant or key client words used to describe the problem, and light-blue can be used to highlight the second most important key client words. (Margulies, 2002; Buzan, 1984; Gelb, 1995).

Because 80% of our brain's activity is involved in visual processing at any given time (Ostrander, Schroeder, & Ostrander, 1994), we tend to learn faster and remember longer by using pictures of things. Therefore, pictures in mind mapping serve as "memory anchors" for key word associations and help us to be more imaginative in our thinking (Gelb, 1995).

Besides simply mind mapping the problem alone, which in some cases generates useful solutions for the client's presenting problems (see Figure 4.1), I use mind maps in four other ways for creative problem solving. Sometimes I map the *opposite* of a client's presenting problems. A map can also

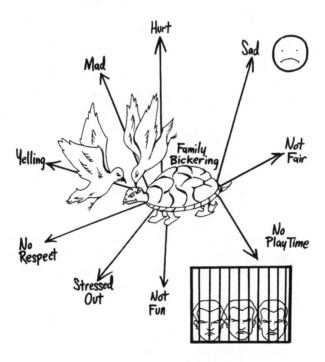

FIGURE 4.1. Mind map of a family bickering problem.

be constructed of the words that family members use to describe their ideal treatment outcome pictures. Sometimes I think of metaphors for the client's presenting problems and mind-map them. Finally, when stuck, I may pull out the dictionary and randomly pick a word to mind-map to see whether this exercise triggers some useful ideas for solving the client's presenting problems (DeBono, 1992). The following case example illustrates how mind mapping a problem can help generate potential solutions.

> Fanny, a Caucasian mother, brought in for therapy her two sons, 6-year-old Albert and 8-year-old Harry, for "constantly arguing" with each other and not responding well to her "rules." Fanny reported that "the boys will not listen" to her unless she "yells" at them at the "top of her lungs." Both boys also voiced their upset feelings about the family's bickering problem, particularly not liking their mother's "yelling" at them "all the time."
>
> Fanny was a single parent; the boys' father disappeared when they were toddlers. Fanny was at her wits' end in trying to manage her sons' behaviors. She had taken all their toys away and prohibited them from going outside for a few weeks. It appeared that the more Fanny yelled and imposed lengthy punishments, the more out of control and oppositional the boys became. This was the destructive interactive dance the family was locked into.
>
> I provided some parenting education for Fanny regarding the need for us to move away from yelling and inadvertently reinforcing the very behaviors she wanted to eliminate with her sons. She could not identify any past successes she had had in resolving other behavioral problems with her boys. Together, we broke down Fanny's main problem concern area—the boys' oppositional behavior—into more concrete outcome terms: "not bickering with me" when asked to do things or follow her rules. When I attempted to externalize (White, 1995) the family bickering problem, I got strange looks from all the family members, as if they found this new construction of the problem to be bizarre. We also discussed the importance of Fanny having more timeouts away from the boys. As an experiment, I gave Fanny an observation task to keep track on a daily basis of what the boys were doing when they were not pushing her buttons. At the intersession break, I constructed a mind map of the family's bickering problem (see Figure 4.1), which at root was contributing to the boy's oppositional behavior.
>
> To symbolize the problem, I drew a picture of a snapping turtle in the center of the page. I connected lines from the turtle to the key words that family members used to describe the problem: "mad," "sad," "no respect," "stressed out," "not fun," "no play time," and so on. I drew pictures of two angry birds pecking on the turtle next

to the word "mad," a face with a frown on it next to the word "sad," and three heads behind prison bars in a window next to the words "not fun" and "no play time." I then highlighted in yellow marker the words "mad," "not fun," and "no play time." After mind mapping, I came up with four ideas to present to the family: (1) Fanny should go out with a friend or on a date when she needed a break from the boys; (2) each boy could throw up a timeout hand signal with each other when conversations were escalating into possible arguments; (3) the boys, with their mother's permission, could go outside to play and take a break from being with the family; and (4) the boys could be put in charge of planning a fun family outing, as it had been more than a year since the family had gone out together. From this menu of intervention ideas, the family selected the first, third, and fourth tasks with which to experiment.

As this case example illustrates, mind mapping can offer therapists a quick and effective method for generating creative solutions. I ended up seeing Fanny and her family four times over a 6-month period. All family members reported changes in the bickering and oppositional problem areas by the second family session. Fanny discovered that once she stopped screaming and reinforcing negative behaviors with her boys, they became more cooperative and compliant with her rules and expectations. Family members found that having periodic timeout periods from one another and going on fun family outings contributed to everyone getting along better when together.

Imagining You Are the Problem

Gordon (1992), in his creative problem-solving research, found that the most important element in innovative problem solving was "making the familiar strange" because breakthroughs depend on "strange" new contexts by which to view a "familiar" problem. One way of making the familiar strange is for the therapist to imagine he or she is the client's problem. Empathically, the therapist identifies with the problem. For example, if I became a child's lying problem, I might ask myself the following questions:

- "How do I think?"
- "How do I feel?"
- "What keeps me going in this family?"
- "What am I scared of?"
- "Why do I prey on this child?"
- "What's funny or absurd about me?"

- "What has to change in this family for me to go away?"
- "What are the pros and cons of being this problem?"

Imagining ourselves as the problem not only can help us better understand the client's problem but also can generate creative ideas for problem resolution. Jonas Salk, the polio vaccine pioneer, imagined himself as an immune system and contemplated how to fight the polio virus from that perspective (Gelb, 1995). The following case example illustrates how to use this idea-generating strategy in clinical practice.

Simon, a Caucasian 10-year-old, was being oppressed by a chronic encopresis (soiling) problem. His parents were both professors at a major university. The parents, particularly the father, expected Simon to excel academically in school, and therefore he was constantly putting pressure on Simon to do his homework and to study. Simon's grades had dropped from straight-A's to A's and B's. The frequency of Simon's soiling problem increased from four times a week to almost daily. No physical or medical problems were contributing to the soiling problem. Prior to being brought to me for therapy, Simon had seen several social workers and psychologists. The parents and Simon were very pessimistic.

The miracle, coping, and pessimistic questions (Berg & Miller, 1992; de Shazer, 1988; Selekman, 2005, 2009) failed to produce any exceptions. When meeting alone with Simon, he disclosed to me how mad he was at his father for putting so much pressure on him at school.

At my intersession break, I imagined that I was Simon's encopretic problem. In self-reflecting as the problem, I thought about how I was getting even with Simon's father by shitting on him and how absurd it was because it did not change him but just made Simon's situation worse. As encopresis, I was feeling mad and frustrated. I wondered whether, if I stopped preying on Simon, he could tell his father directly to back off a little on the school pressures. Simon had never confronted his father about this issue. Rather than giving this family a task, I decided to voice these specific questions as encopresis during the editorial reflection. Suddenly, Simon took a risk with his dad and voiced his angry and frustrated feelings about the school issue. This proved to be newsworthy to the parents, particularly the father, and some useful dialogue followed between Simon and his father. In facilitating the dialogue, I got the father to agree to back off on the schoolwork pressures, provided Simon did the best he could in school. Also, we decided to reinstate father-and-son outings on Saturdays, which had stopped because Simon's grades had declined. Simon and his parents were very pleased with the outcome of our meeting. The encopresis problem was completely resolved in six sessions. The father also committed to stay-ing off Simon's case about school matters.

Attacking the Problem from Different Angles

When feeling stuck with a case or unsure about which therapeutic tasks may be useful with a family's problem situation, it can be advantageous to attack the problem from many different angles. Sometimes I hop into my imaginary helicopter to gain an aerial view of myself and the family to help generate some new ideas. Wujec (1995) recommends looking at the problem situation as if it were "a statue to be examined from several points of view" (p. 64). Wes "Scoop" Nisker, a Buddhist and author of the book *Crazy Wisdom,* emphasized the importance of approaching problems from different angles:

> Crazy wisdom gets wise and crazy by gaining many perspectives: by changing points of view, getting into another place or a distant space and looking at things from there; by finding an odd angle, climbing high for an overview, seeing what is behind it all or underneath it all, stepping outside or going inside. There are many ways of looking at things. (1990, p. 12)

The following case example demonstrates how suddenly taking leave of a family session in progress can sometimes stimulate the therapist to come up with new ideas. An added bonus for the therapist was that abruptly leaving the session prior to taking his intersession break, thus altering the therapy agenda, also helped disrupt destructive family interactions.

> Kit and Maggie, Caucasian 6- and 7-year-olds, respectively, were brought for therapy by their parents for "always fighting over every little thing." The parents reported that they habitually "destroyed" each other's toys and "kicked and hit" each other constantly. When asked about their attempted solutions, the parents start blaming each other in the session, the mother complaining that her husband was "too strict," and he countered with the "too lenient" charge for her. While the parents were embroiled in this give-and-take, both children started fighting over the toys they were playing with. As the father yelled at the children, their behavior escalated. I dismissed the children and met alone with the parents. Attempts to elicit from them an initial treatment goal proved to be futile, for the couple could not agree on anything. They began to blame each other again for the children's behavioral problems. I decided to ask the miracle question (de Shazer, 1988) as a way to break up the blame–counterblame pattern of interaction. In the middle of the miracle inquiry, the couple began to lock horns again. I

decided at this point to get up and check my mailbox as a way to do something dramatically different and to disrupt the couple's destructive interaction pattern. While at my mailbox, I came up with two potential therapeutic tasks that I thought might work for the couple. When I returned to my office, both partners began to laugh and the husband said, "You needed a break from us, right ... huh! huh!" The parents seemed to have mellowed out in response to my improvisational move. I decided to present the two tasks to the couple so they could choose which one they would like to try.

The first task option was for both partners to observe on a daily basis what the other was doing in relationship to the children that they liked or thought was good and to write those things down and bring the information in to our next session. They were not to compare notes until our next appointment. The second option was the "structured family fighting task" (de Shazer, 1985; Selekman, 2005). The couple was instructed to get a kitchen timer and find a quiet room in the house to perform this task. The partners were to flip a coin and select heads or tails to determine who goes first. For 5 minutes the heads partner can argue with the other partner, who is patiently listening and making direct eye contact. Anything left over to complain about must be written down on a piece of paper and used for the next scheduled fighting session. Once both partners have had a turn, they are not allowed to fight again until the next scheduled fighting session time. The couple opted to try both tasks. They also began to take responsibility for their poor role modeling for their children. I provided support and encouragement to the couple and got them fired up to do the tasks.

I ended up seeing this family five more times. The parents returned to our second session reporting a wealth of changes. Both parents reported a lot of parenting qualities and behaviors that they appreciated about each other. After the first scheduled fighting session, they experienced difficulty in arguing with each other in session. The children's fighting behavior problem and sibling conflicts were resolved by our fourth family session.

Using Direct Analogies

Another useful idea-generating strategy is to think about what a particular family or problem situation reminds us of. Some of the families I have worked with have reminded me of a family on a TV show or in the movies. I once worked with a family that reminded me of the family in the movie *The Great Santini,* which starred Robert Duvall as a general who ran his family like the military unit. Over the years, I have worked with a number of Italian families that reminded me of Cher's family in the movie *Moonstruck.*

Not only can analogies take the form of popular TV or movie celebrities, but also family members or particular presenting problems can be compared to comic strip or book characters and animals, insects, and other aspects of nature. Many famous historical figures successfully used analogies to solve problems. Nobel Prize winners Crick and Watson compared DNA molecules to a spiral staircase, which helped them come up with their double helix theory of genetics. Physicist Niels Bohr thought of an atom as being like a miniature solar system (Prince, 1992).

I may use the direct analogy idea-generating strategy to help me get more playful with a family. For example, I think of a name of a new situational TV comedy show to call a particular family in my head. Sometimes I think of a headline in a major newspaper that would best describe a particular family with which I am working.

> Rhonda, the mother, and Harold, the stepfather, a Caucasian couple, brought in 10-year-old Stuart and 9-year-old Liza for therapy because they would not respond to Harold's limit setting and "tried deliberately to push his buttons." Rhonda's children were reportedly "pulling pranks" on Harold and sometimes "trying to hurt" him. Both Stuart and Liza were bitter about their physical and verbal mistreatment by their biological father. The parents had been divorced for 3 years. According to Rhonda, she was "battered" and "psychologically abused" by her "alcoholic" ex-husband as well. Because this was a war-torn family, I decided to give family members plenty of room to tell their painful past stories. While listening to Rhonda and Harold's present concerns about the children's pranks and their aggressive acts, an image flashed in my head that these children reminded me of Pugsley and Wednesday of the *Addams Family*. The family also seemed therapeutically ripe for externalizing the "anger" and "mistrust" problems that ran rampant in this family. All family members were being pushed around by these problems, including Harold. I decided to tap into the children's strong ability to be aggressive and mischievous in helping them and their parents defeat these problems that were haunting them from the past. Both children got very excited about drawing on paper the clever ways in which they could defeat these problems. By the end of our first session together, Harold and Rhonda began viewing the children and the presenting problems in a new light.

Having "Famous Guest Consultants" Visit the Therapist

If you were working with a difficult family and you felt the treatment process was at a standstill and were at a loss for what to do next, what three famous people might you wish to visit you during your intersession break to offer you some inspiration and novel ideas? This out-of-the-box idea-generating strategy can be quite effective in altering our narrow and unproductive ways of trying to make sense of and resolve the client's presenting problems and may spark some fresh and novel ideas and new directions to pursue in the treatment process. We can select famous historic figures, philosophers, artists, architects, scientists, musicians, popular bands, composers, authors, chefs, sports stars, movie and TV celebrities, and popular cartoon characters.

The following case example of Vanya and her parents illustrates how this idea-generating strategy can help pave the way to a new direction in treatment.

> The school social worker had referred Vanya, a precocious Romanian 11-year-old, to me because of her dramatic academic decline. In our collaborative strengths-based family assessment session, the parents spent the first 20 minutes of our session berating Vanya about how "lazy and irresponsible" she had been with regard to "doing her homework" and "studying for her tests" at school. The father was like a steamroller, flattening Vanya out with his criticisms, and the mother was quite anxious or worried about her never making it to college. They felt she had allowed such distractions as "boys" and being both on her "cell phone texting friends" and "on the Internet" to become "more important than her studies." My use of the miracle, coping, and pessimistic categories of questions went absolutely nowhere. Whenever Vanya attempted to say anything, her father would ask her to be quiet or her mother would go off on long monologues about her "failing out of school." When I met alone with the parents, it ended up being more of the same in spite of my determined efforts to redirect the conversation.
>
> Prior to meeting alone with Vanya, I decided to take my mini-intersession break earlier than usual, about 35 minutes into the hour. I closed my eyes and imagined that the realist painter Diego Velazquez, the great jazz trumpeter Dizzy Gillespie, and the southwestern cuisine-inspired and *Iron Chef* TV show star Bobby Flay had decided to pay me a visit during this intersession break period. Velazquez first asked me if I was familiar with one of his greatest paintings, *Las Meninas,* and I acknowledged to him that it is my favorite painting of his (the painting is unique in that Velazquez painted himself in the picture; there is a lot of activity in the painting, such as a person in the distant background going through a doorway and children, dwarfs, and a dog in the foreground—all in all, there is great depth to the painting). The point Velazquez was trying to make with me was that there was great depth and multiple levels of meaning to Vanya and her parents' story that needed to be explored, particularly all of the parents' anxieties and

fears of their daughter not being successful in school and in life, their immigration story and reasons for coming to the United States, and the clash between the Americanization process and Vanya's falling prey to material trappings versus the family's cultural and traditional values. Being the true "realist" he was as an artist, Velazquez also felt that I needed to take the parents' concerns about Vanya's academic problems "real" seriously and empower them to resolve this problem any way that I could, such as by actively collaborating with her teacher.

"Diz" first recommended that I needed to *lighten up* in the session with the family because the atmosphere in the room was much too serious. He stressed that I needed to improvise, such as using my trusty imaginary time machine and have Vanya go back in time to a year or two earlier when she was doing great academically. While blowing the notes in this direction, I was to secure all of the details about what she did individually and her parents did that helped her to perform with excellence.

Chef Bobby Flay recommended that I needed to spice up our family sessions more by throwing some chopped serrano and habanero peppers into the conversational mix because, as it stood now, the family sessions were tasting very bland. Flay thought an interesting and surprising move would be, together with Vanya, to meet with each parent separately to see if that would be more productive and less negative. He also felt I needed to meet alone with Vanya to hear her story directly, and this would prove to be as tasty an experience as eating his chocolate-coconut bread pudding with passion fruit sauce.

Thanks to my famous guest consultants, I ended up trying all of the ideas they helped spark in my mind. After dramatically changing my therapeutic direction with this family, I was able to build solid therapeutic alliances with all family members and eventually to resolve the school academic problems. This idea-generating strategy can also be used as a family play therapeutic experiment (see Chapter 5).

Resorting to "Crazy and Absurd" Ideas

Albert Einstein once said, "If at first an idea does not sound absurd, then there is no hope for it." With very difficult and entrenched family situations, we may need to stretch well beyond our preferred therapy models and really try to generate some seemingly off-the-wall and provocative ideas to share or therapeutic tasks to test out. By listening carefully to the humorous twists and absurdities of the clients' stories and occasionally observing some really strange and unproductive family interactions, elements of what we have heard and seen may ultimately be exploitable in a positive way. The "crazy and absurd" idea-generating strategy can be used during intersession breaks or between visits to generate some off-the-wall and provocative ideas and therapeutic tasks that may be applicable in future sessions.

The first step is to generate a list of all the things that normally you would never say or do with a family in your office. The list has to consist of highly unorthodox or really crazy and absurd ideas. After you have come up with five to six ideas, you then circle or highlight those ideas that may have the best shot at working with the clients in question. Often this novel idea-generating strategy produces some useful ideas that can be tweaked and developed into high-quality creative solutions for empowering the clients to resolve their difficulties.

> Byron, a Caucasian parent, brought his three sons, Tim, 14; Jackson, 12; and Taylor, 8, in for family counseling. According to Byron, they were "lazy, irresponsible, disrespectful, and lived like pigs!" He went off on a long monologue about how since he had separated from his wife Cindy because of her extramarital affair (2 years earlier), the boys had been "on strike and uncooperative" with him. The more Byron would complain about his boys' behavior, the more they bickered with one another in the room. After many attempts at playing traffic cop and trying to steer our conversation in a more productive direction, I decided to ask the miracle question. Although the boys had some great miracles to share, Byron continued to be negative and pessimistic about their making the needed miracle changes happen. I used both coping and pessimistic questions to align myself with Byron's pessimism, and yet it went absolutely nowhere. At this point in the session, I needed a breather from playing traffic cop and sounding board in the room and took my intersession break.
>
> I generated the following list of "crazy and absurd" ideas:
>
> 1. Ask Byron to switch chairs with me, and I would say, "You think you have problems—you want to hear some of mine!"
> 2. As a radical therapeutic experiment, have Byron pack his suitcases and have them by the front door of their house. When asked by the kids where he was going, he was to say, "I am running away from home because you don't need a father and want to live your lives your way. You don't appear to need my guidance and leadership any more."
> 3. Have Byron stage a contest with the boys to see who can be the biggest slob. Byron and the boys could decide jointly what the specific scoring criteria would be in order to be crowned "the king of slobs."
> 4. Suggest that Byron take his boys to the local city dump, observe

garbage at its best, inhale the different aromas, and also spend a little time educating them about how waste is being used environmentally these days.

5. Throw my hands up in the air and fire myself as their therapist. Explain that I had missed the boat with them and maybe they could benefit from having fresh blood in a new therapist.

I decided to meet alone with Byron and, of the various unconventional ideas that I listed, present him with ideas 2–4. Much to my surprise, he laughed (a new response) and really liked the third and fourth ideas the best, saying he would try them out during the following week. After my individual session time with Byron, he was more upbeat and less negative, and the atmosphere in the room changed dramatically when his boys rejoined us. This humorous approach is best reserved for drastic occasions when a radical change in the mood of sessions is desperately sought.

Imagining the Problem Is Solved

When I am at a loss for ideas or feeling stuck in a family session, at my intersession break I pretend momentarily that the family's presenting problems were miraculously solved after they left my office. I allow my mind to run wild with the many possibilities now available to the family and to me since the problems were solved. Not only do I visualize what the changes would look like with the family, but also I watch myself doing things therapeutically differently with them that would be contributing to and maintaining the solution patterns. The following case example illustrates this idea-generating strategy in action.

Joshua, a Caucasian 8-year-old, was brought for therapy by his parents for "low self-esteem" and "withdrawn" behavior and because he "isolated himself" from family members. The parents appeared to be very concerned and committed to helping Joshua. I asked the imaginary wand question to try to generate some possibilities and treatment goals and to better engage Joshua. Although the parents had no problem coming up with their ideal outcome pictures, Joshua had little to say. The parents also shared with me that Joshua was a "very shy child" and that it "takes a while" for him "to trust new people." The parents' attempted solutions consisted of "not allowing him to isolate himself in his bedroom," "forcing Joshua to participate in social activities," and "making him go out to play with his friends." When the parents backed off in the past, Joshua tended to isolate himself in his bedroom or not to go outside after school. The parents could not think of anything that they were doing or had done in the past that helped Joshua be less withdrawn and more sociable. When I met alone with Joshua, I gave him plenty of space to talk and choose what play or art activity he would like to try. Joshua would not talk to me or invite me into his play activity. I was feeling very stuck at this point in the session and took my intersession break.

I closed my eyes and imagined what Joshua and his family would look like when I reconvened with them and all of their problems were solved. I had this mental picture of the parents playing a game or drawing pictures with Joshua on the floor, then offering him choices of what game he would like to play in the session or asking him what team sports activity he would like to get involved in through their local recreational board. I saw Joshua smiling and happier now that he had more of a voice in his family. I saw myself in this session and in future sessions being more playful, asking fewer questions, and putting Joshua in charge of choosing a family art or play activity for his family.

When I reconvened the family, I found myself more relaxed and optimistic about change happening with this family. The parents welcomed the idea of giving Joshua more room to make choices. In future sessions, Joshua was put in charge of selecting the in-session family and art play activities. By our eighth family session, Joshua was not isolating himself any more, was much more verbal, and appeared happier. The parents also discovered that Joshua responded well to their giving him the "responsibility ball" for making choices rather than forcing him to do things or deciding for him.

Solution-Focused Brief Therapy Tasks: Old Standards That Work

The three therapeutic tasks presented in this section are like old jazz standards that aficionados never get tired of listening to. A classic tune, whether played by a jazz great or a young new musician, will work for most listeners. The same is true for all three of the therapeutic tasks discussed here, which were developed by Steve de Shazer and his colleagues at the Brief Therapy Center in Milwaukee, Wisconsin. de Shazer and his colleagues have repeatedly demonstrated that these experiments are highly effective with a wide range of client presenting problems (de Shazer et al., 2007; de Shazer, 1988, 1991, 1994; Gingerich & de Shazer, 1991). Gingerich and de Shazer (1991) found, through their expert system computer program BRIEFER, that these tasks have a high probability of working when accurately matched with clients' unique cooperative response patterns. After describing each therapeutic task, I provide a case example.

The Prediction Task

The prediction task (de Shazer, 1988, 1991) is particularly useful with child cases in which the reported exceptions occur on a random basis and are not deliberate (i.e., the exceptions just happen arbitrarily). I use the prediction task to help increase the frequency of exceptions and to assist family members in becoming more aware of what works.

> Rico, a 9-year-old Puerto Rican boy, was brought for therapy by his mother, Marcella, for "bad temper tantrums," which occurred, on average, "four times per week." Marcella was unaware of what she or Rico was doing on the other 3 days of the week that made them "good days." The two typically fought over Rico's doing his schoolwork, watching too much TV, and buying toys Rico wanted. Rico was very athletic and was a Michael Jordan basketball fan. I could tell he was a real competitor. I gave Marcella and Rico the prediction task. Separately, Rico and Marcella were to predict each night whether the next day would be a "good day" (no temper tantrums) and try to account for what made it a good day. I requested that they both play good detectives for me so we could figure out what worked.
>
> The family came back 1 week later and reported a number of changes. There were fewer power struggles, "only one temper tantrum" occurred, and Marcella was so pleased with Rico's changes that she bought him the "Nike Michael Jordan T-shirt he wanted." Marcella found that "yelling less" and "avoiding power struggles" seemed to prevent temper tantrums. Rico discovered that when he didn't give his mother a hard time "she yelled less" and they got along better.

The "Do Something Different" Task

In child cases where the parents' goal is not related to the reported exceptions, the parents' superresponsible behavior is contributing to the child's superirresponsible behavior, or the parents are stuck trying to win power struggle battles with their child, I utilize the *do something different task* (Selekman 2005, 2009; de Shazer et al., 2007; de Shazer, 1985, 1988, 1991). I explain to parents that their child has "got their number"—he or she knows every move they are going to make. After this short rationale for their need to be less predictable, the parents are given the following directive: "Between now and the next time we meet, I would like each of you to do something different—no matter how strange, weird, or off-the-wall it might seem" (de Shazer, 1985, p. 123).

Kip, a Caucasian 10-year-old, was brought for therapy by his mother for "constantly swearing," "talking" to her in a "disrespectful way," and "not doing his chores." Kip and Charlotte, the mother, were also having "daily arguments" about neglecting his homework. Charlotte did report that Kip was a "good student" and "can be a big help" to her "at times" around the house. Charlotte was at the "end of her rope" with Kip and was "seriously thinking about sending Kip to live with his father" out of state. I met alone with Charlotte and gave her the do something different task (de Shazer, 1985) to perform as an experiment.

In 1 week's time, Charlotte came up with seven things that she did differently around Kip. One day she walked around the house all day in an ape Halloween mask that she had found in a drawer. She bought a squirt gun and "squirted Kip" every time he would "swear at" or "talk back" to her. Once Charlotte began changing her parental "dance steps" around Kip, he had to change his behavior to accommodate to his mother's oddball changes. Charlotte became "less stressed out" and discovered that "parenting" could be "fun." We also successfully implemented the compliment box strategy.

The "Pretend the Miracle Happened" Task

If the family is unable to identify any exceptions or the exceptions that have occurred are not newsworthy, I use the *pretend the miracle happened task* (de Shazer, 1991). I meet alone with the child and have the child pick 2 days over the next week to pretend to engage in the parents' sought-for miracle behaviors—to blow his or her parents' minds! I also ask the client to watch carefully how his or her parents respond when he or she is pretending.

Tabitha, an African American 9-year-old, was brought in for therapy by her mother for what their "pediatrician" diagnosed as "school phobia." For 2 months, Tabitha had refused to go to school. No matter what her mother did to try to get her to go to school, Tabitha would either "say she was sick" or "refuse to get out of bed." Despite the present behavioral difficulties, Tabitha had begun the school year by going to school without any problems. Other than Tabitha's willingness to attend school back then, neither the mother nor her daughter could account for what had made the difference then. After I ask her the miracle question (de Shazer, 1988), Tabitha had little to say about her ideal miracle picture. Her mother, on the other hand, reported several miracle behaviors, such as "Tabitha would get up in the morning and go to school without any battles," she would have a "better attitude about school," they would be "getting along better," and she would "not hear any excuses about not going to school." I used scaling questions (de Shazer, 1988, 1991) to help establish a well-formed treatment goal with the mother. The mother's goal was for Tabitha to go to school at least 1 or 2 days over the following week. Although neither family member gave me any clues about how the school refusal problem had developed, I did find out from Tabitha that she was upset with her mother because her mother had taken her "computer away" from her for the "past 2 months." I met alone with Tabitha to see if I could use the computer as a bargaining chip. Tabitha quickly warmed up to my proposal of trying to win back her computer for her, provided she would be willing to try an experiment of mine. Tabitha was now on the edge of her seat. I asked her to pick 2 days over the next week to blow her mother's mind by pretending to engage in her mother's miracle behaviors. For the first time in the session, I felt that I had gained therapeutic leverage with Tabitha. She desperately wanted her computer back.

In 1 week's time, Tabitha went to school for an entire week! The mother was totally thrilled that Tabitha agreed to go back to school without any battles. I was able to negotiate with the mother to get Tabitha's computer back. A verbal contract was established between the mother and Tabitha that Tabitha would lose the computer again if she started to refuse to go to school again.

Another therapeutic option is to have the parents pretend to engage in their child's ideal miracle behaviors that he or she would like to see with them over 1 week's time. While pretending, they are to carefully notice how their child responds to them. I have them keep track of specific child-identified miracle behaviors that seem to produce the best responses with him or her and use them more and more frequently.

In my solution-oriented parenting groups, parents are given this therapeutic experiment to do at the end of the second group session (Selekman, 2005, 2009). Parents often report in their third group session that they had great results in using this experiment.

Positive Psychology Therapeutic Experiments: Soloing and Playing with Passion and Meaning

There are four positive psychology therapeutic tasks, or experiments, that I regularly use with clients, all of which not only increase children's awareness levels of their key strengths but also greatly reduce negative emotions and help them find more meaning and fulfillment in their lives. An added bonus is they all have been found to reduce the risk of the client's developing depression and anxiety difficulties (Selekman, 2005, 2009; Peterson, 2006; Peterson & Seligman, 2004; Seligman & Dean, 2003; Seligman, 2002). The age of the child and the nature of his or her presenting difficulties determine which of these positive psychology therapeutic experiments I assign to him or her.

Plan Out Your Perfect Day

The beauty and power of the *plan out your perfect day* therapeutic experiment is that it heightens children's awareness and insight about what activities they need to increase in order to trigger positive emotions, bring them pleasure, and create meaningful experiences and what toxic activities, people, and places they need to steer clear of (Selekman, 2009; Peterson, 2006). The night before the appointed day, they are asked to plan out and create a list of what they think they need to do to have what they would consider a perfect day. On the following evening, they then rate the day on a scale from 1 to 10, with 10 being "the best day of my life" and 1 being "the worst day of my life" (see Figure 4.2, which provides the full rating scale developed by Peterson, 2006). It is beneficial to have clients do this experiment each day over a 2-week period so that they can perceive clearly what patterns of behavior work best for them. Once a child is able to identify what specifically he or she needs to do to achieve "6 and above" days, we want to have the client increase doing more of what works for him or her.

Before sending children off to begin this experiment, we need to prepare them for the likelihood that some days will inevitably not go their way or may take a negative turn. I like to come up with Plan B options to save the day and quickly get back on track after any temporary derailments. It is helpful to have children discuss and write down the concrete steps they can take and carry this paper around with them in case they are confronted

10 = The best day of my life
9 = Outstanding day
8 = Excellent day
7 = Very good day
6 = A good day
5 = An average day
4 = A sub-par day
3 = A bad day
2 = A terrible day
1 = The worst day of my life

FIGURE 4.2. Rating scale for the "plan out your perfect day" experiment. Based on Peterson (2006).

with toxic peers and other aversive developments. Another useful problem-solving method is to role-play with them certain situations that they anticipate may occur with toxic peers at school so that they are well aware of how to constructively manage these situations. The following case example illustrates how this therapeutic experiment can be used effectively with depressed children to decrease negative emotions, engender positive emotions, raise hope and optimism levels, and co-create positive self-fulfilling prophecies for them.

Alicia, a depressed and very bright African American 10-year-old, was referred to me by her school social worker for "depressed mood," a decline in her grades, and social withdrawal from her peers. According to the school social worker, Alicia used to be "a very popular social butterfly." She recently experienced two painful losses: her parents divorced, the father moving out of state, and her maternal grandmother died from a sudden heart attack. In the first session, Alicia was quite courageous and shared all of her painful thoughts and feelings regarding these significant losses, voicing a strong desire "to be happy again." Of all the therapeutic activities I had offered Alicia and her mother to try out, she really liked the sound of the "plan out your perfect day" experiment the most. Before we ended the session, I gave Alicia a copy of the rating scale for the experiment so she could rate the quality of each day over the following week.

Alicia came back smiling the next week, reporting mostly 6- and 7-rated days, with one 8-rated day. I explored with her what specifically she was doing to pull off her 6- and 7-rated days, and she said that she spent a lot of time hanging out with her two closest friends, Carolyn and Samantha, both in and outside of school—both of whom are "funny" and share similar interests with her. She steered clear of Liz, whom she described as being like "a poisonous spider." Alicia came up with some "new dance steps" for the upcoming talent show at school, which gave her more confidence that she had a great chance of winning. Her sole 8-rated day was a combination of getting an A grade on her difficult math test and receiving a call from her father, who was flying in for the weekend to spend some quality time with her. Alicia reported feeling much less depressed after having such a great week. Since this therapeutic experiment had worked so well and Alicia was eager to shoot for higher-rated days over the next week, we mutually agreed for her to continue using this experiment.

One week later, Alicia came in beaming, sporting a big smile. She reported that she had all mostly 8-rated days except for one day that ended up being a 6. Alicia had one day that she rated 9. On the 8-rated days, she continued to socialize, mainly with Carolyn and Samantha, who put her in a good mood. She was doing better in all of her school subjects; during her free time she played her flute, and she went shopping with her mother a few times. Her 9-rated day consisted of a combination of winning the school talent show and spending time with her father. Knowing that Alicia loved hip-hop dancing so much, the parents split the costs for a hip-hop class that they thought she would enjoy; naturally, Alicia was thrilled about this turn of events.

"You at Your Best" Story

Children who are strong in the linguistic intelligence area (Gardner, 1993) especially enjoy doing the *you at your best story* (Selekman, 2009; Peterson, 2006). However, I have had similar success in using this experiment with children that possess other major strengths or that are strong in other intelligence areas. The act of simply writing about our past personal achievements triggers positive emotions and memories, which can help neutralize negative emotions. The client is asked to write a short story (only three to four paragraphs) about something he or she accomplished in the past that he or she was proud of. After they write the short story, I have the clients underline with different colored ink or markers both their agency thinking (examples of useful self-talk or positive cheerleading friends that get them fired up) and pathway thinking (effective problem-solving steps) that helped them to achieve their positive accomplishments. I take the time to clearly and concretely define for them what I mean by these two types of thinking and write the definitions down for them as well.

After they have completed their stories, I have the children bring them in, read them to me, and then we discuss how we can tap their agency and pathway thinking to help them achieve their current goals for themselves. Children discover that their stories of success can serve as road maps for future successes. Peterson (2006) has even found that individuals who read their you-at-your-best stories before they go to bed sleep better. The case example below illustrates how this therapeutic experiment is not only emotionally uplifting but also operationally instructive.

Sally, a depressed and anxious Caucasian 11-year-old, was having a hard time fitting in with her peers both at her new school and in her neighborhood. Her father's company had transferred him to their Chicago office, which led to the big family move. However, this move was devastating for Sally, in that she had to leave her close friends and in the past had had a hard time making new friends. Sally felt like a stranger in a strange land at her new school and as though she was "invisible." Two of Sally's passions in life were playing tennis and writing. I discovered that she was a nationally ranked junior tennis player. Since she also liked to write, I proposed that she try out the you-at-your-best story experiment over the following week.

One week later, she brought in her two-page story of her winning a big national tennis tournament prior to the family's move to Chicago. In great detail she wrote about how she fired herself up with self-talk (agency thinking) to beat some of her arch rivals on the junior tennis circuit. Her pathway thinking was reflected in her references to using an aggressive "serve and volley game" and "really concentrating to nail down her hard first serves." While reading her story to me, she was smiling and sounded very confident about her game. Summoning up her tennis playing language and metaphors, I recommended that she experiment over the next week by pretending that making one new acquaintance or friend at school would be comparable to winning a tennis match at a national junior tennis tournament. I shared with her that I was confident that, by not sitting on the baseline and concentrating on getting those first serves in and getting up to the net, she would be able to successfully initiate at least one conversation with a peer at school and begin to establish a new friendship.

One week later, not only had Sally made two new friends, but one of them had played tennis competitively as well. Sally was very proud of her accomplishment and was feeling more confident about being able to connect with other peers as well.

Three Good Things to Be Grateful for

One way we can help neutralize negative emotions that children are grappling with and help improve the quality of their lives is to have them daily, before they go to bed, keep track of positive things happening in their lives that they are grateful for (Selekman, 2009; Emmons, 2007; Peterson, 2006). As an assignment they can accomplish quickly each day right before they go to bed, clients can write down three things that they are grateful for in their lives in a diary or journal book. They should then read their daily entries of three positive things or blessings right before they lay their heads down on their pillows, which often leads them to sleeping better when they do (Emmons, 2007; Peterson, 2006). Regularly honoring what one is grateful for in one's life and acknowledging gratitude to others is strongly associated with life satisfaction (Peterson, 2006; Peterson & Seligman, 2004).

Using Your Top Strengths in Creative Ways

Peterson (2006) has developed a creative therapeutic experiment that he calls *using your top signature strengths in novel ways*. This exercise grew out of having adults first take the online *Values in Action (VIA) Classifica-*

tion of Strengths questionnaire and then having them experiment with using their top five signature strengths in novel ways to improve the quality of life for both themselves and others. I have found that with older children I can use a modified version of this experiment after children take the *Values in Action (VIA) Inventory of Strengths for Youth* (or, if this is too difficult for them to do, I simply have them identify what they think their top three or four strengths are and have them experiment with using them in creative ways). Not only do children find this experiment both fun and interesting to do, but it also expands their horizons by further developing their interest and skill areas and enables them to experience the benefits of reaching out to others.

> Tom, a Caucasian 11-year-old, was referred to me for ADD and get-ting caught at school drinking a can of beer in the boys' bathroom. Although Tom was quite popular at school, he had a history of clown-ing around in class and testing his teachers' limits. On the positive side of things, Tom was respected as a talented athlete, leader, and come-dian by his peers. He had lots of friends, both in and outside of school. The beer incident at school resulted in his having several detentions and spending periods of time in the principal's office. The parents were quite upset with Tom about the beer incident and grounded him for a month. It turned out that this was not the first time he had taken beer from his father.
>
> In the first family meeting, I built an alliance with Tom by spend-ing a lot of time having him share with me examples of his natural leadership and athletic abilities. He seemed to take pride and joy in taking charge and serving as the captain a lot in gym class sports activi-ties and helping his team win. Tom and I discussed how he was now on the "hit list" at school because of the beer incident and the steps he thought he could take to work his way off. He thought it would be best to "be cool" with his teacher, which meant not clowning around in her class. I then asked him about how he thought he could use his great sense of humor and social skills in positive ways over the next week that could help get him off the hit list. Tom came up with two really brilliant ideas. The first was for him to reach out to a new student who was being teased and bullied. Just to make sure that Tom was not planning to defend this new student by fighting the bullies and getting himself in further hot water, I asked him what he planned to do. Tom was first going to try to establish rapport with this boy and then recom-mend that he ignore and try to walk away from the bullies. If this did not work, he was going to recommend that the boy "hang close" to him. His rationale was that the bullies would think the new boy must

"be cool" since he was associating with Tom, which would lead to their "backing off." I complimented Tom on his great idea.

Next, we discussed how he could use his great sense of humor and natural stand-up comedian abilities in a creative way. One of his ideas was to use his humor in his relationship with his 8-year-old brother. Tom openly admitted that he was not very nice to his younger brother, Will, usually bossing him around and yelling at him a lot. He decided to experiment with "making Will laugh with gentle clowning around" and to tell him some "simple clean jokes."

In a collaborative meeting the following week at the school with Tom's teacher, the school social worker, the principal, Tom's parents, and Tom, Tom's altruistic outreach act to the new student in his class was the big news of the day! All the adults in the room were impressed by Tom's kindness and positive actions. Tom was smiling and soaking up all of the compliments he received. His teacher, Mrs. Fish, shared with the group that Tom was having a great week in her class. In fact, usually she would send him to "the principal's office at least one to two times per week." Not only did this not happen, but also Tom was refraining from being "the class clown" and "working harder in class." The parents also acknowledged that Tom was treating his younger brother much better and they were actually "laughing together," which the parents were really pleased with. I gave Tom a big high-five for his outstanding job.

Conclusion

When selecting or constructing therapeutic experiments for a family, it is important for therapists to have the family perform the same experiments in the second and subsequent sessions if it continues to work for them. Therapists and clients get into trouble when they stop doing what is working. Any therapeutic experiments selected or constructed for a family should be appropriate to the family's problem definition; capitalize on their strengths, language, beliefs, and stages of readiness to change; tap into the unique cooperative response patterns of family members; and be in line with their treatment goals. In this chapter, I have presented several specific ways that therapists can generate creative ideas for effective problem solving and designing and selecting appropriate therapeutic tasks and exercises. It is my hope that therapists will find the idea-generating strategies discussed in this chapter to be useful in stimulating their own creative juices, thereby aiding in developing unique and original therapeutic exercises for their client families.

5

Curious George Meets Dr. Seuss

Family Play and Art Therapy Strategies

The world of reality has its limits; the world of imagination is boundless.
—JEAN-JACQUES ROUSSEAU

One day, after reading *Curious George Takes a Job* to my daughter Hanna, 3 years old at the time, I began to wonder what would happen if Curious George got lost and somehow stumbled into a Dr. Seuss story. Being an avid Dr. Seuss fan, I wondered how well Curious George would get along with Marco in *And to Think That I Saw It on Mulberry Street,* or with Horton the elephant in *Horton Hatches the Egg,* or the moose Thidwick in *Thidwick the Big-Hearted Moose.* Would Dr. Seuss try to rescue Curious George if he got lost in the Desert of Drize by providing him with a Crunk-Car or a Zumble-Zay? Finally, I wondered whether Dr. Seuss would want to try to teach Curious George a lesson about the dangers of being too curious. I came to the conclusion that Curious George would get along quite well with Marco, Horton, and Thidwick, that he would make it out of the Desert of Drize unscathed, and that, by the end of the story, Curious George would be quite a bit wiser about when to take risks and when not to.

Like Dr. Seuss, I want to coauthor stories with families that are filled with adventure, laughter, and surprises; stories that stimulate wonder and imagination. In each session, I want family members to learn something new about themselves that can make a difference in their thinking and doing. I want to banish any unhelpful beliefs held by the child and his or her family that keep them stuck and help them see that all they needed and wanted was already inside them. As Milton H. Erickson has pointed out, "We know a lot more than we think we do; we have vast, untapped reservoirs of ability" (in Ostrander et al., 1994, p. 178).

In this chapter, I present several family play and art therapy experiments that are Dr. Seuss-like in that they can successfully help family members step outside their familiar rational worlds and enter a world of imagination, where anything is possible. The unique needs of the family and what makes the most sense therapeutically dictate whether to select one or a combination of family play and art therapy experiments to implement in the second and subsequent sessions. For example, for rigid families that have forgotten how to play together, the *family portrait, imaginary time machine, invisible family inventions, the famous guest consultants, child as the director of a new family drama,* and *child as mentor for his/her parent* experiments can be most beneficial.

I conclude the chapter by discussing three highly effective visualization tools and several mindfulness meditation practices that can be used with children.

Major Family Play and Art Therapy Experiments

In this section, I present eight major family play and art therapy experiments, describing each and offering helpful guidelines about when and how to utilize them in the treatment process. Case examples help demonstrate the utility of each of these therapeutic experiments.

The Family Squiggle Wiggle Game

Winnicott (1971a) originally developed the *squiggle wiggle game* as an effective therapeutic tool to assess the child's problem situation, his or her thought processes, and emotionally laden material about his or her family, as well as to help build rapport with the child in a fun and playful way. When working one-on-one with a child, the original squiggle wiggle format can be modified and used as an indirect method to introduce to the child new ideas or potential solutions to his or her presenting problems. These ideas can be embedded in the therapist's squiggle picture and story and reflected back through the child. The family squiggle wiggle game is particularly useful with young children or children who have difficulty expressing their thoughts and feelings with family members.

With younger children, I invite them to select a family member to draw a squiggle on a sheet of paper and then ask them to create a picture out of the squiggle and try to tell a story to the best of their ability to the family and me about the picture. The child's picture and story can be quite newsworthy to the family, helping them to better understand what the child is going through and how the child views him- or herself, and it can reveal individual or family secrets or how the child views the family or its social world. Once the child's picture and story are adequately discussed, he or she then draws a squiggle and has the whole family create a picture and tell a story about it. Most families tend to create a picture and story that incorporate the child in a positive way. Sometimes family members gain valuable insights from the child's picture and story or are so shocked by it that they request the opportunity to change the child's picture and the ending of the story to have a better outcome. The case example described next is a good illustration of this clinical situation.

> Luis, a 6-year-old Puerto Rican boy, was brought to the family session by his parents, who were very concerned about his "withdrawn" behavior, not socializing with "other children" in the neighborhood, "day dreaming in class," and looking "very sad" all the time. Luis's 14-year-old sister, Wanda, also accompanied the parents to this session. After multiple relocations, the family now lived in a gang-dominated neighborhood, and intense feuding was going on between Luis's father, Carlos, and Carlos's cousin, Ricardo. Recently, Luis had witnessed his father embroiled in a fistfight with Ricardo. The mother, Victoria, was on Prozac for her own "clinical depression." For the bulk of our first family session together, I had great difficulty engaging Luis. The imaginary magic wand question, trying to engage him in a board game, and using humor all proved unproductive with Luis. However, I remembered that earlier in the session Victoria had said Luis liked to draw. So I decided to try the squiggle wiggle game with him. I drew a squiggle on the construction paper, which not only elicited a smile from Luis but seemed to spark his curiosity. His parents and sister had their eyes fixed on Luis's paper. Suddenly, after Luis drew a picture of himself crossing the street and about to be run down by a truck, Carlos voiced his concerns about wanting to save his son and asked Luis if he could draw a "stop sign" on the street and a "police crossing guard." Victoria and Wanda also got on the floor and asked Luis's permission to draw their additions as well. The mother drew an "underground walkway" so that Luis would be able to "cross safely" to the other side of the street. Wanda drew a "police car with flashing lights" knifing in between Luis and the truck to save his life.
>
> Family members were totally shocked by Luis's picture. They had no idea that he wanted to die. Although Luis remained very quiet, nonverbally he appeared to appreciate his family's concerns about him, which he indicated by smiling and showing interest in what family members had to say and what they were drawing. When the family returned 2 weeks later, the parents and Wanda reported numerous changes. Luis was socializing more with family members and peers, appeared to be in "happy spirits," and was "much more talkative." I was quite shocked

by Luis's many changes as well—this was not the same boy I had seen 2 weeks earlier! The parents attributed Luis's seeming transformation to his expressing himself fully in our last session. Luis disclosed that he was "happy" now because his father and cousin were "friends" again. I ended up seeing the family for one more session 6 weeks later to assess the family's progress; they reported no further problems.

Marshall McLuhan once observed that "art as radar acts as an 'early alarm system,' as it were, enabling us to discover social and psychic targets in lots of time to prepare to cope with them. Art, like games, is a translator of experience" (1964, p. 214). Through the use of the family squiggle wiggle game, Luis was offered a platform on which to express his sad feelings about the chaos in his life and to successfully rally his family around him in a display of support. Like an "early alarm system," family members could graphically see in Luis's drawing his crying out for their help.

The Imaginary Feelings X-Ray Machine

For children who are not at all verbally inclined or have difficulty in expressing their feelings, the *imaginary feelings X-ray machine* can be quite helpful (Selekman, 2005, 2009). The client and family members are asked:

- "If I had an imaginary feelings X-ray machine that could show me what your feelings look like inside, what would I see in the X-ray pictures?"
- "Where in your body would those feelings live?"
- "If you were to draw scenes from times in your life when those feelings were really present and alive in you, what would you draw?"

I then have the client lie on his or her back on some thick-grade paper rolled out on the floor and select a family member to draw an outline of his or her body on the paper. Once the outline is complete, the child is asked to draw within it (with magic markers or crayons) scenes or feelings from his or her life, as depicted in X-rays taken of them. When the child is done, the X-ray results are discussed by the family and the child. Other family members can do this experiment as well. This experiment is particularly useful with children presenting with somatic complaints and/ or growing up in high-stress home environments where their voices are not heard, they are reticent to express how they feel, or they have a hard time articulating their thoughts and feelings. The experiment also can be used in children's groups, particularly with children who have alcoholic or substance-abusing parents. It has been my clinical experience that children find this family art experiment to be fun, and it definitely increases their awareness of their emotions. Family members also are often surprised by what the child expresses about him- or herself and the family situation through the visual representations. The added bonus is that this activity often sparks empathy from the parents and the older siblings, helping to open up new lines of communication.

> Robbie, a Caucasian 9-year-old, was brought for therapy by his mother, Phyllis, for "school behavior problems," "getting into fights" with peers, and breaking his mother's rules. Robbie's parents had been divorced for 3 years. The father, Conrad, was an "active alcoholic" and used to be verbally abusive toward Robbie and Phyllis. Conrad was inconsistent with visitations, and Robbie was "very difficult to manage" for Phyllis when he returned from a weekend visit with his father. Phyllis's prime reason for bringing her son in for treatment was that she felt that he needed to "talk about his feelings about his alcoholic father." Apparently, Robbie always ran out of the room when Phyllis tried to get him to talk about his father. Phyllis called herself an ACOA (adult child of an alcoholic) and was actively involved in Al-Anon. Her father had died from alcoholism. In the first session, I connected well with Phyllis, and we worked on some parenting strategies. Robbie and I failed to click even after several attempts to get "in the door" with him.
>
> In our second family session, I decided to try the imaginary feelings X-ray machine experiment with Robbie, and he responded with excitement. Robbie's X-ray picture proved to be quite revealing. He drew a volcano erupting on the left side of his chest area. After drawing his heart, he put a padlock on it, so nobody could get inside. With the help of the imaginary feelings X-ray machine, Robbie was better able to talk about his anger toward his father (the erupting volcano) and how his father had repeatedly "hurt" him by forgetting promises to take him to baseball games or to buy him things. The padlocked heart was symbolic of Robbie's unwillingness to allow himself to be hurt by his father anymore. Another important change was Robbie's seeking out his mother to talk about his "bad" feelings when upset at home or when thinking about his father. With the help of the imaginary feelings X-ray machine, we were able to better open up the lines of communication between Robbie and his mother.

The Family Portrait

Most art therapists use family drawings as an assessment tool for eliciting from children how they view themselves in the context of their families. By means of family drawings, children can teach us about family interaction patterns, coalitions, conflicts, and how they view themselves in their families. DiLeo (1973) identified two common observations of family dynamics in children's family drawings: *omission of a family member* and *omission of self*. In the first instance, the child may omit from the drawing a family member with whom he or she is in conflict, whom he or she is rejecting, or whom he or she feels rejected by. Omission of self is characterized by the child's placing him- or herself at the very end of a line of family members (i.e., self-perception as having low status in the family). It is most telling about their negative self-perceptions when children place a younger sibling before them in the chronological sequencing of family members (DiLeo, 1973). Similar to the previously discussed family art therapy tasks, the family portrait can be used with younger children and children who are not very verbal and as a therapeutic means of challenging family patterns and beliefs. In some cases, if the child wishes to get the parents involved in this activity, the parents could be invited to draw themselves in the family portrait or add background drawings capturing important themes about their family. The following case illustrates the power of the child's family portrait drawing in challenging family patterns and for opening up space for possibilities.

> Jacob, a Caucasian 7-year-old, was brought by his mother, Amanda, for counseling for his "low self-esteem," "spacing out in class," "ADD," and isolating himself in the family. Jacob's 6-year-old sister, Jeanette, was described as a "gifted child" by her teacher. The father, a successful businessman, could not attend this initial family session due to his work schedule. Jacob was very shy and did not open up much to me. To get a better impression of how he viewed himself in his family, I invited Jacob to draw a family portrait. Amanda was totally shocked by Jacob's drawing. Not only did he place himself at the very edge of the drawing, but also he positioned himself slightly *behind* everyone else. Unfortunately, Jacob had little to say about his drawing. In our next family session, the father was also very concerned about Jacob's drawing. The father's presence at the session, however, appeared to bring Jacob to life. He was better able to talk about not seeing his dad that much because of business trips and how he felt that "Jeanette always gets her way." The family was referred to a neurologist for the "spacing-out" problem, whereupon it was discovered that Jacob had a seizure problem. Jacob's teacher had mistaken this problem as a symptom of ADD. After Jacob was placed on the right medications and his father set aside more weekend time to spend with him, his symptoms both at home and at school rapidly stabilized.

The Imaginary Time Machine

The *imaginary time machine* therapeutic experiment can be used at any stage of treatment (Selekman, 2005, 2009). It is particularly useful when a therapist is faced with an impasse because it can propel the treatment system into new, uncharted possibilities. The therapist begins: "Suppose I had an imaginary time machine sitting over here, and I asked each of you to enter it and take it wherever you wished to travel in time. Where would you go? Who would you be with? What would you do there? What difference would that make in your life?" It is important to instruct the children to use all of their senses—and take note of colors and motion—while time traveling, which makes the experience more vivid. Clients can allow their imagination to run wild in terms of where they want to transport themselves or their family in time. When using this playful and fun experiment with children and their families, I have been impressed with their tremendous creativity. Family members have come up with the following time-traveling scenarios: one family transported its members back in time to a fun and marvelous family vacation; one child transported himself and the family into the year 2500, where they lived on a spaceship orbiting Mars; an 11-year-old African American boy transported himself back to World War II to secure a Sherman tank to bring back to the present to help defend himself against a neighborhood gang that had been hassling him on the streets; and an 8-year-old Mexican girl transported herself back to the neighborhood where her family used to live and she had lots of friends—unlike her present reality, where in the new suburban community she had few or no friends.

What is most powerful and effectual about this therapeutic experiment is its great capacity to immediately lift up family members from their oppressive problems and help galvanize imaginative solutions. Traveling into the past allows family members to instantly summon up past successes, such as useful coping and problem-solving experiences, times when they were more emotionally close, and fun things their family members used to do together. After going back to a place in history, a child may want to bring back the creative ideas and wisdom he or she learned while with a famous historic figure of those times, or to make the experience more fun, have this historic figure join us as a special guest consultant sitting in an empty chair in my office. Alternatively, by transporting oneself into the future, *anything* is possible because it has not happened yet. Osborn (1993) pointed out that "when we look forward to something we want to have come true, and we strongly believe that it will come true, we can often make ourselves make it come true" (p. 33). In cases where the parents are at wits' end and feeling highly frustrated with their child, we can have the child hop into the imaginary time-travel machine and suddenly he or she is now 19 or 20 years old, visiting the parents at home on holiday break from college. We can explore with both the parents and the child how things have changed in their relationship now that he or she is a responsible and mature adult. We can ask the parents what kind of questions they will be asking their son or daughter during this pleasant visit. The child can be asked to guess what the parents will be most curious about in his or her future life as a young adult. Often this use of the imaginary time-travel machine can help instill hope in the parents and open up space for possibilities in their relationship with their child (Selekman, 2009).

Finally, another way the imaginary time-travel machine can be used is having the child serve as the fearless leader for his or her family on an adventure trip in the future. Some children take their family down the Amazon River, others climbing through the Himalayan mountain range, and yet others on an African safari.

The two case examples below demonstrate the effectiveness of the imaginary time-travel machine for co-creating compelling individual and family changes:

> Charlie, an adopted Guatemalan 11-year-old, was school-referred for family counseling by his social worker for problems with "anger management, fighting with peers, mouthing off to his teacher and mother, and oppositional behavior." Charlie was on the "school hit list" for his verbal and physically aggressive behaviors. Although Charlie had serious behavioral difficulties, he was an excellent student with many intellectual gifts. Charlie had three adopted siblings from different birth parents—a 7-year-old sister, and 10- and 15-year-old brothers. The parents had no difficulties with their other adopted children.
>
> My first two family sessions proved to be unproductive. Even when I met alone with Charlie, I found myself doing most of the talking in an effort to engage him. Ellie, the mother, had a tendency to bring up everything that Charlie had done wrong. David, the father, was more laid back and pointed out that he rarely had arguments with Charlie when they were together. He shared that Charlie was "very athletic" and "strong for his age." When asked what he did to prevent arguments with him, he was unable to identify any specific parenting strategies that seemed to work when they were together. In both of our family sessions, the use of the miracle, coping, and pessimistic questions failed to produce any realistic treatment goals, to identify useful coping or problem-solving strategies that were working for the parents, or to help me foster a stronger cooperative relationship with them.
>
> In our third family session, I decided to try to inject more playfulness and fun into our meeting by introducing the imaginary time machine. I invited Charlie to hop into my imaginary time machine and take his parents on an adventure trip anywhere in the world that he was

longing to visit. He decided to take his parents with him to the "Great Barrier Reef" off the northeast coast of Australia. They went "scuba diving" and saw "beautiful tropical fish," were dropped into the heart of "reef and bull shark" territory in "a special cage," and Charlie and his father went "deep-sea fishing for a day" and reeled in "a few huge marlins." Charlie lit up with excitement and great enthusiasm while describing the details of their family adventure trip. The parents also appeared to enjoy hearing the details about Charlie's family adventure dream trip. However, Ellie felt quite uncomfortable with the shark cage part of the adventure vacation. I asked Charlie which of his strengths and talents his parents would come to know on their family adventure trip. He replied, "That I am fearless, I can be a great leader, and to trust me." I asked him how he would help his mother get over her fears about going down below in the shark cage. Charlie would offer "to hold" his "mom's hand" and reassure her that she was "completely safe" in the cage with him. Ellie smiled and thought it was "real sweet" that Charlie would "reach out to comfort" her. This was a side of Charlie that she had not seen a lot of lately. David shared with Charlie that he was impressed with his "family leadership abilities."

Although the parents could not afford a family trip to Australia, they decided to put Charlie in charge of planning a "fun Florida Keys family trip," which would include snorkeling and a day of deep-sea fishing. He did all of the research on the Internet and went with his mother to a travel agent as well. We also came up with other ways Charlie could have a leadership role around the house, like helping his younger sister with her challenging schoolwork. The parents also enrolled Charlie in wall-climbing and strength-training classes at their local YMCA so that he could channel his aggressive energy into positive activities.

The next case example involves a depressed Caucasian 10-year-old girl who was underachieving in school and lived in a chaotic home environment. Her father had been incarcerated for armed robbery.

Melinda was brought for therapy by her mother for "failing three subjects in school," "looking depressed," and "testing" her mother's limits. Melinda's parents were divorced as a result of her father's "alcohol and drug abuse problems," "violent" behavior toward her mother, and "yelling" problem. Melinda really missed her father and had a tendency to defend him when her maternal uncle and cousins would "say bad things about him." In the first session, I had great difficulty engaging Melinda, particularly in eliciting from her what she would like to get out of family therapy. Her mother, Alice, did most of the talking and appeared to be overly concerned about Melinda's academic performance problem. My use of the miracle question (de Shazer, 1988) and humor failed to lighten up the atmosphere in the therapy room or create any possibilities with the family. After introducing the imaginary time machine task to Melinda in our second family session, she came to life! Melinda transported herself back to the days of Pocahontas. Pocahontas took Melinda "through the woods" and taught her about nature and how to make clothing out of animal hides. Pocahontas and Melinda became "close friends." Melinda seemed as though she were in a total trance state when describing her special encounter with Pocahontas.

To further capitalize on their special relationship together, I had Melinda and Pocahontas hop into the imaginary time machine and ride it forward to the present day. I explored with Melinda what advice Pocahontas would give her and her mother to help them get along better. According to Melinda, Pocahontas would tell her and her mother to "stop arguing" so much, for her mother to come to her defense whenever the uncle and cousins would put down her father, and for both of them to "listen better" to one another. When asked about how Pocahontas would be helpful to Melinda at school, Melinda pointed out how she would be "paying more attention" in class, "concentrating better" on her work, and "taking home and completing" her daily homework assignments.

With Pocahontas as my co-therapist, I was able to open the door for possibilities with this family. We were able to improve communications in Melinda's relationship with her mother, particularly by getting Alice to defend Melinda when the uncle and cousins would put down her father. Melinda also brought her failing grades up to a "C" level.

Invisible Family Inventions

Similar to the imaginary time machine experiment, the *invisible family inventions* experiment stimulates creative problem-solving abilities with family members and invites them to play together, which may be a novel experience for families plagued by entrenched negative patterns of interactions and fixed beliefs about their problem situations (Selekman, 2005, 2009). This experiment can be used at any stage of treatment, by asking the family, "If you as a group were to invent something that could benefit other families just like you, what would that be?"

I try to avoid giving the family any ideas, leaving the imagination process up to them. Once they or the individual child come up with their gadget or invention, I like the family or the child to draw on paper with colored markers or crayons a prototype of what they think the gadget or invention would look like. Once they achieve success with this experiment, family members discover that they can work together as a team without conflicts or problems, which proves to be a newsworthy experience for them.

Some examples of patented invisible family inventions are a "chilling-out" cylindrical tank into which family members can go when they have an "attitude problem" or are ready to "blow their stack" with other family members; family jet packs to transport the kids around more quickly, thus freeing up the mother to run errands or do things for herself; and a special TV with a screen the family can walk through to join the cast of their favorite TV shows or movies or to become a new character in a video game.

> Samantha, a bright Caucasian 10-year-old, was brought in by her mother for "constantly arguing about everything." Raquel, Samantha's 6-year-old sister, accompanied them to the session. Samantha's parents had recently divorced after a 1-year separation. Samantha was "refusing to do her chores" and was starting to associate with "troublemakers" in their neighborhood. Despite all the behavior problems, Samantha managed to get "B" grades in school. I had discovered earlier in the session that her favorite subject was science. As a way to lighten up the atmosphere in the room and move the conversation away from the complaints the mother and Samantha were exchanging with each other, I presented the invisible family invention experiment to the family. Samantha took the lead in trying to brainstorm ideas with her family, coming up with a highly creative idea. She invented a "pill that families could take" whenever they are plagued by chronic "arguing" problems. According to Samantha, once the pill was ingested, family members would be unable to "swear," "yell at," or "blame" one another. Instead of negative responses, family members could utter only "compliments," "praise," and low-volume positive responses to one another. The positive effects of the pill were mostly contributed by the mother, with some help from Samantha. They both agreed that such a pill would "make families stronger" and probably would "make the world a better place to live in."
>
> By the end of our session, the atmosphere in the room had lightened up considerably. Samantha and her mother resolved to take the invisible pill on a daily basis as an experiment, to see if it would help them "communicate better." Two weeks later, the family returned in better spirits, reporting that the pill had helped them "get along better." In closing our session, I suggested that they try to market their new pill and get the Food and Drug Administration to approve the pill for other families to help them with their problems.

The invisible family inventions experiment is wonderful in that it helps families generate their own unique solutions for their presenting problems by having them come up with creative ways for helping other families. Samantha's creative pill invention served as a pattern intervention strategy and a constant reminder to both Samantha and her mother that they constantly strive to interact with each other only in a positive way, particularly under the influence of the pill. Interestingly enough, whenever Samantha and her mother were tempted to push each other's buttons, an image of the pill would flash before their eyes and prevent them from being negative with each other.

Another case example demonstrates the high level of creativity and inventiveness that children are often capable of.

Eleven-year-old Chris was brought in for consultation by his physically handicapped maternal grandmother, who recently was granted total guardianship rights for him. Chris's mother had been in jail for murder since he was a toddler, he did not know his father or older brother, and he had been living in and out of group and foster homes for most of his life. Chris's presenting problems included violent behavior toward his maternal grandparents (kicking and hitting them when frustrated), ADD, and suspected Tourette syndrome, possibly accounting for his tics and excessive swearing.

At the beginning of the family consultation, I prevented Chris from kicking his grandmother after he discovered he had been brought to a counseling session instead of what was supposed to be a fun family outing; she had told him that they were going to run errands and then were all going to drop by his favorite department store. As a way to prevent an incipient crisis from escalating further, I got Chris to agree to meet with me alone; I had learned that in previous counseling sessions with numerous therapists the grandmother would typically spend most of the session time talking about how "crazy and ill" he was.

To open up my individual session time with Chris, I wanted to come to know what his key strengths were. He bragged about being a "great Pokemon game player," "real good with Game Boy," "great on the computer," loved to "build things," and was "good at sports." After discovering that he was into computers and Game Boy, I thought he would really enjoy trying out the invisible family inventions experiment. Chris came up with a really creative and interesting invention that he called "The Cyclops." It was a virtual reality helmet with a dark visor. Users of the Cyclops would charge it by plugging it into their turned-on TV sets. The Cyclops was a highly versatile device. If he were mad and tempted to try to kick or hit his grandmother while wearing the virtual reality helmet, "metal chains would come out" that only he could see that would pull his "legs and arms back." Also, there was a "lip lock device" that would operate if he "started to swear at" either one of his grandparents while wearing the helmet. He was really concerned that if the Cyclops had "a short-circuit" or malfunctioned his "lips might get permanently locked together!" I shared with him that—knowing that could possibly happen—he really should think twice about swearing at his grandparents. Chris made a really beautiful drawing of the Cyclops.

Another "cool feature" of his virtual reality helmet was that while wearing it you could transport yourself to the set of a Harry Potter movie. Chris was a big Harry Potter fan. I asked him, "While on the set of a Harry Potter movie, what would you be dying to ask Harry Potter about?" Chris shared, "How to give a Patronis Charm." I asked what else would Harry Potter teach or say to him, and Chris responded with "Get off the set! You're disrupting our movie!" We both laughed.

At the end of our enjoyable time together, I strongly recommended to Chris that he pretend to put the Cyclops helmet on at home when mad with his grandparents to help him not cave into trying to hurt them. The grandmother thought this was a good idea and would give him a cue to grab the Cyclops helmet whenever he would start to get mad and lose control to help him not get into trouble. Chris agreed to try this strategy out and thought it was a "sweet" (cool) idea.

The Child as Director of the New Family Drama

When working with families that have been chronically oppressed by their difficulties, in which the child appears to be locked into the family's scapegoat role or in which there is a lack of playfulness and family fun, I will do the following: I put the child in charge of one or more therapy sessions, to act as if he or she were the director of a TV drama or sitcom about his or her family. From behind a video camera, the child directs family members how to behave and converse with one another. The therapist can play the role of the child or an absent family member. As the director, the child can be as creative as he or she likes with the themes, story lines, family role behaviors, and humorous elements of the new family drama/sitcom. The therapist and the family review the videotapes of each episode that the child directs and produces, and the child takes the lead in offering editorial comments.

The benefits of this family play therapy experiment are threefold. First and foremost, the child's competencies shine through when given a voice and empowered. Second, outmoded family beliefs about the child and unproductive family interactions are changed. Finally, family members become much more playful and spontaneous with one another, helping them to liberate themselves from their oppressive problems.

The following case example illustrates how this family play therapy strategy can create possibilities with a stuck case.

Pedro, an 11-year-old Mexican boy, was brought into therapy for constantly testing his mother's limits, not doing his chores, and underachieving in school. His mother, Maria, was at her wits' end with Pedro. She had a stressful managerial position with a company and was tired of coming home from work and having to "yell at Pedro about everything." Her other child, Theresa, 10 years old, was an honors student at Pedro's school and "never misbehaved."

The first and second sessions proved to be highly unproductive in identifying a realistic and readily achievable treatment goal as well as in trying to break up the blame–counterblame pattern of interaction between Maria, Theresa, and Pedro. When meeting alone with Pedro, I discovered that he felt blamed for everything and that his mother favored Theresa over him.

In my third family session, I decided to improvise and capitalize on one of Pedro's strengths and main interest areas, filmmaking. At school, Pedro was considered to be the most talented member of the school audiovisual crew. I showed Pedro how to use my video camera and explained the director's task to the family. For the first time, the mother and Theresa began to respond to Pedro in a more positive way. While filming and directing his new TV show, he had me pretend that I was Pedro preparing dinner for his mother, with Theresa's assistance, in the kitchen. They made spaghetti and a salad for dinner. When Maria came through the front door, she was greeted at the door with hugs and kisses by the children and was escorted over to the nicely set dining room table for dinner. Throughout the filming of this first episode of the new family drama, there was much laughter, smiles, and comments from the mother like "How nice," "That was so sweet," and so forth.

Needless to say, this family session proved to be highly successful at disrupting the long-standing blame–counterblame pattern in the family and altering outmoded family beliefs about Pedro. I ended up seeing the family four more times and collaborated closely with concerned school personnel. Besides consolidating gains and amplifying changes, we implemented many of the creative ideas for improving family communications that Pedro had come up with while directing and producing the new family drama.

The Child as Mentor for His or Her Parent

In situations where one or both parents appear to be emotionally or physically disconnected from the child client and he or she has voiced a strong desire to get closer or spend more time with the most disengaged parent, I introduce the *child as mentor for his or her parent* experiment (Selekman, 2006, 2009). Most importantly, we have to first secure the disengaged parent's commitment to spending the time doing this meaningful and fun family connection-building activity. Next, the child needs to identify some specific skill he or she possesses that he or she will attempt to teach the disengaged parent in 1 week's time. Many children are quite savvy with computers and other technology, are skilled artists, good at building and fixing things, and may be good athletes. For 1 week's time, I have the parent and child come up with a daily schedule of minimally one half-hour of protected time a day where the child will teach his or her parent how to master his or her skill. No cell phone usage or other interruptions are allowed during the child's mentoring session times with his or her parent.

By the end of the week, not only does the disengaged parent make some important discoveries about how competent, patient, and skilled his or her son or daughter is, but also their relationship is strengthened and they grow closer together.

Diego, a 10-year-old Puerto Rican boy, was brought for therapy by his mother, Adela, because of his oppositional defiant behavior and fighting in school. According to Adela, Diego frequently challenged her household rules and authority. Diego's behavioral difficulties began after Adela had divorced his father, Alberto, when he was 8. Since the divorce, Diego had limited contact with his father, who now had a new girlfriend that he was spending most of his free time with. Prior to the divorce, Alberto used to spend lots of high-quality time with Diego.

After I made a strong connection with Diego and his mother in our first family session, Adela voiced a strong desire to have Alberto more present in her son's life. Diego had shared many times how much he missed not seeing his father more. Adela pointed out to me that she and Alberto used to argue a lot and had a stormy divorce, which might be contributing to his keeping his distance from them. However, the family thought it would be a great idea for me to try to engage Alberto to participate in Diego's family therapy.

I met with Alberto one time alone to balance out the amount of times I had seen all family members, to build an alliance with him, and to gain his commitment to participate in future family sessions with Diego. In the next family session, I met alone with Diego and Alberto. Diego did a courageous job of sharing with his father how much he missed not seeing him more often. Since Diego's passion and major skill was playing soccer, I introduced the child-mentoring-his-father experiment to them. When Alberto was in both junior and senior high school, he had played soccer competitively and still loved kicking the ball around with his adult friends and watching soccer on TV. One of Diego's soccer playing skills was ball movement and control. It turned out that this happened to be a weakness in Alberto's soccer playing abilities. For one week's time, we all mutually agreed that Diego would serve as Alberto's coach/mentor and teach him how to have better ball movement and control skills. Both Diego and Alberto were quite excited about wanting to try this experiment out and came up with a daily schedule to do it together.

In 1 week's time, Alberto began our family session by sharing what an "excellent coach" Diego was. Thanks to Diego, he had improved his ball movement and control skills. They also had a lot of fun doing this experiment, planned to kick the soccer ball around together on a more regular basis, and intended to see each other more often for other activities. The end result of this experiment was that it paved the way for Alberto to make a commitment to being more present in Diego's life.

Famous Guest Consultants' Family Experiment

In the preceding chapter, I discussed how a similar approach could be used by the therapist as a powerful idea-generating strategy when feeling stuck in the treatment process. When working with families that have difficulties with family communications and problem solving, the *famous guest consultants' family experiment* can in a playful way bring them together as a team to generate creative solutions for their presenting problems. In the session, each family member is to come up with the names of two or three famous people they admire and have been inspired by. The famous people can be historic figures, philosophers, artists, architects, scientists, musicians, rock stars, composers, authors, chefs, sports stars, movie and TV celebrities, or popular cartoon characters. After family members come up with their chosen sources of inspiration, they are told to put themselves into the heads of these famous people—that is, to try to think like them, what they are famous for, and the types of steps they would take to resolve the family's difficulties—and then write down on paper the ideas they come up with. Next, the family as a whole decides which ideas to experiment with for 1 week. Often family members laugh together at the options suggested and find this in-session exercise a fun diversion that also yields insights.

Cortez, a 10-year-old Puerto Rican boy, and his parents were referred to me by their pediatrician because of his oppositional defiant behavior, family conflicts and arguing, and poor parental management skills. The mother, Fernanda, and the father, Rubin, were hard-working parents who put in long hours at their jobs, Fernanda working in a plant and

Rubin as an auto mechanic for a foreign car dealership. Fernanda's sister, Rosalita, watched Cortez after school and into the early evening until the parents got home. In our first family meeting, all family members were in agreement that the "power struggles" and "arguing" had to stop. I could feel the tension in the room, and it was clear that the family had forgotten to try to make room for some fun family playtime together. Cortez even said that he missed not spending more time with his father throwing the baseball around and playing soccer together.

At this point in the session, I introduced the famous guest consultants' family experiment to the family. Fernanda's famous people were Secretary of State Hillary Clinton, actress Penelope Cruz, and Los Angeles Dodgers baseball player Manny Ramirez (formerly with the Boston Red Sox). Rubin's famous people were New York Yankees baseball star Alex Rodriguez, Spanish film director Pedro Almodóvar, and former Real Madrid soccer star Carlos Alonso González (aka "Santillana"); he is reputed to be Spain's all-time best player. Cortez's famous people were Philadelphia Phillies homerun hitter Ryan Howard, the Cavaliers basketball star LeBron James, and rapper Jay-Z. Next, I had family members pretend to put themselves in the minds of these famous people.

Fernanda wrote down that she admired Hillary Clinton for being a strong woman with good values who believed in "diplomacy and negotiating, not the use of aggression to resolve conflicts in the world." With Penelope Cruz, she admired both her "beauty and dynamic acting abilities," particularly "her range and versatility in movies." Since the family used to live in Boston and go to a lot of Red Sox games, Fernanda's favorite player was Manny Ramirez. She loved the fact that he was such a "clutch hitter" and would get the big home run when his team really needed it. After sharing why she chose her famous people, Fernanda went back and shared with us what ideas were sparked from the experiment. First, as a family they should "stop arguing so much" and instead "try to listen to one another, using negotiation and compromise to reduce the conflicts and clashes." Second, and closely related to her first idea, she felt they all needed to be "more flexible and patient with one another" and "improvise when necessary." Third, in the spirit of Manny Ramirez, "concentrate and get yourself fired up to provide what your team needs in the moment."

Rubin wrote down that, like Manny Ramirez, Alex Rodriguez was good at delivering under pressure for his team. Rubin loved going to and renting Almodóvar movies because they were so entertaining and humorous, and Almodóvar explored the depths of the relationships of the leading characters in the movie. Having been a soccer star himself in high school, he closely followed the soccer teams in Spain. His all-time favorite player was the Real Madrid striker and master header Santillana. Apparently, when Real Madrid had their best seasons in the past it was often due to Santillana's great teamwork and goal scoring. In reflecting on the ideas that were sparked by his famous people, he felt that everyone needs to be flexible and sensitive to "the stress they are under with work" and give each other some "chilling-out time." Rubin felt that they needed to create together a new atmosphere at home where it is "more playful and fun" and "eliminate the fighting." One quality that he highly respected about Santillana was his strong desire to be a team player. He felt that they all needed to "commit to being team players," which would help them have "more respect for" and "get along with" one another.

Cortez then shared why he selected his famous people and new ideas that were sparked for him. He not only admired Ryan Howard for his "homerun-hitting" abilities but his "strong desire to help the team win." Cortez pointed out that thanks to Howard, his team was now "one of the top National League teams." In common with Ryan Howard, he selected LeBron James because of his "great leadership" and athletic abilities. Cortez shared that he "really liked Jay-Z's music" and admired him for being such a "great rapper."

Next, the family put their heads together to determine which of their ideas they planned to experiment with over the coming week. Clearly, they all agreed that there needed to be more "teamwork," to be "more flexible and patient with one another," to "negotiate and compromise" with things that family members wanted from one another, and to build in "more family fun time." Cortez requested that his dad try to make more time "to play catch together." Rubin agreed to set aside some weekend time for that.

In our next session, the family reported considerable improvement in their communications, having had only one argument, and said they went on some fun family outings together. Rubin got some tickets through his car dealership to a Cubs game and took the whole family. Also, Rubin shared that "Cortez's throwing arm" was "getting much stronger" and he actually "stung" his "hand with one of his fastball pitches."

Stuffed Animal Team

With very young children, ages 3 to 5, I utilize their favorite stuffed animal friends as co-collaborators in the solution construction process. As part of the engagement process with children, I explore with them who their favorite book, TV, cartoon, and movie animal characters are. I then inquire whether the child has stuffed animal versions of these characters at home.

Finally, I share with children that Winnie the Pooh, Barney, Clifford, Curious George, and their other favorite stuffed animal friends can be a big help to us while we are working together by helping to make them "happier," "less mad," "not scared" anymore, and so forth. Because most children are at the peak of their imagination and pretending abilities during the toddler and preschool years, typically they are quite excited about the idea of having their stuffed animal friends participate with them in therapy sessions.

I generally pursue this therapeutic strategy midway into the session after I have a clear understanding of the presenting problem and what the parents' goals are. I meet alone with the child and have the child introduce me to each of the stuffed animals, telling me what he or she likes best about each one. In a highly concrete way, I talk about the presenting problem and then inquire with the child what each of the stuffed animals would do to try to resolve his or her problem. I ask the following kinds of questions:

- "If Winnie the Pooh were sad, what would he do to make himself happy?"
- "If Curious George were scared, who would he go to for a hug?"
- "What would Clifford the red doggy tell you to do to make you happier?"

To the best of my ability, I also represent the voices of the celebrity stuffed animals and share with the child the various creative ideas and solutions each of the animals whispered in my ear. If the child wishes to be the voice of each of the stuffed animals, he or she can do that as well. Some children tend to have better imaginative abilities with this experiment than do others. Often, with the help of the stuffed animal team, the child can generate some creative problem-solving strategies and solutions. Before ending the family session, I have the child bring the stuffed animal team in to meet the parents and have him or her share with the family what creative problem-solving strategies and potential solutions the stuffed animal team came up with.

Rodney, a bright Caucasian 4-year-old, was brought in for therapy by his parents for "trying to hurt" his baby sister, Lisa (9 months old), on several occasions. Ever since Lisa arrived in the family, Rodney had "mishandled" her in a "rough" way, "thrown things at her," and engaged in "attention-seeking" behaviors with his parents. The parents had tried everything from "timeouts" to "modeling" to teach Rodney how to handle Lisa in a "caring and gentle" manner, but he continued to "misbehave." The parents were feeling totally stuck and "frustrated." They could no longer leave Rodney alone with Lisa.

Throughout the first session, the parents were highly pessimistic. I normalized for the parents some of Rodney's attention-seeking behaviors as being a typical response to having to "share center stage with a new sibling." I further pointed out how the firstborn child often feels "dethroned" by the baby. The parents agreed and disclosed that they might have "spoiled Rodney," which did not help either.

Rodney was fairly quiet throughout the bulk of our first family session. Earlier in the session, I found out what Rodney's favorite toys were. Besides his Tonka trucks, his two most favorite stuffed animals were the Cat in the Hat and Tigger of Winnie the Pooh story fame. I suggested that Rodney bring the Cat in the Hat and Tigger into our second session to see whether they could help us out with the Lisa situation. In the second session, when meeting alone with Rodney, we discussed the problem and I asked him to talk to both the Cat in the Hat and Tigger to see what they would suggest to help him not hurt his sister. Rodney decided to pretend to talk for each one of them. When pretending to be Tigger, he hopped around the room and said, "Be funny for Lisa." I asked Rodney if Tigger thought he should "be a clown for Lisa to make her smile." Rodney thought it would be nice to be a clown for Lisa. As the voice for the Cat in the Hat, Rodney could also be a clown and sing songs for her. Rodney's favorite song was the "The Hokey Pokey." With the help of the stuffed animal team, Rodney was able to generate two useful solutions that helped him get along better with his baby sister. The parents were very supportive of the ideas that Rodney and the stuffed animal team came up with.

I ended up seeing Rodney and his parents three times. Rodney greatly enjoyed being a clown and singer for Lisa, especially when she would smile and giggle. He also enjoyed all the positive attention he was getting from the parents by changing his behavior. His parents reported no further aggressive behavior toward Lisa.

Externalizing Family Play and Art Therapy Strategies

In this section, I present three family play and art therapy experiments to use with children and families when it makes sense therapeutically to externalize their presenting problems (Freeman et al., 1997; Freeman & Lobovits, 1993; White, 1995; White & Epston, 1990). In challenging child cases in which the client is young or not very verbal, integrating art and play therapy methods with the narrative therapy approach (White, 2007; Freeman et al., 1997; White & Epston, 1990) can empower these children and their families to conquer their oppressive and chronic presenting problems in a fun way. Externalizing the presenting problem through drawings on paper summons up both the child's sense of courage and spirit of playfulness, which helps lead his or her family in the direction of change.

The Family Mural

Historically, art therapists have used the family mural art task as a diagnostic tool to assess such family dynamics as communication problems, coalitions, and parent–child conflicts (Malchiodi, 2003; Oster & Gould, 1987; Riley & Malchiodi, 1994; Sobol, 1982). Typically, the family is invited together to draw or paint a picture of themselves on a large sheet of paper. Sometimes the family is asked to illustrate themselves involved in an activity together (Kwiatkowska, 1978; Sobol, 1982). Although these two uses of the family mural can offer valuable insights about family roles, relationships, and perceptions of one another, outmoded family beliefs and entrenched patterns of interaction may remain intact. Therefore, I have found it to be more effective to use the family mural art experiment as a visual therapeutic tool when engaging families in externalizing conversations. Through the use of externalizing questions (White, 1995, 2007; Epston, 1998; White & Epston, 1990), I first have the family co-construct the presenting problem into some objectified beast or archenemy, describing it in graphic detail (shape, color, demeanor, facial expression, etc.) and how it pushes all family members around. Sometimes the child and his or her family describe the problem in human form. Once there is some consensus about what the externalized problem looks like, I have the family draw a mural that depicts the various ways each family member interacts with the problem and how it gets the best of each of them. To help guide the family with the task, I might have them depict a recent scenario in which the problem was victorious over all of them. A second family mural can be drawn or painted that either depicts the various ways individual family members have achieved victories over the problem or illustrates in mural form their strategy for defeating the problem. What is most remarkable with this family art therapy experiment is the resultant rapid and dramatic shift from the family's viewing the identified client as the problem to the family groups rallying around the child to prevent him or her from being further oppressed or victimized by the problem. The following case example illustrates the effectiveness of the family mural experiment with a difficult case.

> Peter, a Caucasian 9-year-old, was brought for therapy by his mother, Marne, for chronic "stealing" and "lying." According to Marne, Peter had been "stealing money" from her since he was "5 years old." The lying behavior was a relatively "new problem." Peter had also stolen coins from his 10-year-old sister's piggy bank. Peter and his sister, Wendy, fought frequently, sometimes getting quite physical with each other, leading to one of the children getting hurt. Marne felt "totally frustrated" with Peter, for none of her "consequences" for Peter's acting-out behaviors worked. Prior to coming to see me, Marne had

taken Peter to "five other therapists," and nothing had changed with his behavior. Seeing me was a "last-ditch effort" before trying to get Peter "placed in a group home." Peter was also feeling frustrated by his stealing and lying habits.

I introduced the "habit" frame as part of the externalization process and as a new way for the family to view the stealing and lying problems. At a conference table, on which a large piece of poster board was lain, I had the family brainstorm together how they would envision the stealing and lying habits if they were to draw them with magic markers on the poster board. I also shared with the family that I wanted them to draw a recent scenario in which the stealing and lying habits were pushing all of them around. None of the family members could come up with an image for the lying habit. Both the mother and Peter came up with the idea of drawing a bandit-like man with a mask covering his nose and mouth sneaking into Marne's and Wendy's bedrooms and stealing money from them. Each family member had already drawn him- or herself, so the mother's drawing of the stealing habit was a separate picture from Peter's drawing of himself, which was already on the poster board. Wendy drew herself yelling at Peter. Marne drew herself standing next to her children with her hands on her head, which was to indicate her frustration with the situation. As we discussed the family mural, all family members could clearly see how the stealing habit had a life of its own and was making them all feel frustrated and mad, including Peter. Peter talked about how he felt like the stealing habit takes him over and brainwashes him to steal money from his mother and Wendy. By the end of our discussion about the family mural, both Wendy and Marne began to view the stealing habit as the real family villain. The family interactions changed as well. Family members stopped blaming Peter and offered their support instead. Wendy came up with the idea of hiding her piggy bank in a place where the "stealing habit will never find it." Marne thought this was a great idea for "tricking the stealing habit" and said that she would find a new hiding place for her money too.

I ended up seeing Peter and his family for four more sessions over a 6-month period. By our second family session, there had not been one stealing or lying incident or any fighting between Wendy and Peter. All family members talked about how they were not going to allow the stealing and lying habits to push them around anymore. The new family story that was evolving about Peter was that he was a "responsible young man." As the changes had occurred so rapidly with the family, I cautioned them to be on their toes because stealing and lying habits "do not die easily." The family saw this as a challenge to unite as a group and take measures to prevent themselves from becoming vulnerable prey to the habits. Wendy's idea about outsmarting the stealing habit by changing the location of her piggy bank proved successful. The mother also found this same solution useful in thwarting the stealing habit.

Drawing Your Problems on Paper

Another useful externalizing art therapy exercise is to have the child draw his or her problem on paper (Selekman, 2009). It is crucial with the mechanics of this art task to give the child plenty of time to create an image or symbol to represent the oppressive problem that is pushing him or her around. To help guide the child with the art experiment, I ask the following questions:

- "If you were to draw a picture of 'anger,' 'the attitude,' fears [or whatever], how would you make it look on paper?"
- "What colors would it be?"
- "Would it look mean, happy, sad, scary, or what?"

These questions can be particularly helpful if the child is having trouble coming up with an image or symbol to represent the problem. Once the child has drawn his or her problem on paper, the therapist can invite the child to come up with a combat plan for defeating the problem on either the same or another sheet of paper. Children often feel empowered by this art therapy exercise, in that their problem is no longer controlling them from within their minds and now they feel more in control of the problem after externalizing it on paper. I use this approach with a child who is not very verbal or who tends to shut down when the whole family is present. The parents can be called in to hear the child's story about his or her drawing and the child's strategy for taking back control of the problem. Typically, parents find it newsworthy to learn about how the child views the problem and its effects on him or her and the rest of the family. The parents can also be invited to help support the child's plan of attack and offer any additional ideas to help the child defeat the problem. The parents can draw their ideas on the child's paper or on a separate sheet of paper.

Raymond, a Caucasian 8-year-old, was brought for therapy by his parents for "bad nightmares." According to Meredith, the mother, the nightmares had been pushing Raymond around for the past year. Apparently, Raymond would "wake up screaming in the middle of the night and run into" his parents' bedroom crying and seeking their comfort. The parents were totally perplexed by the nightmare problem. They could not identify any family crisis or changes, or anything else, that could have caused the nightmare problem.

When meeting with the whole family group, Raymond hardly talked and appeared very shy. His two sisters, 9-year-old April and 12-year-old Melanie, talked up a storm about themselves. My use of the imaginary wand question and humor failed to engage Raymond.

I decided to meet alone with Raymond and attempt to have him draw his nightmares. Using crayons, Raymond drew two different pictures of the "monsters" that were in his dreams. The first monster looked like a "ghost with big sharp teeth." The second monster was "big and hairy" and looked like a wolf man. We discussed what each of these monsters would try to do to him when he was sleeping. The ghost monster would drape his sheetlike body over Raymond's head and try to "make it disappear." The other monster was more aggressive and would start "taking bites" out of him. I asked Raymond if he was getting scared talking about these monsters, and he confidently answered, "No." I shared with him that I was getting scared hearing about these awful monsters. Raymond responded, "Don't be scared—they are only in my house."

Toward the end of the session, I had the parents come in to see the monster pictures. The parents could now understand why Raymond was having the bad nightmares. Knowing that the mother had a talent for crafts, I suggested that she and Raymond make a "dreamcatcher" together to place over Raymond's bed to prevent the evil monsters from pushing him around during the nighttime. I drew a picture on paper of what dreamcatchers look like and shared with the family how Native American parents made dreamcatchers to trap evil spirits that were trying to scare their children at night. By the end of our discussion, Raymond was much more animated and looking forward to making the dreamcatcher with his mother.

I ended up seeing Raymond and his family three more times over a 4-month period. In our second session, Raymond was eager to show me the beautiful dreamcatcher he and his mother had made together. Raymond also reported that he had not had even one nightmare over the 2-week period. After consolidating and amplifying the family changes, I predicted that the monsters might try to stage a surprise attack over the next-session interval. To help safeguard against the potential sneak attack, I recommended that every morning Raymond and his mother carry the dreamcatcher outside to let it air out after doing battle with the monsters the night before. I pointed out that monsters cannot survive outside the house and the smell of fresh air and the sunlight on the dreamcatcher is lethal to these monsters. I further added that often the monsters disappear for good after performing this ritual even just once.

The Habit Control Ritual

Once the child's presenting problem has been externalized, the habit control ritual (Selekman, 2005; Durrant & Coles, 1991) can be used to empower family members to liberate themselves from the problem's reign over them. After externalizing the problem, I have the family members keep track on a daily basis of the various things each one does to achieve victories or to stand up to the problem and not allow it to push him or her around. At the same time, I want family members to keep track of the various ways they accept invitations from the problem to be pushed around by it or to lock horns with one another. I recommend to families that they keep a daily record of both their victories and the problems on a large piece of poster board. Additionally, I encourage family members to work out together, to interact more and be better fit to defeat the problem.

In the session, I encourage the parents to serve as supportive coaches to the child when they see him or her accepting invitations from the problem to get into trouble. For example, a parent could say to her son, "It looks like the Temper is trying to make you not do your homework ... Are we going to let it take away your TV time tonight, or are we going to get the homework done?" I have the parents be their own coach for their relationship as well, particularly when the problem is trying to make them argue with each other about how to manage the child's behavior. A father might say to his wife, "Why are we allowing the Temper to divide us again?" I also encourage family members to meet as a group after dinner to evaluate how well they are doing at achieving victories over the problem and where they need to tighten up their defenses to be less vulnerable to the problem.

> Sidney, a Caucasian 7-year-old, was brought for therapy by his parents for "severe temper tantrums," fighting with peers, and "attention-deficit/hyperactivity disorder" (ADHD). Sidney was adopted at the age of 1 by the Petersons, who had no other children. Ever since he was adopted, the parents had described him as being "difficult" and a "behavior problem." The mother described him as being like the Looney Tunes cartoon character, the Tasmanian Devil, in that when Sidney had temper tantrums, he would "leave a pathway of destruction from room to room." "Plates, pencils, books," and other projectiles would typically end up being "thrown into walls" and sometimes at the parents when Sidney had "bad temper tantrums." The parents had "tried everything under the sun" in the way of consequences, but nothing had worked. The pediatrician had placed Sidney on Ritalin, which did seem to help him perform and behave better at school.
>
> I decided to externalize the temper tantrum problem into "the Temper." After mapping the influence the problem had over Sidney, his

parents, and the day-care instructor, it was clear that they all had been victimized by the Temper. Sidney did "not like the battles" with his parents, and he wanted his family to be "happy." The parents disclosed that they had been "arguing a lot more lately" with each other. When I asked unique account questions (White, 1995), not one family member could identify anything he or she was doing that helped achieve victories over the Temper. In fact, the parents reported that more than half the time the Temper was victorious over them. I gave the family the habit control task as a way to help them become more aware of what they were doing daily not to allow the Temper to push them around as well as to keep track of how the Temper got the best of them. We discussed the importance of physical training as a family and the parents' supportive coaching of Sidney to avoid accepting invitations from the Temper; I suggested they work together as a team to achieve victories over the Temper. Like a football coach before the big game, I got the family fired up to do team battle with the Temper.

Three weeks later, the family returned and reported a variety of changes: about 70% of the time they were victorious over the Temper, Sidney's behavior greatly improved at home and at the day-care center after school, and the parents were "arguing less." Sidney found that "forgetting" about the Temper worked for him at home and at the day-care center. However, a new Temper had invaded this family: the "Homework Temper" was now pushing them around.

The Homework Temper was not only sabotaging Sidney when he started to do his homework, but it was making Sidney and his mother lock horns. We brainstormed possible strategies that could help us defeat the Homework Temper. The parents decided that the father would monitor the homework situation and the mother would "back off." Also, Sidney decided to experiment with the "forgetting about the Temper" strategy that had worked so well for him.

At the end of the session, I had family members clasp hands in a team circle to get them fired up to defeat the Homework Temper. Five weeks later, the family came back reporting that "88% of the time the Temper was out of here!" Sidney was "doing his homework without any battles" and reported improvement in all areas of his life. Sidney and his father were also spending more quality time together. Mutually we decided to stop therapy because of the numerous changes that had occurred and the family's expressed desire to "test the waters" on their own.

What was most remarkable about Sidney and his family was the way they worked so well as a team to quickly defeat both the Temper and the Homework Temper. Based on the family members' descriptions of the temper tantrums and their effects on them individually and collectively, the family seemed ripe for externalizing the problem (White & Epston, 1990). I had begun therapy by using a fairly pure solution-focused approach; however, the exceptions elicited by the miracle and coping questions (de Shazer, 1988; Berg & Gallagher, 1991) were not newsworthy to the parents because they did not fit with the dominant story that Sidney was the problem. Once the temper tantrums were externalized, the new construction or frame for viewing the problem proved to be congruent with the family's beliefs about it. Sidney was also tired of being pushed around by the Tempers and the resulting "battles" that followed with his parents. Sidney was most impressive in spearheading the family's counteroffensive and subsequent victories over the oppressive Tempers. He thereby successfully helped his family embark on a "happier" lifestyle.

Creative Visualization

During creative visualization, individuals use imagination to create what they want in their life. According to Parnes (1992), the "Visionizer," when pursuing his or her dream, "proceeds from examining 'what is' to exploring 'what *might* be,' to judging 'what *ought to* be,' to assessing 'what *can presently* be,' to deciding 'what I *will commit to do now*,' to action that becomes a new 'what *is*'" (p. 3). Visualization pioneer Wenger (1985) and Wenger and Poe (1996) stress the importance of describing "the dickens out of" the images when visualizing. Buzan (1989) has found in his research that people are more likely to attend to and remember something if it moves, is colorful, imaginative, exaggerated, and absurd. Bonny and Savary (1973) and Gordon and Poze (1981) have provided empirical support for the importance of describing images in comprehensive detail in their imagery research. This mental process combines the analytical powers of the left brain with the imaginative powers of the right brain (Parnes, 1992). Ostrander et al. (1994) contend that if individuals imagine something vividly enough and determinedly bring their senses and emotions into play, their deep mind stops calibrating the differences between the imagined event and an actual one. The more of themselves they engage in the imagining process, the stronger the desired effect will be.

Two studies with children who experience learning difficulties have empirically demonstrated the efficacy of visualization techniques in improving their academic performance. In the first study, Dr. Robert Hartley of the University of London took a group of children growing up in poverty who did poorly academically and gave them the following directive: "Think of someone you know who is very clever. Now, be an actor. Close your eyes and imagine you are that very clever person, and do the picture-making test the way he or she would." The children were successfully able to imagine they were clever and became clever. Their test scores rose considerably. Imagining they were someone else—in this case, someone bright and clever—became a shortcut to expertise for them (in Ostrander et al., 1994, pp. 149–150).

Rosella Wallace, an educational psychologist, used the "head of the careful observer" technique with children to help improve their sense of self-awareness, articulation, and writing (in Ostrander et al., 1994). Wallace had the children in her study imagine fitting a head of a careful observer over their own heads. She asked them questions to get them to describe aloud, with their eyes closed, this special observer:

- "How does he act?"
- "How does he approach objects, people, and events?"
- "Make him part of your imaginary world."

The children in her study found that they became superversions of themselves, using the observer's eyes, senses, and mind to perceive scenes as richly and vividly as the careful observer does. Wallace put it best: "It's virtual reality without the equipment" (in Ostrander et al., 1994, p. 155).

Some of the most famous people in history were great visualizers. Einstein once said, "Imagination is more important than knowledge." He attributed his scientific acumen and genius to what he called "vague play" with signs, images, and other elements, both visual and physical (in Wenger & Poe, 1996). This "combinatory play," he wrote, "seems to be the essential feature in productive thought" (in Dilts, 1994, p. 48). One day Einstein visualized what would later become his famous theory of relativity simply by wondering what it would be like to run alongside a light beam at the speed of light (Dilts, 1994; Wenger & Poe, 1996).

Other noteworthy visualizers include Michelangelo and World War II hero General George Patton. Michelangelo imagined his sculptures as living beings, patiently awaiting his hammer and chisel to free them from material confinement. He also derived ideas for new artworks by studying the shapes of cracks in building walls. General Patton imagined that he was the reincarnation of celebrated military leaders from the past, seeking to apply many of their time-tested warfare strategies and tactics to modern-day combat (Ostrander et al., 1994; Wenger & Poe, 1996).

Children make excellent visualizers for a number of reasons. Young children in particular like to pretend, have a keener sense for wonder, and are highly open to suggestion. Children have very sensitive and thin-boundaried brains, which makes them unusually sensitive to people, forces, and external stimuli in their environments (Ostrander et al., 1994; Wenger & Poe, 1996). "Children's imaginations roam freely because they are not constrained by adult rules of thinking" (Wujec, 1995, p. 20). Their use of approximate thinking and undying curiosity provides them with a world of enchantment and possibilities.

In this section, I present three different ways I utilize creative visualization techniques with children. The case examples illustrate these techniques in action.

Imagine Yourself as . . .

For children who experience learning difficulties and behavioral problems, one highly effective visualization strategy to help empower them to resolve their difficulties is for them to imagine becoming someone they greatly admire (e.g., a famous person in history, a close friend they respect, a TV or movie star, music celebrity, or sports star) (Ostrander et al., 1994). Once the child has been able to access a crystal-clear image of the person he or she will become for a designated period of time, I have the child apply all his or her senses while visualizing. I ask the child to describe out loud, in the present tense, with his or her eyes closed, the following:

- "Where is the conversation taking place?"
- "How is he or she dressed?"
- "What is his or her facial expression?"
- "What do you see him or her doing?"
- "How does his or her voice sound?"
- "What is he or she telling you?"
- "What do his or her clothes feel like?"

The next step is to have the child access an image of him- or herself merging with the ideal other and becoming the other. Again, I have the child close his or her eyes and visualize him- or herself shaking hands with the admired ideal other and watching the latter disappear while the child becomes that person. Often, when the child becomes that admired ideal other in the session, the therapist can observe shifts in his or her voice, posture, and confidence level.

Before applying the *imagine yourself as . . .* visualization strategy to the child's presenting problem, I have the child practice becoming his or her selected ideal other a few times a day for a week, with the rationale that "the better you get at acting as if, the more easily you will become the person you want to be." After 1 week of solid practice, I have the child show me how quickly he or she can become the ideal other while visualizing. I then have the child see him- or herself, as the ideal other, taking constructive steps to resolve his or her presenting problem. For example, one child I worked with averaged C grades on quizzes and at times was disruptive in class. During our session he "became the smartest kid in his class." The next day he went to school and not only got A grades on two class quizzes but also behaved well for the whole day. His teacher called his mother to share her amazement at how well he had performed on the quizzes and gave the child great praise for his behavior.

The following case also demonstrates the imagine yourself as … visualization strategy.

LaTisha, a 10-year-old African American girl, was brought for therapy because of her "fears" of having to "talk or sing in front of others." According to the parents, LaTisha always got "panicky in class and at church" when she would have to give a talk or "perform with the children's chorus." Sometimes LaTisha would get so nervous that she would "start to cry or run off the stage" at church when performing. The parents were totally perplexed by LaTisha's fears, which began when she was 8 years old, for, to their knowledge, nothing had happened that could have caused this problem. LaTisha could not explain why she was having this problem either.

Out of respect for cultural differences, I explored with the family how they felt about working with a white therapist. The parents appreciated my asking them about this and acknowledged that they did not have a problem with it. I asked them if they had been praying hard for LaTisha to help her conquer the fear problem. Her mother in particular was praying daily for LaTisha. I got the parents' permission to meet alone with LaTisha to try the imagine yourself as … visualization strategy.

Because LaTisha loved the arts and was a very visual person in general, I was confident that this technique would work. LaTisha selected the pop music star Whitney Houston as her admired ideal other. LaTisha proved to be an excellent visualizer; she had no difficulty accessing a clear image of seeing herself become Whitney Houston. I had her practice becoming Whitney Houston daily for a week.

When the family returned for our second session, the parents reported that LaTisha seemed "more self-confident." LaTisha appeared more relaxed to me and happily reported that she found the visualization technique "helpful." However, the real challenge for LaTisha was 2 weeks away. She had to sing in a choral concert at another church in front of a large crowd. I had LaTisha continue to visualize herself daily performing as Whitney Houston, giving a great performance in the upcoming choral concert. As she had been to this church before and had a clear image of what it looked like, it was fairly easy for her to transport herself to that church and to see herself being a singing success.

Before I saw the family for our third session, I received a phone call from LaTisha's parents. According to the parents, LaTisha did an "outstanding job," and they were "so proud of her" performance in the choral chorus. Apparently she had "held her head up confidently," singing throughout the whole concert. I complimented LaTisha on the phone and told her I too was very proud of her. We mutually agreed to get together in 1 month, as there were no more signs of fears either at school or at church and things were going so well. The third session ended up being our last session.

Visualization as an Aid in Cognitive Management and in Disputation Skills Training

Visualization strategies can be quite effective in disrupting the unhelpful thought patterns that are driving the symptoms of depressed and anxious children. The visuals can take many forms, such as having children visualize the problem as an icicle in their hand, a giant hand karate chopping the "bad" thoughts, or a stoplight turning red. As part of the visualization process, I may access some of the children's other senses, such as seeing themselves listening to their favorite song being played at a high volume whenever they begin to think negatively or are overanxious.

When teaching children disputation skills, I like to use visualization as an aid in helping them grasp in their minds what these skills look like in practice. For example, when teaching children how to *search for evidence* supporting a particular way of perceiving a *negative* experience, I urge them to imagine themselves as detectives gazing through their magnifying glasses, looking for clues to support their views. When having them think about two to three *alternative explanations* why something upsetting happened to them, I have them think of their minds as being like kaleidoscopes. Children have acknowledged to me in our work together how these visual images helped them to master these two disputation skills. These visualization strategies are particularly useful when the parents have changed and are doing things differently around the child but the child is still symptomatic or plagued by intrusive negative thoughts.

Visualizing Movies of Success

Another way I use creative visualization with a child is to have him or her visually capture a past achievement or personal triumph when performing at school, in the arts, or in a sports event and use this internal movie as a road map for success in the presenting problem area. It is most important to have children close their eyes, picture in their minds a blank movie screen, and then engage all their senses in the visualization process and for them to describe to the therapist what they see, hear, feel, touch, and taste, including color and motion (Selekman, 2005, 2009). Children can practice accessing their visualized movies of success a few times each day. The following case example illustrates the efficacy of the visualization of success strategy with a challenging case.

Levon, a 10-year-old African American boy, was brought for therapy by his mother, Ayeisha, due to "acting out in school," "problems with authority," an "attitude problem," and "not following" Ayeisha's "rules." Ayeisha was a single parent; Levon's biological father had "walked out" on her. She had two other children, LaTonya and Heather, who were at home being watched by Ayeisha's adult sister. Levon had not seen his father since he was 2 years old. Although Ayeisha described Levon as being a "talented athlete," she was quite upset with his "poor performance in school" and "lack of respect" for her and her rules.

Early in the session, I checked out with Ayeisha and Levon how they felt working with a white therapist. Neither Ayeisha nor Levon reported any concerns about our racial differences. I divided the session up and spent some individual session time with both Ayeisha and Levon. Ayeisha was very pessimistic about the likelihood of Levon's ever changing. We agreed to work on some new parenting strategies together, and I gave her an observation task as an experiment. I had her keep track of anything she was doing daily to keep the situation with Levon from getting worse, even if it helped only a little bit. Levon was a little more challenging to engage than his mother. He was somewhat guarded with me in the early part of the session. I joined best with Levon when I had him talk about how he became the most valuable player for his football team 2 years in a row.

Levon had been playing on his public football league team for the past 3 years. He had led the league 2 years in a row in scoring the most touchdowns. He proudly shared with me that he had "scored 20 touchdowns" to cap off his most successful year as a running back. I asked him what his formula for success was, and he replied: "Stay low … keep your legs moving … spin when you get hit." I shared with him that "I thought I was listening to Walter Payton," the former Chicago Bears star running back. Levon laughed and shared with me that he liked "Walter Payton a lot!"

At this point, I decided to have Levon close his eyes and take me on a visual journey back in time to his best football game ever. He described for me a fairly recent game in which he had scored "three touchdowns" and had "gained 150 yards" on the ground. His graphic detail of this game literally put me right on the sidelines, watching him perform with excellence. Levon was animated, he could taste the sweat coming down his face, he could hear the crowd, and he saw clearly the corner of the end zone toward which he was running to score a touchdown. While heading for his third touchdown, he broke three tackles. It was quite clear that Levon greatly enjoyed this visual trip back in time.

Using football metaphors, we talked about various ways he could "score touchdowns" both in school and at home with his mother. Levon admitted that he was tired of "fumbling" in school (getting poor grades) and that he needed to "stay low" and focus on his reading more. On the home front, I suggested that he work on "spinning off" of his mother's "nagging" him and keeping his "legs and feet moving" toward getting his chores done. Finally, I prescribed for him to practice his visualization of his best game on a daily basis. I also asked him to notice how his teacher and mother respond differently to him when he is breaking tackles and scoring touchdowns with them.

By our next session, Levon had made considerable progress. Levon found that the visualization of his best game greatly helped him perform and behave better at home and at school. Ayeisha was very pleased with Levon's progress as well. The observation task helped her discover that not nagging or yelling at Levon seemed to help them get along better. We had two follow-up sessions to further consolidate gains, and treatment was completed.

The Mind as a *Guest House:*
The Use of Mindfulness Meditation and Related Practices

Another powerful and effective set of coping tools and strategies we can teach children as young as 6 years old is mindfulness meditation and related practices (Selekman, 2005, 2009; Lantieri & Goleman, 2008; Hanh, 2003, 2007). By helping children learn how to embrace and tolerate everything that happens in "the miraculous moment," they will be less reactive to emotional distress, oppressive negative thoughts, and frustrating life events. When teaching children about mindfulness, I like them to capture in their minds the image of having close friends and guests over to their house for a visit. I ask children the following questions:

- "Do you usually tell them as soon as they walk through the front door that they can only stay for a certain amount of time, or are they free to stay as long as they wish?"
- "Are you usually a gracious, warm, and friendly host toward them, or do you treat them in a rude way?"
- "Do you experience happiness and joy inside, or do you feel sad and can't wait for your friends to leave?"

Children are readily able to imagine having friends over to their home, urging them to stay for long periods of time, making them feel warmly welcomed, and feeling inside a strong sense of happiness and joy in being strongly connected to their friends. Next, I share with them the importance of learning how to embrace *their own thoughts and feelings* as if they were invited friends and new guests visiting their homes. For older children and adolescents, I like to read to them the Persian poet Rumi's notable poem *The Guest House*, which serves as a nice introduction to mindfulness and embracing one's thoughts and feelings, treating them as if they were guests in your home.

> This being human is a guest house.
> Every morning a new arrival.
>
> A joy, a depression, a meanness,
> some momentary awareness
> comes as an unexpected visitor.
>
> Welcome and entertain them all!
> Even if they are a crowd of
> sorrows, who violently sweep
> your house empty of its furniture,
> still, treat each guest honorably.
> He may be clearing you out for
> some new delight.
>
> The dark thought, the shame, the
> malice, meet them at the door
> laughing, and invite them in.
>
> Be grateful for whoever comes,
> because each has been sent as a
> guide from beyond. (Barks, 2004, p. 109)

Most children and adolescents to whom I read this wonderful poem not only enjoy it but more easily begin to grasp the idea of being compassionate with one's negative thoughts and feelings and treating them like friends rather than trying to escape from or fight them as though they are enemies. They also embrace the idea that if you view your negative thoughts and feelings as friends it is hard to be afraid of or be pushed around by them. For children and adolescents that do not understand the meanings of some of the words in the poem, I further clarify for them what Rumi was trying to say.

Three simple mindfulness meditations that can be taught to children as young as 6 years old are *watching your breath, the sound meditation,* and *taking a trip to popcorn land.* Prior to teaching the meditations and related practices, have the child get as comfortable as possible in a chair or lie down on your office floor. Each step of the meditation is to be presented concretely and performed slowly by the child. The meditation should be practiced once or twice in the office before having the child perform it daily in a quiet place in his or her home. Ideally, if the children are able to practice daily for a minimum of 10–12 minutes in a quiet room in their homes for a few weeks, over time they will become proficient at using this coping strategy to help center themselves and soothe themselves when they need it. To cover possible contingencies, I tell children that sometimes while meditating we are visited by rowdy new guests who may try to upset us or push our buttons in the form of worrying thoughts or down moods; rather than letting them ruffle our feelings or push our buttons, I advise the children to just simply label or acknowledge their presence and treat them with loving kindness and compassion—and then refocus on meditation.

In order for children to become really skilled at meditating, we have to secure the parents' support for ensuring that they are given daily quiet time to engage in this healthy activity. I like to educate parents about all of the physical and psychological health benefits of having their children meditate daily. Once parents are on board with their children having meditation practices, they will monitor it as a daily routine. In some cases, parents will ask to be taught these meditations as well and may at times meditate with their children.

Finally, I present two additional mindfulness exercises that also are easy for children to grasp and fun to do, namely, *cloud watching* and *wave watching*.

Watching Your Breath

Once the child is in a comfortable seated or prone position, he or she is instructed to carefully observe his or her chest expand while inhaling and contract while exhaling. When the exercise is done slowly and focused on the breathing process, children often report feeling very relaxed after trying this mindfulness meditation. The child should practice doing this meditation for 10–12 minutes daily.

The Sound Meditation

After getting comfortable, the child closes his or her eyes and carefully tunes in to the various sounds in the ambient environment. The child is told not to try to figure out the source or dwell too long on a particular sound he or she hears but to simply label the different sounds mentally. Many children and adolescents whom I have try this meditation often fall asleep while doing it. The child should practice doing this meditation for 10–12 minutes daily (Selekman, 2005, 2006, 2009).

Taking a Trip to Popcorn Land

Most children like popcorn, and hence, enjoy doing this simple food meditation. After getting the child into a comfortable and relaxed position, the therapist places a piece of popcorn in the child's left palm. The child is told to carefully study the popcorn's coloring, shape, and inner contours and shadowing for 2–3 minutes. Then the child is asked to shift the piece of popcorn to his or her right hand and carefully roll it around, allowing it to touch all of his or her fingers and to close his or her eyes while doing this. Next, the child is to place the piece of popcorn in his or her mouth, rolling it around with the tongue, and be careful not to bite down on it yet. After doing this for a few minutes, the child is to slowly and finely chew the piece of popcorn without swallowing it. The final step is for the child to swallow the ground-up piece of popcorn and describe silently to him- or herself any sensations he or she experiences as it slides down the throat into the stomach. For 12 minutes, the child has been in popcorn land! Many of the children I have worked with enjoy doing this popcorn meditation more than any other one. Our jobs as therapists are made easier when children enjoy doing meditation and are able to practice it daily at home (Selekman, 2005, 2006, 2009).

Cloud Watching

Cloud watching is a fun mindfulness experiment that children can use as a coping strategy when being pushed around by powerful negative thoughts and feelings (Selekman, 2009). Children are instructed to get out of their heads, go outside, and look up at the sky and try to identify as many cloud shapes that resemble animals, human heads or faces, and other familiar object shapes as possible. After they have finished studying the clouds and feel more centered and less stressed out by their negative thoughts and feelings, I have them write down what animal, human head, or familiar object cloud shapes they discovered. In our next sessions, I have them bring in their lists of all of the different cloud shapes they discovered to talk about. This mindfulness experiment becomes like a fun and relaxing game for children. They also become like explorers discovering new territory. Their parents can be encouraged to recommend this activity to their children as one possible strategy to help them cope with emotional distress or some recent stressful life event.

Wave Watching

Wave watching is another relaxing mindfulness experiment we can have children do to cope with emotional distress and stressful life events. Unlike cloud watching, where children can do this alone in their backyard or front yard, parents will need to accompany them while doing this exercise to either a beach, a river bank, or the waterfront of a lake. Children are instructed to carefully watch waves as they come ashore and return back to their source. I educate children about how problems and life challenges are like waves, in that they are not fixed but rather are in constant motion. Most older children can grasp this idea about the impermanent nature of problems and life challenges, which can then free them up from worrying or ruminating about their difficulties. To make this exercise into a multisensory experience for them, we can have children pay close attention to what they smell, feel on their skin, and hear while watching the waves. This heightened concentration helps them to better immerse themselves in the wave-watching experience while further relaxing them.

Interpretation: A Cautionary Note

When engaging in family art therapy activities, the therapist must be careful not to present his or her reflections about family members' artwork as authoritative pronouncements carved in stone. Gestalt art therapist Janie Rhyne cautions therapists to avoid "either/or dragon thinking" that leads to "putting clients into diagnostic boxes." As a corrective, she recommends that therapists who become stuck in this way of thinking consider the following: "The either/or dragon is a robot construction; he can be dismantled and reduced to powerlessness if we, person to person, can accept all of us as being in different places on the road of discovery and recognize that we can all learn some new directions from each other" (Rhyne, 1996, p. 29).

Tinnin (1990) suggests, when interpreting clients' artwork, that "the therapist must be careful when converting a message from pictures into words to avoid unintentional distortion by his or her own verbal censorship" (p. 9). Typically, I invite family members to reflect on their own art products first and offer my own interpretations or reflections after each member's "voice" has been heard. My reflections are usually presented as "crazy ideas that just popped into my head" or with qualifiers of uncertainty, such as "I wonder if … " or "Could it be … ?"

The therapeutic power in family art therapy experiments is that the art representations of the family or self within the family provide an opportunity for family members to look at their problem situation "once removed." The family art experiments offers families a new lens for observing their situation and themselves as if they were outside their family system. Processing their collective art products with other family members enables them to discover new themes and new histories, create an alternative view of their problem, and invent a new reality (Malchiodi, 2003; Riley & Malchiodi, 1994).

Conclusion

In this chapter, I presented several family play and art therapy experiments and creative visualization techniques that can be utilized with a variety of children's presenting problems. All these therapeutic experiments and techniques can be used at any stage of treatment. Most of these experiments or activities not only address the child's individual issues but produce changes throughout the family as well. Therapists will find in general that using the various therapeutic experiments and techniques discussed in this chapter livens up their therapy sessions and makes their clinical work with families more enjoyable.

6

Bringing Out the Best in Children
A Solution-Oriented Parenting Approach

We see the brightness of a new page where everything yet can happen.
—RAINER MARIA RILKE

What qualities and skills do children need nowadays to help them thrive and flourish throughout their lives? What tools and strategies do parents need to employ to help their children be more resilient, compassionate, creative, and good moral citizens? Along these same lines, some important questions to ask parents in critically reflecting on their parenting practices are: What kind of adult do I want my child to grow up to be? How do my current parenting methods contribute to or hinder my child from developing into this kind of adult? My guess is that a lot of the parents we work with in our clinical practices do not ask themselves these questions or critically evaluate their parenting styles and methods. Furthermore, many parents we work with tend to forget about their past successes at managing their children's challenging behaviors and, too, what they are doing presently that helps contain current difficulties or even helps alleviate them. One reason parents often lose sight of this critically important information is that current problems loom so large before their eyes that their children's positive nonproblematic behaviors go relatively unnoticed. Another reason for this selective amnesia is that parents often get stuck clinging to narrow ways of viewing their children's problematic behaviors and therefore begin anticipating trouble even before it happens. This perceptual problem can set in motion a negative self-fulfilling prophecy in their relationships with their children.

In this chapter, I reflect and further elaborate on why these future-focused questions are important, based on empirical research, what parenting experts think, my 28 years of professional experience working with parents, and my own personal experiences as a parent. Parents' formidable challenges are magnified by today's tough economic times, loss of savings (and in some cases employment) and having to raise children in a toxic, materialistic, and technologically driven world of extremes characterized by the proliferation of electronic screens that compete for children's attention at the possible expense of contact with family and friends. I address these wider societal and cultural issues and offer practical strategies of what parents can do to provide their children with the emotional insulation they need to cope with all of the stressors in their lives and not lose their core personal perspective amid all the material electronic trappings and potentially negative peer influences of modern society.

First, I present an overview of the *solution-oriented parenting approach,* which is a highly effective and practical method of parenting that taps both the child's and the parents' expertise to bring out the best in the children and to rapidly resolve any challenging behaviors that parents may encounter with them (Selekman, 2005, 2009). Next, I list and discuss 11 key qualities and skills that can help children become more resilient and flourish in all areas of their lives. Finally, I present specific parenting therapeutic experiments and strategies that are designed to foster cooperative relationships with children, accentuate both parents' and children's strengths and natural gifts, and rapidly resolve even the most challenging of children's behavioral difficulties.

Guiding Principles of Solution-Oriented Parenting

There have been many parenting self-help books written and parenting prevention-based models developed that are overly focused on parental skill deficits and children's problem behaviors—versus *what is right with both the parent and the child* and how to utilize their respective strengths, natural gifts, and resourcefulness to increase what is presently working or had worked in the past to construct *future* solutions to a wide range of children's problems. Solution-oriented parenting is not just a positive and resiliency-enhancing parenting method but also a philosophy about how to bring out the best in children.

There are essentially eight guiding principles of solution-oriented parenting. Let us discuss each in turn.

1. *There are always "spaces in between" the problem behaviors.* Solution-oriented parents believe change is happening all of the time and are skilled detectives at focusing their main attention with their imaginary magnifying glasses on the *spaces in between* or nonproblematic times

when their children are being cooperative, responsible, displaying caring and affectionate behavior toward them and others, exhibiting good self-discipline, and demonstrating positive problem-solving behaviors. Solution-oriented parents are aware of or strive to expand their awareness of what specifically they may be doing that is contributing to their children's positive behaviors, such as using humor, being flexible, being respectful with how they talk to and treat them, offering choices, being affectionate, and spending quality time with them.

2. *All children want to cooperate with their parents, and it is only a matter of* when. Solution-oriented parents speak the *language of change* with their children. This is not only conversing in their children's language, especially using their key words (the words they use a lot and are meaningful to them), their metaphors (from popular books they like to read, sports, dancing, music, and other hobbies they enjoy engaging in), and their beliefs, but it is also confidently conveying to their children that further changes *will* happen with them and it is only a matter of *when*. With older children, the use of an *illusion of alternatives* can be quite effective at gaining their cooperation, particularly with chore completion. A child can be asked, "Which do you prefer to do first—clean under your bed or the floor of your closet?" Another example of a parent's using the language of change with his or her child would be as follows: "When you empty the garbage, which would you prefer to play together—a board game or ping pong?" By speaking the language of change with their children, parents can rapidly foster cooperative relationships with them and not have to deal with power struggles.

3. *Solution-oriented parents are skilled detectives at catching their children at their best.* Not only do solution-oriented parents become quite skilled at catching their children at their best, but also they like to honor these sparkling moments with compliments, hugs, high-fives, engaging in a fun or meaningful activity with them, or even leaving nice notes in their bedrooms regarding their positive and responsible behaviors. They strive for the daily goal of three to four compliments per child per day and limit criticisms or "No's" to one a day. A great alternative option that solution-oriented parents make maximum use of is "*Yes, and ...* " instead of saying, "No!" The "Yes, and ... " approach nicely combines what the child and parent alike both want, both parties feel heard and validated, and they get their needs met. The parent is modeling for the child flexibility, good problem solving, and how to negotiate a win–win arrangement with a person who may have a different viewpoint or agenda.

4. *Solution-oriented parents are optimistic and view parental challenges as opportunities.* Despite their best efforts, at times all solution-oriented

parents run into a brick wall and lose their temper with their children. However, solution-oriented parents are persistent and resourceful and maintain their optimism even in the face of adversity and feeling stuck. Seizing the opportunity to model for their children how to make amends and resolve conflicts, solution-oriented parents are quick to apologize about yelling, swearing, or talking to them in a disrespectful way.

When stuck about how to best manage challenging behavior, solution-oriented parents first seek out past strategies they used to resolve the same child's or siblings' past problematic behaviors, to consider whether something similar might work with the current difficulties. They should also allow their imagination to run wild and consider how things will look differently when the problems no longer exist. While visualizing this future of a problem-free reality in their relationships with their children, they might in the process identify new steps to promote more positive behavior.

5. *Solution-oriented parents keep an open mind and believe there are many possible explanations for their children's most challenging behaviors.* When they find themselves adopting too restricted a way of viewing their children's problematic behaviors, solution-oriented parents actively summon up the curiosity to come up with three or more possible explanations for their children's behavior. One way is by positively reframing it in their minds. For example, a parent who formerly viewed his or her child's difficult behavior as "an attitude problem" might view it instead as being *dramatic*. Similarly, a "defiant" child might simply be an *assertive* one. Once solution-oriented parents make this shift in their minds, they begin responding more positively and constructively to their children's challenging behaviors. Kazdin (2008) has found in his research that when parents can see the *positive opposites* in their children's negative behaviors, they are then on the pathway to building new patterns of interaction. Solution-oriented parents are sensitive to the fact that they need to carefully match their responses to the unique temperament of each child. For example, with a highly sensitive child the parents should automatically modulate their tone of voice and scrupulously refrain from yelling in order to gain the child's cooperation (Taffel, 2009).

6. *Solution-oriented parents are flexible, and they improvise whenever necessary.* With behavioral difficulties that seem intractable, solution-oriented parents first consciously determine whether they are persistently stuck doing *more of the same*, which may not only be maintaining but further exacerbating the very behaviors they want eliminated. If so, they will actively experiment with novel ways of responding to their children until change occurs. Once they find strategies that seem to have a positive effect

on their child's negative behavior, they will continue to use them until this behavior is stabilized.

7. *Only a small change is necessary.* Solution-oriented parents set small and realistic goals for their children. They realize that goals are the start of something new, not the end of something. The parents also try to make the journey on the path to achieving their goals with their children an enjoyable and meaningful ride. Because they are practical thinkers and realists, solution-oriented parents prepare themselves and their children for the hard work and inevitable bumps in the road as they pursue their goals.

8. *Solution-oriented parents give priority to establishing and maintaining strong and meaningful relationships with their children.* Solution-oriented parents savor and protect their relationships with their children by setting aside daily uninterrupted quality time with them. They strive to keep the lines of communication open with them, engage them in meaningful growth-producing activities, take pride and joy in their accomplishments, validate and reassure their children when they experience setbacks or are upset, and honor their voices in decision making. They regularly solicit from their children feedback on the quality of their parenting relationship and are open to and willing to make needed changes to show that they care and are committed to improving their relationship with their children.

The Resilient Child: The Key Qualities and Skills Children Need to Flourish

In this section, I present 11 qualities and/or skills that need to be cultivated in children to help them to be resilient and to flourish throughout their lives. Solution-oriented parents strive to cultivate and accentuate these important qualities and skills in their children. After describing each one, I provide recommendations of what parents can do to help optimize it for learning and development. When modeling and teaching children specific skills and/or offering them tasks geared to develop or strengthen particular skills, parents need to be sensitive to their unique learning styles, temperaments, and what they are capable of grasping at their developmental stage. The 11 qualities and/or skills are:

- Emotional awareness and flexibility
- Empathy
- Self-esteem
- Curiosity
- Social intelligence

- Creativity
- Problem solving
- Self-discipline
- Optimism
- Moral intelligence
- Gratitude

Emotional Awareness and Flexibility

Parents can develop and strengthen their children's proclivities for emotional awareness and range by creating a home environment where they and other family members feel safe and free to express the full spectrum of their emotions. Parents need to be transparent in their actions, ever ready to explain their emotional reactions to their children in response to a wide variety of events or triggers. By doing so, they increase the child's awareness that we possess many emotions and there are certain environmental or life situations, or thoughts, that trigger them. This helps them to develop "mindsight"—that is, the capacity to genuinely and accurately experience others' thoughts and feelings (Siegel, 2007; Siegel & Hartzell, 2003). When children grow up in family environments where it is not safe to express one's feelings, where they are repressed or silenced, not only does one's capacity for mindsight fail to develop, but also one is at greater risk for developing psychosomatic, substance abuse, and self-harming difficulties.

Finally, parents need to model for their children how to constructively and positively manage their negative emotions. Parents can model this through appropriately verbalizing their upset feelings to their partners, meditating, jogging, going for a walk, or engaging in a meaningful hobby or activity. Through imitation, children will learn how to appropriately handle their negative emotions when they are triggered by stressful and frustrating family and social situations.

Empathy

A child develops empathy for others primarily through witnessing his or her parents being empathically attuned to their children and reassuring them constantly when they are experiencing emotional distress or life disappointments. When children can consistently count on their parents to soothe them when they need it, eventually they internalize these comforting experiences and not only develop a cohesive sense of self and the capacity to soothe themselves but also are able to provide empathy and support to others needing it (Siegel & Hartzell, 2003). Taffel (2009) observes that inculcating empathy in children summons up the best hidden parts of their selves, which all parents would like to see more of. The pioneering child psychiatrist D.W. Winnicott contended that the child's increased capacity for empathy, especially toward his or her parents, was an indicator of good mental health (Winnicott, 1971b, 1985).

A common way that parents can encourage their children's capacity for empathy is to purchase a pet for them. Parents can model for them how to love, be kind to, and care for the pet. Children also thereby learn how to be responsible for something dependent on them. When the experience is successful and they find this responsibility rewarding, their enhanced empathy can be further generalized to relationships with friends and peers.

Self-Esteem

Children develop genuine self-esteem by successfully mastering developmental and environmental tasks or challenges and through the parents taking pride and joy in their accomplishments. As children get older, they not only can take pride and joy in their own accomplishments but also can identify their strengths and weaknesses as well. The stronger their sense of self-worth is, the less likely they are to have a major emotional meltdown when they fail at something, are rejected, feel let down by their peers or parents, or experience other frustrating situations. Children with high self-esteem celebrate their successes and are able to identify without feelings of inadequacy skill areas in which they need further development. Parents, in addition to celebrating with them their children's successes, can support them in their quests to overcome weaknesses by providing them with tasks and opportunities to develop their skills in these areas. While trying to develop proficiency in these skill areas, parents can share their own personal stories as children and adolescents about how they struggled with learning and mastering similar skills. This sharing conveys that they understand what their children are going through and helps normalize the experience for them.

Curiosity

According to Sylvan Tomkins, a well-known social psychologist:

> The importance of *curiosity* to thinking and memory are so extensive that the absence would jeopardize intellectual development no less than the destruction of brain tissue. There is no human competence which can be achieved in the absence of a sustaining interest. I am, above all, what excites me. (in Kashdan, 2009, p. 6)

Tomkins's quote underscores the significant role curiosity plays in helping to make one's life more meaningful and fulfilling. Research indicates that children who are curious tend to have greater intelligence and stronger cognitive functioning abilities, do better on tests, and get higher grades in school (Kashdan, 2009).

Children by nature are inquisitive and enjoy exploring their environments and discovering the world. With younger children, the word "why" is often the lead word that they begin their questions with to their parents and their teachers. Parents should encourage their children to ask lots of questions and critically reflect on both their ideas and those of others. They can share examples of how, as children, they used their curiosity with their parents, such as the kinds of questions they asked them or the kinds of things they were interested in exploring and learning more about. To help further cultivate curiosity and thirst for knowledge, parents should provide in their home environments and outside their homes many rich learning opportunities for their children. This initiative can take the form of going to aquariums, planetariums, or art, historical, natural history, and science museums; taking trips to a wide variety of cultural and ethnic community events; nature walks; reading together science- or history-related children's books; playing board games that tap the child's curiosity and problem-solving abilities; or studying a drop of pond water under a microscope or looking at the stars with a telescope. While engaging in these activities with their children, parents can ask them questions about their opinions, reflections, what they are experiencing, and what they want to know more about. It is important that parents listen carefully and observe what *sparks* their children's interest the most—whether discovered on their own or through an activity together. This spark may have been ignited at school or by participating in a field trip with peers. Once parents discern an area of special interest to their child—whether art, dancing, theater, a specific hobby, or a social cause—they should investigate where their child can learn more about it and become more expert or adept. Besides contributing to a more balanced life, cultivating a key interest with a child gives him or her additional meaning and purpose in life as well as affording the child a positive outlet to counteract school and other life stresses.

Finally, another way parents can encourage curiosity in their children is to help them perceive the unusual in the usual, whether in doing chores, homework, or babysitting a younger sibling (Kashdan, 2009). Parents can make such mundane tasks into a game by having their children come up with three novel ways of accomplishing the tasks in fun, or at least more interesting, ways. Devising new ways of doing a chore or exploring offbeat aspects of a subject for a paper or book report both stimulates one's curiosity and widens the mind.

Social Intelligence

Many parenting experts and researchers regard one's ability to establish and maintain relationships as one of the most important life skills that children can acquire (Goleman, 2006; Kohn, 2005; Taffel, 2009; Kazdin, 2008; Peterson, 2006; Peterson & Seligman, 2004). Positive psychologists have found in their research that an individual's ability to make and sustain social connections is strongly associated with life satisfaction (Kashdan, 2009; Peterson, 2006; Peterson & Seligman, 2004).

Developing relationship skills begins at home with how well parents model expressing their thoughts, feelings, desires, and intentions as well as in being playful, genuinely listening to, and sharing their stories with each other. Children need to observe their parents displaying affection and respect toward each another and constructively resolving conflicts as they arise. These kinds of positive observations serve as a template or framework for how children should interact with their peers and with adults outside the home. Parents constantly need to encourage their children to maintain strong connections with extended family members and to nurture and protect their close relationships with their friends.

Once children start feeling more competent socially, they take more risks in establishing new relationships with peers and seeking out support from friends and even adults outside the home when they need help in coping with certain stressors. They also gradually develop the capacity to self-observe, that is, to step outside themselves and notice the effects of their behavior on others.

For older children who have difficulty with this skill, it may be helpful to have them practice role playing or pretend to put themselves in the place of a child whom they had mistreated in some way and try to experience what he or she was thinking and feeling when they behaved this way. The parent can pretend to be them in this role-play exercise. This skill-building exercise can help them to develop an *observing ego*. Kohn (2005) recommends that parents should also use role playing with their children to try to gain a better grasp of how the children are thinking or feeling about the way the parents interact with them. In the role play, the child can play the role of the parent whose behavior is most troublesome to him or her. Through creative role play, the parent has the invaluable opportunity to experience firsthand the thoughts and feelings of the child and how parental behavior is really perceived by him or her.

Creativity

Parents can develop and maximize their children's creative capacities by exposing them to a wide variety of activities that tap their imagination and powers of inventiveness—running the gamut from art, music, theater, dance, and literature to even cooking cuisine. Depending on what sparks an appreciative interest in the children, parents can build things with them, tour museums, or take in a Saturday movie or ballgame. Parents need to give their children ample opportunities to play and to constantly move in and out of their worlds of imagination (Taffel, 2009).

Unfortunately, many of the popular computer games and gadgets that children claim as "must-haves" (mostly out of envy that their friends possess them) rob children of their own creativity and inventiveness. This is why it is so important that parents enforce firm guidelines regarding their children's resort to mindless "high-tech." Technology is never an adequate replacement for direct one-to-one contact with family members and friends—nor should it be used as a babysitter.

In a study of talented high school students who had been consistently engaged for over 4 years in meaningful flow state activities associated with their creative capacities and key interests, Czikszentmihalyi, Rathunde, and Whalen (1993) found that these students reported less anxiety, better physical health, more life satisfaction, and greater achievement in the activities that tapped their creative talents than the control group of adolescents who discontinued their involvement in the key flow state activities. The more flow state activities that parents can encourage their children to get involved in, the more likely the children will enjoy meaningful outlets and protective offsets to their curricular disappointments. Thus, there are many long-term benefits of parents providing their children with as many activities both within and outside their homes that provide their children with the opportunity to expand their horizons in tapping their creativity, imagination, and inventiveness.

Problem Solving

Parents need to increase their children's awareness of their key strengths and talents and educate them about how specifically to tap their expertise to master or resolve challenging situations they are faced with. They can pose the following questions to their children:

- [a child with football skills] "What will you do today in class to *score a touchdown* with Mrs. Brown [the teacher]?"
- [a child who is a good gymnast] "If Mary starts to tease you again, how will you *keep your balance* and not allow her to upset you?"
- [a child who is talented in art] "How do you *picture* in your mind what your science project presentation poster will *look like*?"
- [a child who is a good dancer] "How will you *stay on your toes* and *move to the beat* if some of the questions on the science test today end up being harder than you thought they would be?"

By using the language and metaphors associated with the children's key talent areas, parents can help trigger positive emotions in them and raise their self-confidence levels. Once children discover the benefits of tapping their own expertise to be successful, they can continue to use this strategy when faced with future challenging situations.

In addition to providing children with ample opportunities to master tasks, recognize patterns, and solve puzzles, parents need to teach them that there are multiple ways to interpret and resolve difficulties they may encounter in family relationships, with peers, at school, or in the neighborhood. When it comes to interpersonal problem solving, it is important for parents to teach their children that conflict is inevitable and can be a great opportunity for change. In fact, recent research indicates that it is good for children occasionally to observe their parents disagree, as long as it is well-regulated and they model constructive resolution of their disagreements and conflicts (Cummings & Keller, 2007). Parents can in concrete ways try to help their children understand that change begins with them, in that we cannot always count on the other person or people they are having difficulties with to make the first move. This is why I believe it is important that parents teach their children the importance of adopting a mindset and stance of loving kindness and compassion for everyone, even those people they would consider mean, or their enemies. My strong belief is that if we taught more children loving kindness and compassion, not only would there be less bullying in our schools but also less violent crimes committed by youth in our society as well.

Parents need to model for their children constructive ways of managing stress and frustration, such as meditating, doing yoga, walking, jogging, bicycling, lifting weights, and the like. To add to the learning experience, they should ask their children to join them in these healthy activities. Children learn from their parents that there are many positive ways to cope with stress. They may also discover that, far from being just fun and pleasurable, these activities can become a daily ritual involving high-quality time spent together. Once children discover the psychological and physical benefits of engaging in regular daily exercise, they will come to regard it as an invaluable coping mechanism.

One useful problem-solving tool that parents can teach their older children is *incubating* (Hall, 1995). Such famous scientists as Albert Einstein, Thomas Edison, and Charles Darwin found it useful, when mentally "stuck" or blocked on finding the solution to a problem, to step back from the problem, deliberatively will in out of mind for a period of time, and then come back to it later with a fresh perspective. Learning a similar approach with their problems helps children keep an open mind and gain new perspectives, be less impulsive with their tentative solutions, stimulates curiosity, and affords them the opportunity to have initial ideas or possible solutions gradually evolve into higher-quality solutions.

Self-Discipline

From early childhood onward, parents have ample opportunities to teach their children how to be well disciplined and responsible. The typical regimen might include everything from establishing firm guidelines about putting toys and belongings away, keeping bedrooms clean and orderly (depending on age), doing their chores, and completing and turning in their homework. Parents need to help their children learn how to stay focused on a task, take the initiative to follow through with their intentions and commitments, think through the options and choices they face in the challenges they confront, and persist in their actions until the task is complete (Brooks & Goldstein, 2007).

Parents need to have clear expectations for their children's behavior and to provide consequences for noncompliance, viewing this as a loving act that provides internal self-control when their children are challenging their authority, have broken a rule, or have gotten into trouble. After children have paid the consequences, a great opportunity exists for parents to explore with them the wisdom gained from having had a behavioral setback or made a bad choice that they can put to use when faced with a similar situation in the future. Consistent parental limit setting, paired with sympathetic counsel in the wake of reasonable but tempered punitive consequences, helps children develop better impulse control and an internal wise voice of reason, which enables them to make better choices in the future as well.

Optimism

Optimism has been found to be one of the key traits of individuals who flourish and report satisfaction with their life (Peterson, 2006; Peterson & Seligman, 2004; Murray & Fortinberry, 2006). In their Penn Depression Prevention Project Seligman and his colleagues (1995) found that teaching children disputation skills to challenge their pessimistic thoughts immunized them from developing depression and anxiety difficulties. Learning how to adopt an optimistic mindset also enabled these children to perform better academically than students who were more pessimistic. Seligman and Dean (2003) has concluded that *disputation skills* are the most important life skill that therapists and parents can teach their children, including how to challenge their pessimistic and other self-defeating thoughts and how to avoid dwelling too long on disappointing outcomes. In our family sessions, we can teach parents disputation skills and have them practice using them, both at work and at home, in response to their children's challenging behaviors. Once they develop some proficiency in using these valuable tools, we can put the parents in charge of teaching their children how to use them in the context of our family sessions, encouraging them to work with their children at home to further hone these skills.

At home, parents can practice responding to their children in an optimistic manner. For example, when the child experiences a disappointment, such as getting a poor grade on a test, the parent can respond by saying:

- "I know this must be hard for you, but I am confident that you will be better prepared for the next math test."
- "What steps do you see yourself taking to be better prepared for the next test?"
- "Are there any problems that you remember from the test that you would like me to try to help you with?"

This kind of optimistic way of responding as a parent will lead to the child's being empowered to bounce back and take responsibility to do better on the next test.

Moral Intelligence

Moral intelligence includes not just a child's sense of right and wrong but also his or her values relating to family, cultural background, religion, ethics, and social justice. It encompasses having a strong sense of compassion and respect for others who are struggling or less fortunate than oneself. According to Weissbourd (2009), parents need to be *moral mentors,* adding, "The parent–child relationship is at the heart of moral development, including parents' modeling of honesty, kindness, loyalty, generosity, a commitment to justice, the capacity to think through moral dilemmas, and the ability to sacrifice for important principles" (p. 2).

One way parents can help their children commit to being moral people is to involve them in regular service work in the community that they can do together. The age of the child determines what specific work tasks they are capable of handling. My daughter Hanna and I made a commitment together to help prepare meals for homeless adults at a church-run community shelter once a month. As a result of this service work, she not only cares deeply about these homeless adults' well-being but also feels good about herself as a person for doing this work. Also, caring about the less fortunate has led her to involve herself in such other causes such as wildlife protection and environmental conservation.

Parents have an obligation with older children to raise their consciousness regarding such key social injustice issues as human rights and genocide. Again, depending on age and intellectual capacity, the parents can engage them in dialogue about social injustice in general or can expose them to specific issues by viewing television specials and documentaries together or even attending meetings and rallies on specific social injustice issues together. Parents, of course, need to use discretion in what they choose to expose their children to and be sensitive to their emotional maturity levels in terms of what they are capable of handling. They can also have their child sponsor and regularly write to a child his or her age from a developing country. These kinds of experiences can assist children in developing their moral intelligence and greatly contribute to their becoming caring, compassionate, and respectful citizens of the world.

Another helpful way parents can advance their children's moral development is to share stories about themselves as children and some of the moral dilemmas they faced, providing firsthand examples of moral development. Every child likes a good story, particularly their parents' own stories about how they made good choices when faced with challenging situations.

Children who are strong in moral intelligence will not be bystanders when a peer at school or in their neighborhood is being bullied. They will take a stand and try to defend the person being victimized or immediately seek out adult intervention. My own view is that, if parents and early educational programming focused more attention on moral development, children would learn to be compassionate advocates for their peers who are struggling to fit in, thereby helping to eliminate bullying problems in the schools.

Gratitude

A final personal quality that parents should try to inculcate in their children is *gratitude*. Positive psychology research has consistently found that gratitude is strongly correlated with life satisfaction. Regularly acknowledging and writing down all that we are grateful for, past or present, in our lives increases our optimism and happiness levels, decreases negative emotions while increasing positive ones, helps us be more empathetic and socially connected to others, can calm our nerves, and improves the quality of our sleep (Emmons, 2007; Peterson, 2006; Peterson & Seligman, 2004; Seligman, 2002).

Teaching gratitude to children begins with parents having their children invariably say "thank you" verbally or in written form to persons who help or support them, or give them love, wisdom, valuable life skills, or gifts on special occasions. Parents should urge them to savor what they possess or have experienced in their lives versus what they do not have—another reason that parents should avoid at all costs buying something whenever their child desires it (usually because their "friends have it"). As discussed earlier (in Chapter 4), having children keep a gratitude log or journal and daily write down what they are grateful for has many psychological benefits.

When their child is having a tough day or feeling down, parents can encourage him or her to look for extraspecial entries in the gratitude log to trigger positive emotions and lift sagging spirits.

As another helpful way to cultivate gratitude in their children, parents can regularly share with them significant people and experiences in their own lives that they are grateful for, and why. Children like to hear stories from their parents about positive things that their parents, siblings, close friends, extended family members, or adult inspirational others have said and done that made a difference in their lives.

Major Solution-Oriented Parenting Therapeutic Experiments and Strategies

In this section, I present 12 solution-oriented parenting therapeutic experiments or strategies (some of which are previously discussed therapeutic experiments) that can be used with a variety of challenging behavioral difficulties. Concrete steps on how to implement each strategy are provided.

Parental Presence and Mindfulness

When parents are truly engaged in *parental presence* with their children, they are consciously living in the present moment—not just aware of what they are thinking and feeling but also empathetically attuned to their children's inner thoughts. Siegel and Hartzell (2003) refer to this parental ability as *mindsight,* which allows parents to focus on the thoughts, feelings, perceptions, sensations, memories, beliefs, attitudes, and intentions of their children and others, as well as their own inner emotional and sensory experiences. In their interactions with their children they are transparent, that is, they make their intentions and the full spectrum of emotional reactions available to their children—for example, modeling sadness and crying in response to an important loss. When their child experiences sadness or frustration, mindful parents genuinely and deeply listen to him or her, use empathy and validation, and then soothe the child before offering any explanations or suggestions. Mindful parents model for their child the importance of showing others that are experiencing emotional distress *loving kindness* and *compassion* (Hanh, 1998). They also model for their children how important it is to use loving kindness and compassion with oneself by engaging in meaningful, healthy, and constructive activities for coping with stress and frustration—such as by meditating, doing yoga, jogging, lifting weights, playing an instrument, dancing, singing, or engaging in artwork. Observing the psychological and physical benefits of engaging in these activities may ultimately prompt the children to learn how to do some of these activities from their parents.

Increase Your Dance Steps That Work

Solution-oriented parents believe in *keeping things simple* as a starting point for resolving any difficulties their children may be experiencing. Once parents find something that works, they need to do more of it and keep using this particular solution-building strategy or other effective strategies until the difficulty is resolved. However, where some parents err is that, when a crisis occurs or there is a stressful family life cycle transitional change, they stop doing what was working and the child returns to former challenging behaviors or new ones. It is helpful in session when parents get temporarily derailed like this to explore with them what steps they need to take to get back on track with the methods that worked in the past. To further empower the parents, I bring out my imaginary crystal ball and have them gaze into it, seeing themselves back on track 1 week from the day of our session successfully managing their child's behavioral problem. I have them describe in detail the specific steps they are taking—the time of day and for how long—to remedy the situation.

The Compliment Box

In family situations where there appears to be a lot of blaming, negativity, and criticism, the *compliment box* (Selekman, 2006, 2009) is a useful tool. The parents get an old shoebox, cut a slit in the top, and on a daily basis write down compliments for each child. They compliment the children on what they like about them as people and things they have done that they really appreciated. Parents who regularly share with their children their appreciation of who they are as people and what they have done generally have one thing in common, namely, a strong family (Stinnett & O'Donnell, 1996). After dinner each night the box is passed around, and the children reach in and read their compliments out loud. With young children, the parents can read the compliments that they pull out for them. Once children come to appreciate the benefits of the compliment box and start warming up to their parents more rather than defying or stressing them out, they can be asked to join in on the compliment writing process and generate some compliments for their parents or siblings, as well. This therapeutic exercise models for children the importance of sharing one's gratitude or appreciation with others and can greatly improve family communications and the emotional climate at home.

Ignoring Skills

Some parents we work with become highly reactive emotionally to everything that their children do that does not conform with their multitude of unrealistic expectations and rules. When children constantly feel micromanaged and are being reprimanded all of the time, they become resentful or rebellious toward their parents, or—conversely—become overly compliant and devoid of self-confidence and the ability to self-regulate. The bottom line is that some battles are not worth fighting, and parents need to pick and choose when to stand their ground (Taffel, 2009; Kazdin, 2008; Kohn, 2005). Research indicates that, when dealing with strong-willed children or children with oppositional defiant disorder, *ignoring skills* can be quite effective. According to Forehand and Long (2002), parents should ignore the following behavior by their children:

- Demanding attention in an inappropriate manner
- Demanding that you immediately do something you do not wish to do
- Crying for attention
- Temper tantrums
- Whining
- Sulking
- Screaming
- Arguing
- Acting irritable

Why ignoring is so effective is that initially it may be a new behavior for the parent to engage in, which takes the child by surprise. Even afterward, though, the parents' refusal to be an audience for manipulative ploys or to serve as a sparring partner to the child has the effect of neutralizing, or deflating, the child's obstreperousness in a potential power struggle.

The Imaginary Time Machine: Bringing Back the Best from the Past

Throughout a child's development, certain periods of time will be especially difficult, when family stress seems to peak and parents find their roles totally unenviable. During such stressful times, parents might find themselves having shorter fuses, overcontrolling, and being more authoritarian, which can lead to more limit testing and even brazen power struggles. One effective tool I like to employ in such adverse conditions is the *imaginary time machine,* "to bring back the best from the past" (Selekman, 2009). The parents are told to pretend to hop into my imaginary time machine and take it back in time to when the child was younger and they were thoroughly enjoying his or her company and their own parenting roles. Using all of their senses, extending even to details of color and motion, they are to respond to the following questions:

- "How old is your child?"
- "Where are you?"
- "What are you doing together?"
- "How are you thinking and feeling?"
- "What are you enjoying the most about your child at this moment?"
- "How is his [or her] presence in your lives making your lives more meaningful and special?"
- "Now, if you were to bring back any aspects of this past experience with your child and implement them in your current relationship with him [or her], which aspects or parts would you choose, and how, by reinstating them, would they make a difference for you now in your relationship?"

Often, this time-traveling experience triggers positive memories and emotions for the parents and suggests some useful ideas that they can then put into practice immediately. They may come up with a former activity they used to enjoy with the child that he or she would really appreciate doing with them again. Most importantly, the parents' negative ways of viewing the child and interacting with him or her in the present are at least temporarily transformed.

Use of Positive Consequences and Service Work

A great alternative to the use of punishments or such traditional parental consequences as timeouts, taking favorite objects away from the child for periods of time, or grounding older children, are *positive consequences* (Selekman, 2005, 2009). Positive consequences might take many forms for a variety of accomplishments, for example, a parent's giving a child a big hug or high-five for completing a chore without being reminded, doing a good deed for a neighbor, doing something positive for someone less fortunate, or participating in the community's cleanup drive. Children greatly benefit from their parents using positive consequences because they help build self-esteem, give them the opportunity to practice loving kindness and compassion, and teach them the importance of generosity and altruism. In the spirit of the great humanitarian Mahatma Gandhi, it provides them with the opportunity to experience how true happiness is about what you can give to or do for others rather than what you get from others (Gandhi, Desai, & Bok, 1993).

Another way parents can foster their children's natural altruistic tendencies is by recommending service projects they and their children can do together in the community. For example, they could work together in a homeless shelter serving meals, help out in a nursing home facility, or participate in fundraising walks or bicycle rides for such causes as AIDS, cancer, violence prevention, and the like. Both positive physical reinforcements and service work involvements can contribute to children's moral development and help them to be more caring, concerned, and compassionate members of society.

The Secret Surprise

The *secret surprise* (Selekman, 2005, 2009) experiment, or strategy, is quite effective in changing parent–child interactions and injecting positive emotion into their relationship. I meet alone with the parents in the context of our family session and have each parent come up with two positive things they could do over the next week that their son or daughter would notice and really appreciate. They are not to tell the child what the surprises are; rather, the child is asked to be like a detective and try to figure out what they are. Eeryone is told that we will discuss the results of the experiment in our next family meeting. Most families really enjoy this upbeat and playful therapeutic experiment.

Pretend the Miracle Happened

Similar to the secret surprise, the *pretend the miracle happened* (Selekman, 2005; de Shazer, 1991) experiment (discussed earlier in Chapter 4) can inject positive emotion into the parents' relationship with the child and improve their interactions. This experiment is particularly effective in clinical situations where the parents cannot identify any pretreatment changes with their child and they are feeling pessimistic. In the context of the miracle question inquiry conducted earlier in the initial family session, parents can learn from their children what specifically they need to do differently that will help them get along better. When meeting alone with the parents, they are to pick two or three of their child's identified miracle-like behaviors he or she would like to see happen with them and then actually implement them a few times over the next week. While the parents are "pretending," they are to carefully observe how their child is responding to them. It is important for them to note which of their miracle-like behaviors seem to produce the most positive responses from their child. The therapist should encourage the parents to continue to engage in these behaviors until the child's objectionable behavior is completely resolved.

Catching Each Partner at His or Her Parenting Best

When working with parents who are constantly undermining or criticizing the other partner's parenting abilities, the *catching each partner at his or her parenting best* exercise can be quite productive in promoting more support and teamwork. In 1 week's time, each parenting partner is to pull out his or her imaginary magnifying glass and carefully observe daily for times that the other partner interacts with and sets limits with the children in ways that the first thinks are creative, helpful, and effective. The parents are not to compare notes until the next scheduled session. What often happens is that each partner ends up spontaneously complimenting the other, and/or they decide to join forces as a team and surprise each other well before I see them again. Once we identify what each of them does individually and as a team, we want to have them increase doing what works in the parenting department.

Do Something Dramatically Different

In clinical situations where the parents are stuck doing *more of the same,* such as yelling, making threats, pleading, overcontrolling, being superresponsible, getting into power struggles, and constantly taking things away from the child for lengthy periods of time, the *do something different* (Selekman, 2005, 2009; de Shazer, 1988) experiment (discussed earlier, in Chapter 4) can be quite effective. The therapist shares with the parents that they have become so predictable to the child that he or she knows precisely which buttons to push, how to make them feel guilty or allow the child to abdicate responsibility for his or her actions. The therapist coaches the parents to respond *differently* to the child when provoked by his or her acting up or attempts to get them to be overreactive or superstrict. Whether off-the-wall or simply different from anything the child has ever encountered from them before, the responses typically confuse the child at first. Next, in order to accommodate to their changes and stop the parents from acting so strangely, the child starts to behave more cooperatively and discontinues the very behaviors that were stressing out the parents. The parents' absurd and outrageous behaviors can run the gamut from, for example, doing a wild dance with their spouse or by themselves, or suddenly humming a song, or dressing in a bizarre manner, or talking about things completely unrelated to what the child is demanding. Four benefits may accrue from this admittedly desperate therapeutic experiment: (1) parents' reflective skills are enlarged so they can step back and both see the big picture and think more clearly about what the best options are for responding to their child's challenging behavior, (2) they abandon parenting methods that have proven to be unproductive, (3) they become flexible, playful, and more readily can access novel responses to their child's behavior, and (4) they find themselves enjoying parenthood more again.

Be Mysterious and Arbitrary

The *be mysterious and arbitrary* therapeutic experiment is best reserved for clinical situations where the child has dethroned the parents and is totally in charge of the family mood. One way parents can take back control of their household and feel less like hostages is to have them, over a 1-week period, spontaneously and randomly engage in mysterious and unexpected ways of behaving—such as retreating to their bedroom to read books; or doing something together elsewhere for a longer-than-expected time; or leaving the house at an odd time for a while without letting the child know where they went. When the child approaches the parents and asks them what they were doing in the bedroom or when they went out together, they are to respond with "Oh, we just felt like being alone together" or "We just felt like going out." The parent is to avoid giving the child explanations. On a cautionary note, I would use the leaving the house strategy only with older children who are self-sufficient and who are not self-destructive. Furthermore, I always have an adult friend of the parents or a relative check in with the child while the parents are out to make sure he or she is safe and okay. In common with the "do something different" experiment, the children are often confused by their parents' strange behavior and feel uncomfortable about their new mysterious lifestyles. They can also become quite intrigued by and curious about what their parents are up to. This will lead them to be more cooperative and to alter their difficult behaviors to better accommodate their parents' more unpredictable ways. Once the child's behavior shows signs of changing, parents can reassume their leadership roles in the family again without explanations as to why they were previously being mysterious and seemingly arbitrary with the child—since everyone is entitled to a little bit of privacy!

Externalizing Oppressive Parenting Patterns

Some parents come to us complaining about how they continually find themselves yelling, blaming, nagging, making threats, micromanaging, and dishing out punishments to their children. They describe these rigid ways of interacting with their children as if these patterns of interaction have a life of their own. Moreover, they describe in excruciating detail the huge psychological and physical toll these patterns of interaction are exacting, complaining of "feeling stressed out all the time," "feeling out of control," "feeling like I have high blood pressure," or even "feeling like a failure as a parent." When asked if these parental patterns are getting the best of them, more often than not they will share with us that it was a problem in their family of origin as well. As therapists, we can point out to parents that the patterns of interaction they practice are largely the same ones that were practiced with them as children. As therapists, we urge them to make a break with the past and begin anew co-creating patterns of interaction with their children that are more satisfying to all. Like an inspirational coach, the therapist needs to emotionally fire up parents to take a stand against the oppressive parenting pattern of the past and to dethrone it. The next step is to ask the parents and the child such externalizing questions (White, 2007; White & Epston, 1990) as these:

- "It sounds like, when you were growing up, 'yelling' really got the best of you and your relationship with your parents. Did it try to brainwash you to resent them and continue to want to push their buttons?"
- "When 'yelling' was making things out of control with you and your parents, what else did it try to make you think and want to do to add more fuel to the fire?"
- "Have there been any times recently or in the past when 'yelling' was making you and Billy [child client] lock horns with each other and you said to yourself, 'Isn't this déjà vu?'"
- "When 'yelling' completely takes control of you and unleashes itself on Billy, what do you think is going on in Billy's mind?"
- "Mary [the mother], has there been any time lately when you found yourself tensing up and 'yelling' was about to take control of you, and yet you stood up to it and frustrated it?"
- "What did you do differently to thwart 'yelling' and put it in its place?"
- "Billy, can you think of any time lately when you were a better wizard than 'yelling' and you did something to outwit it so it could not cast its spell on you to try to make your mom upset?"
- "What courageous steps did you take or what did you tell yourself to stand up to 'yelling's' powerful spells?"

By asking questions like these, both the parent and child can see how they are both being victimized by the pattern, and inevitably they begin joining forces to defeat it. The parent's original—but outmoded—views about the child's presenting problems dramatically change, which leads to the development of more positive ways of interacting.

Rules for Radical Parents:
Gandhian Nonviolent Passive Resistance Tactics

Some of the nonviolent tactics that Mahatma Gandhi employed to liberate India from British rule can be used quite effectively by parents (Gandhi et al., 1993). Omer (2004) utilizes Gandhi's nonviolent passive resistance tactics in his parenting model to empower parents that have been dethroned by a tyrannical child or a child engaging in extreme acting-out and self-destructive behaviors. One powerful Gandhian tactic is to stage a *sit-in* right inside the child's bedroom door. After a child meltdown episode or some other acting-out episode, the parents are to allow the child to go to his or her bedroom to simmer down before taking any further action. As Omer (2004) observes, parents must strike when "the iron is cold." When coaching parents to stage a sit-in, they must agree to not respond verbally or physically to their child's threatening or provocative behaviors once they are inside his or her bedroom. Upon entering the room, the parents announce that they plan to sit in front of the child's bedroom door as long as it takes for him or her to come up with some solutions for the unacceptable behavior. Over time and once the child discovers the parents are not going to budge or be a sparring partner verbally, he or she starts to make some suggestions about alternative ways of behaving when frustrated or angry. The parents are pre-instructed to be encouraging, willing to "go with" any options suggested by the child, and to develop alternatives if available. If the child is sometimes violent and the parents are concerned about this, they can get an adult relative or friend of the family to be in the house at the same time they will be staging the sit-in. Once the child starts behaving better, the parents should reward him or her with affectionate gestures and by spending more quality time together and offering to engage in fun and pleasurable activities he or she would enjoy doing with them. The parents can also help involve the child in meaningful hobbies and activities that the child likes especially.

7

Optimizing Therapeutic Cooperation in the Second and Subsequent Sessions

I don't lead musicians, man. They lead me. I listen to them and learn
what they do best.
—Miles Davis

In the second and subsequent sessions, we typically observe four possible therapist–family member cooperative response patterns: *better, mixed-
opinion, same,* and *worse* (Selekman, 2005). How well family members
manage and succeed with the assigned therapeutic experiments dictates what
the therapist should continue to do or do differently in future sessions with a
particular family. As noted in Chapter 2, therapists need to carefully match
their questions and therapeutic experiments with the unique cooperative
response patterns (de Shazer, 1985, 1991) and stage of readiness to change
(Prochaska et al., 1994) of each family member. It is important to remember
that family members do want relief from their oppressive problem situations, no matter how pessimistic or skeptical they may appear. Therefore,
carefully listening to and observing family members' verbal and nonverbal
responses to the assigned therapeutic experiments provide us with important clues to how they want to change. With children, the therapist needs
to assess whether the best way to cooperate with them and promote change
is through the use of in-session family play and art therapy activities, out-
of-session therapeutic experiments, or a combination of both. Some children do their best therapeutic work when engaged in a board game of their
choice, playing with puppets or toy figurines, or when participating in a fun
and playful in-session family activity that taps their imaginative powers and
ability to dramatize their family stories.

In this chapter, I provide guidelines for how to optimize therapeutic cooperation, amplify and consolidate family members' therapeutic gains, assess assigned therapeutic experiment effectiveness, and constructively manage family member slips or setbacks with each of the therapist–family member cooperative response pattern groups. I also discuss how to empower highly pessimistic families, which are indicative of the *worse* family group.

The "Better" Group

The *better* group typically returns to the second and subsequent sessions looking very different and reporting numerous changes in their problem situation. In general, it is best to begin the second session with confidence and optimism by asking the family, "So, what's *better*?!" Each reported family member solution-building pattern (new ways of feeling, viewing, and doing) needs to be carefully amplified and consolidated. The therapist should highlight differences by making distinctions with family members about old unhelpful patterns of behavior and outmoded beliefs and their new solution-building patterns of behavior and different ways of viewing themselves and their problem situations. Consolidating questions (Selekman, 2005; de Shazer, 1994; de Shazer & White, 1996; White, 1995, 2007) can effectively amplify the family's new solution patterns and make them more *newsworthy* on the meaning level for family members. Following are some examples of consolidating questions:

- "How did you do that?!"
- "How did you manage to take that big step?!"
- "How did you come up with such a great idea?"
- "What did you tell yourself that helped you to do that?"
- "What will you have to continue to do to get that to happen more often?"
- "Is that different for your son to do that?!"
- "Let's say we get together in a month; what further changes will you tell me you made?"
- "Since you have made such great strides, have you gotten any new ideas about yourself as a parent that you would want others to know?"
- "How will I know that you're confident enough for us to stop?"
- "Do you have any new ideas about how you view yourself as a person now, as opposed to when we first started working together?"
- "What would you have to do to go backwards?"
- "How will I know when things are better enough with your situation?"

- "On a scale from 1 to 10, 10 being better enough, what number would you use to rate your situation today?"
- "Let's say this was our last counseling session together; what fun things will you be doing during this time period in the future?"
- "How will you celebrate your victory over the problem?"
- "Who will you invite to your victory party?"
- "What will you say in your victory speeches?"

After adequately consolidating family gains, the therapist should assess with family members whether they feel they successfully achieved their initial treatment goals, how they found the assigned therapeutic experiments, and if or when they would want to come in for a future checkup session. The family members should be in the driver's seat in terms of determining how long they wish to remain in treatment and the frequency of appointments.

If there have been a number of individual and family changes between sessions, it is advisable to give the family a "vacation" from therapy as a vote of confidence. By giving families longer time intervals between visits, we are giving them the empowering message that they have the tools and the strengths to make it on their own. While on vacation from therapy, the ripple effect triggered by the changes they achieved in treatment will be free to reverberate throughout the family system and other social systems with which the family interfaces.

Finally, if family members indicate that they found the therapeutic assignments to be helpful in generating out-of-session changes, the therapist should have them do more of what's working until they are confident enough to stop doing the experiments. In the editorial reflection, I prescribe that the family continue to engage in *exactly the same* therapeutic experiments, invoking the familiar but time-honored rationale that "if it ain't broke, don't fix it." Families and therapists get into trouble when they stop doing what is working for them, which leads them to feel as if they are back to "square one" when they experience even a minor setback.

The "Mixed-Opinion" Group

When families return for their second and subsequent sessions concerned about their failure to make more headway in terms of goals achieved, or with new concerns, I normalize the situation by pointing out that change is a funny thing in that it often appears as "three steps forward and two steps back" (de Shazer, 1985). Before addressing family members' concerns, I first try to amplify, cheerlead, and consolidate the gains they have already made in treatment. I also emphasize to families that we are just striving for incremental changes here, which can eventually lead to bigger changes. If these interviewing strategies appear to be acceptable to family members based on their verbal and nonverbal feedback, I further empower the family by amplifying their changes and utilize a future focus through presuppositional and consolidating questions (Selekman, 2005; O'Hanlon & Weiner-Davis, 1989). For example, I may ask a family: "Let's say we were to get together in 4 weeks; what further changes will you make happen by our next session?" The therapist can expand the possibilities with family members' visualizations of future success and explore with them where they will rate themselves on the scale in terms of goal attainment at this future time.

If some family members still have concerns, I shift gears and ask conversational questions (Andersen, 1991; Anderson, 1997; Anderson & Goolishian, 1988a, 1988b) to give them ample space for storytelling, which may include ventilating emotionally laden material, like an illness in the family or a family secret. I might ask:

- "Is there something we did not talk about in our first meeting that needs to be talked about?"
- "What do you wish we had addressed or tried to resolve in our first meeting together that might have prevented that big argument on Tuesday?"
- "Are there any other concerns you have with your situation or with what led you to contact my office that, unless we resolve them, will come back to haunt us later?"

By showing sensitivity to and respect for the concerns of family members in the second and subsequent sessions, we not only strengthen our therapeutic alliance with the client but also help prevent crises from occurring that could have a deleterious effect on the progress the client has already made.

The use of coping sequence questions (Selekman, 2005; de Shazer et al., 2007; Berg & Gallagher, 1991) helps to create possibilities for more pessimistic or cautious family members, being particularly useful with "yes, but ... " clients. Some examples of coping sequence questions are:

- "I'm curious—how come things are not *worse* with your situation?"
- "What steps have you taken to prevent things from getting worse?"
- "What else seems to help things from getting worse?"
- "How has that made a difference?"

Therapists also need to go back to basics with mixed-opinion families by asking *themselves* the following questions:

- "Do we have a customer here?"
- "Is the treatment goal too ambitious?"
- "Do we need to break the goal down into smaller and more doable objectives?"
- "Are we working on the "right" client's problem?"
- "What experiments might better fit family members' unique cooperative response patterns?"
- "Do I know what the parents' "key question" is about the problem?"
- "Do I know the parents' theory of change?"
- "Does the problem appear to occur on a random basis?"

Guidelines for Therapeutic Experiment Design and Selection for the "Mixed-Opinion" Group

1. If one or both parents continue to be superresponsible around the child and/or participate in frustrating and unhelpful power struggles with him or her, we can offer them the "do something different" task (Selekman, 2005, 2009; de Shazer, 1985, 1991).

2. If the problem or symptoms appear to be occurring on a random basis, prescribe the "prediction task" (de Shazer, 1988, 1991).

3. If one or both parents undercut or put down the other parent's attempts to discipline or manage the children in the family, prescribe an observation task. For 1 week, have each parent observe what parental behaviors the other parent engages in with the children that he or she likes or approves of and write them down on paper. They are not allowed to compare notes until the next scheduled family session.

4. If the previously offered therapeutic experiments from the first or subsequent session were partially helpful, or one or more family members disliked the therapeutic experiments offered, the therapist should explore with them any ideas about how these experiments can be modified or changed to their liking. The therapist can also brainstorm ways to simplify or improve the therapeutic experiments.

5. The secret surprise task (Selekman, 2005; de Shazer, 1985), which is a playful task for helping to generate more exceptions, can challenge the parents' problem-saturated beliefs about the child client. Parents are often pleasantly surprised by the good deeds or nice things the child does to shock them in a positive way in 1 week's time.

6. If still stuck, we can offer the family 2–3 of the family play and art therapeutic experiments to choose from to try out in session or use the idea-generating strategies described in Chapter 4.

Case Example

Mildred, a Caucasian mother, spent the majority of our first family interview complaining about her 10-year-old overweight son, Isaac's, "overeating," "living off junk food," and "refusing to stick with any sports activities" for which she would sign him up. Isaac's father, Sidney, had died from a heart attack and had been quite obese as well. Mildred's catastrophic fear was that, unless she took steps now to help Isaac with his weight problem, he would eventually die from a heart attack, like his father. When I met alone with Isaac, I found out that his mother was constantly nagging him about what he ate and pushing him to participate in athletics at school and through their local recreation board. Isaac reported that his mother's behaviors contributed to his feeling more anxious, powerless, and hopeless about being able to lose weight. When Isaac experienced these feelings, he would "pig out" and eat foods that he knew were bad for him. Isaac could not identify any exceptions to this problem pattern. To assist Isaac with combating unpleasant emotional states and self-defeating thoughts, I taught him visualization strategies and how to decatastrophize (Seligman et al., 1995) his negative thoughts. I also prescribed that Isaac pretend to engage in his mother's miracle behaviors over the next week and observe how she responded to him when he was pretending (de Shazer, 1991). I gave Mildred the "do something different" task (de Shazer, 1988) as an experiment to help disrupt her superresponsible pattern of interaction with Isaac.

One week later the family came back with mixed opinions about their progress. The transcript of the beginning of our second session illustrates how to address this therapeutic situation.

THERAPIST: So, what's better?!!

MILDRED: Not much ... I mean yesterday he ate a whole bag of cookies!

ISAAC: Yesterday was a bad day for me, but I had a much better week!

THERAPIST: What steps did you take to make it a better week?

ISAAC: I ate fruit a few times over the week for dessert, instead of cookies or doughnuts.

THERAPIST: Wow! Is that a new thing for you to do?

ISAAC: Yeah, I think Mom would tell you that I rarely eat fruit or vegetables.

THERAPIST: Is that true, Mildred?

MILDRED: Yes, I was surprised by that, but ...

THERAPIST: Isaac, did you eat some vegetables as well this past week?

ISAAC: I ate salad twice.

THERAPIST: Really? Is that new for Isaac to eat vegetables like salad?

MILDRED: Yes (*smiling*), I almost fell out of my chair when I saw him eat two large portions of salad.

THERAPIST: Isaac, have you gotten any new ideas about yourself in terms of eating better over this past week?

ISAAC: Yeah, I think I'm doing better with my eating and feel happier.

MILDRED: Certainly, I'm encouraged by his progress, especially his starting to eat a little better, but we still have days like yesterday and ...

THERAPIST: I appreciate your cautiousness; this difficulty has been going on for a long time. I'm curious, though; did you observe any other moments or days before yesterday where Isaac was showing you signs of progress?

MILDRED: Yes, in fact 2 days ago he agreed to sign up for Little League.

THERAPIST: Wow! How did you get him to do that?

MILDRED: The funny thing about that was that I didn't force it on him like I usually do. I just left the flyer on the dining room table. Interestingly enough, he approached me with a desire to play this year.

THERAPIST: Really? How did you come up with that clever idea to leave the flyer on the dining room table?

MILDRED: I don't know, I guess I am too pushy with him and need to give him more space to make decisions.

THERAPIST: Is he a good baseball player?

MILDRED: Yeah, when he used to play a few years ago he was a great slugger. Isaac also has a good arm.

THERAPIST: Isaac, were you surprised when your mom gave you space to choose whether or not you wanted to play Little League?

ISAAC: Yeah, usually she tries to force me to do things.

THERAPIST: Besides letting you decide whether or not to sign up for Little League, did you see your mom do anything else differently that you liked over the past week?

ISAAC: Yeah, she didn't nag me as much.

THERAPIST: Were you doing anything else differently that helped your mom nag less?

ISAAC: I've been asking her to go with me on bike rides and to take me to the YMCA to swim.

THERAPIST: Wow! This young man's on a real health kick crusade! There's no stopping Isaac now! He's on a roll! That's worth a high-five! (*Both Mildred and Isaac smile.*)

As readers can clearly see, we made a complete U-turn from Mildred's initial pessimism to spending the majority of the session highlighting important changes that occurred in 1 week's time. Cheerleading was used to help reinforce and amplify family members' important behavioral changes and new ways of viewing themselves and their situation. Because both Mildred and Isaac were heading in the right direction for improving their situation, it made no sense to offer them any new tasks with which to experiment.

The "Same" Group

With the "same" group, some or all of the family members will be eager to tell the therapist that nothing much changed with their problem-saturated situation. However, it is still helpful to explore with individual family members whether there were any periods during which they experienced any slight improvement with the problem. Any reported solution-building patterns of behavior can be used as potential building blocks for solution construction, particularly if increasing their frequency can empower the family to resolve the presenting problem.

If family members continue to be negative and cannot identify any exceptions occurring between visits, I shift gears and ask coping sequence questions (Selekman, 2005, 2009; de Shazer et al., 2007; Berg & Gallagher, 1991). This approach may produce some important solution-building material on which we can capitalize that was not reported earlier in the session. Similar to the process with the mixed-opinion group, the therapist should go back to basics and revisit with the family the following concerns:

- "Are we working on the 'real' or the 'right' problem?"
- "Does the problem need to be restated in more concrete or solvable terms?"
- "Does the goal need to be broken down into smaller objectives that are more doable, or is there a new goal that we should pursue at this time?"

- *(Therapist asks him- or herself)* "Do we have a customer participating in our sessions, or do we need to further assess who the customer is in the client system?"
- "Are there any new helping professionals involved with the case who should be consulted or collaborated with?"

When further assessing customership, I may ask the client or other family members the following question: "On a scale from 1 to 10, 10 being most concerned about you, what numbers would you give absent family members, concerned relatives, and helpers outside the home?" A high number on the scale indicates that we need to expand the treatment system and engage these absent family members and significant others to aid us in the problem-solving effort. When new helping professionals get involved with the family's case, I get consent forms signed so I can begin collaborating with these helpers to try to develop cooperative working relationships with them. The use of open-ended questions and curiosity can be employed to explore family members' concerns.

Guidelines for Therapeutic Experiment Design and Selection for the "Same" Group

1. If the "do something different" task has not been tried and it seems appropriate, prescribe it as an experiment for the parents, particularly if the parents are stuck engaging in "more of the same" attempted solutions (Watzlawick et al., 1974) to manage the child's misbehavior.

2. Track the problem-maintaining sequences of interaction and use pattern intervention strategies (O'Hanlon & Weiner-Davis, 1989; O'Hanlon, 1987), such as adding something new to the context in which the problem occurs, subtracting one element from the problem pattern, exaggerating the problem–symptom pattern, and so on. In Chapter 6, I presented other pattern intervention strategies that can be employed with parents.

3. If the family describes the problem as continuing to be oppressive and out of control or appearing to have a life of its own, I externalize the problem (Selekman, 2005, 2009; White, 1995, 2007; Epston, 1998; White & Epston, 1990) and design a ritual such as the habit control ritual (Selekman, 2005; Durrant & Coles, 1991) to help empower the family to conquer the presenting problem.

4. When the parents have made some changes but the child is still symptomatic or not very verbal and the parents still have concerns, it may

be worthwhile to implement the family play and art strategies such as the imaginary feelings X-ray machine, the mindfulness meditations and practices, disputation skills training, or creative visualization strategies described in Chapter 5.

5. If still stuck, use the idea-generating strategies described in Chapter 4.

Case Example

Stella, a Caucasian mother, brought her 7-year-old son, Horace, for therapy because he walked around "angry all of the time," had "temper flare-ups," and "hit" the neighborhood children with whom he played. The first session with this family was characterized by Stella's complaining about Horace's difficult behaviors and Horace's adamant refusal to let me engage him. Not only did Horace refuse to answer my questions, but also he would not play a board game or draw any pictures when I tried to involve him and his mother in a family art task. At the end of the session, I prescribed Stella an observation task to help me better understand what was working during the times when Horace was not having difficulties.

One week later, Stella came back for our second session with a frustrated look on her face and quite pessimistic. She could not report even one exception to Horace's problem behavior. To better match her pessimism, I asked, "How come you have not thrown in the towel with counseling? What keeps you trying?" Stella responded, "I'm hoping this behavior will pass … I don't know … maybe it's me … I worry a lot." I decided to track the problem-maintaining sequence of interaction between Stella and Horace. It was clear that Stella was stuck nagging and being too overprotective with Horace, which often led to Horace's temper flare-ups and his taking out his anger on a peer or destroying one of his toys. I offered Stella the do something different task (de Shazer, 1985) as an experiment to try over the next week. When I met alone with Horace, he continued to treat me like I had the plague.

When the family returned for their third session, I did not recognize them. Smiles were plastered on both Stella's and Horace's faces. Apparently, Horace was in "good spirits" most of the week. There had been no temper flare-ups and no fights with kids. When I inquired what Stella was doing that produced this miraculous outcome, she disclosed that she decided to stop nagging and "infantalizing" Horace. Stella observed that when she discontinued these two problem-maintaining behaviors, Horace's behavior greatly improved. I prescribed that Stella continue to do more of what was working.

I ended up seeing Stella and Horace two more times to consolidate gains. The biggest surprise for me in this session and the final two was that Horace initiated checkers games with me!

The "Worse" Group

Families that fit into the "worse" group category are often very pessimistic. Some of these families have experienced multiple treatment failures and have a tremendous dislike for therapists. Others have been plagued by multiple crises and problems that have been oppressing them for many years. Therapists typically run into a brick wall with such families when they tend to be too optimistic, do not provide the family with enough space to tell their problem-saturated stories, and fail to cooperate with their feelings of hopelessness and despair. Therefore, it is important to begin therapy sessions with pessimistic families by asking open-ended conversational questions (Andersen, 1995; Anderson, 1997; Anderson & Goolishian, 1988a, 1988b) and operating from a position of "not knowing." To gain access to their beliefs about why their problems exist, and to make sure I have a good handle on what they view as the "real" problem, not what I or other therapists have thought is "the problem" that keeps them stuck, I want to give family members ample space to share their problem-saturated stories about negative past experiences with therapists. It is also quite useful to shift gears and cooperate with the family's pessimism and ask such pessimistic questions (Selekman, 2005, 2009; de Shazer et al., 2007; Berg & Miller, 1992) as the following:

- "What keeps you going with this situation?"
- "How come you have not thrown in the towel already?"
- "What do you suppose is the smallest thing you could do that might make a slight difference?"
- "And what could other family members do?"
- "How could you get that to happen a little bit now?"
- "Can you think of anything you used to do with your son [or daughter] in the past that seemed to be helpful, that we might want to test out now?"

It is also quite helpful to place families that are therapy veterans in the expert position and have them serve as consultants on how to best conduct therapy with them. I ask them the following questions:

- "You have seen a lot of therapists before me; what did they miss with your situation?"
- "What were some of the things these therapists did with you that you disliked the most?"

- "In what ways can I be more helpful to you as a therapist?"
- "In your minds, if you had the most perfect therapist to work with, what would he or she be like?"
- "What would he or she ask you about or do with you that you would find most helpful?"
- "If I were to work with another family just like yours, what advice would you give me to help them out?"
- "If there was one question that you think is most critical to hear from me so that I can best help you out, what would that question be?"

I have found it helpful to have crisis-prone, highly pessimistic families predict what their next crisis is going to be. I elicit the details about who will likely be involved, where it will happen, and what effects it will have on family members. This therapeutic strategy can successfully disrupt their long-standing family crisis-prone pattern, especially if the therapist offers tools for effectively managing the future crisis situation. Also, while brainstorming collaboratively with the family about past successes, we may stumble on problem-solving or coping strategies that once worked and can be revisited or revived as effective tools in achieving future successes. As with families responding with the "same" on progress made between sessions, it is also important to go back to basics with those responding "worse" in terms of revisiting customership, problem definition, and the initial treatment goals that were established. Active collaboration with involved helping professionals is also critical.

Guidelines for Therapeutic Experiment Design and Selection for the "Worse" Group

1. Utilize pattern intervention (O'Hanlon & Weiner-Davis, 1989; O'Hanlon, 1987) strategies to disrupt the family dance that appears to fuel the child client's symptoms/problems.

2. Externalize the problem as a viable therapeutic option with highly pessimistic, stressed-out families that describe their problems as chronic and oppressive in nature.

3. Use the idea-generating strategies described in Chapter 4 to design new therapeutic experiments that can aid in the change effort.

4. Use the mindfulness meditations and practices, disputation skills training, creative visualization strategies, or the family play and art therapy strategies discussed in Chapter 5 if the child's symptoms are not stabilizing.

5. If working solo, recruit a colleague or a few staff members to serve as a reflecting team (Andersen, 1991, 1995). Team members can offer you and the family some fresh, helpful new ideas for viewing the family's problem. The team is free to reflect on key family themes and the unspeakable, such as family secrets that may be driving the child client's symptoms/problems.

6. Another consultation team strategy that can be used when the treatment system is at a standstill is the *therapeutic debate* (Papp, 1983). The therapist remains in a neutral position while two of his or her colleagues debate in front of the family about the disadvantages and dilemmas of changing their situation. One colleague represents the parents' position, and the other colleague represents the child's position. They can speculate aloud about family members' concerns, fears, hidden agendas, and the like. Family members are free to chime in with their thoughts, which can open up space for possibilities.

Case Examples

Three case examples demonstrate my work with highly pessimistic multiproblem families. In all three of the cases, I felt a strong sense of being stuck early in treatment, as well as therapeutic paralysis in response to the parents' hopelessness and despair and the children's chronic and intractable symptoms.

> Lance, a Caucasian 5-year-old, was brought in for therapy at the preschool teacher's request for "severe impulse control problems," "ADHD," "soiling," "bedwetting," and "low self-esteem problems" related to his "severe speech handicap." The parents, both recovering alcoholics, observed a major decline in Lance's behavior after the sudden and tragic death of his younger brother, Tony, following Tony's heart surgery.
>
> Tony had been born with multiple birth defects, including a heart valve problem. Initially, his open heart surgery appeared to go as well as possible. But Tony died in his bed 8 hours after returning home from the hospital. This was a terrible tragedy for everyone in this family. Both parents experienced bouts of depression. Until I began seeing Lance and his family, he had engaged in a daily ritual of "searching through the house for" his deceased brother and "calling out his name."
>
> For the bulk of our session, Lance could not sit still; he crawled under tables and my desk, and I could barely understand what he was saying because of his severe speech problem. One thing I did discover in my first encounter with Lance was that he enjoyed drawing. I made a mental note of this strength. The parents were very pessimistic about

Lance's ever being able to get over the loss of his brother. Of all of Lance's presenting problems, the parents considered the "real" problem to be whether he would ever "get over the loss of Tony." They were slightly less concerned about Lance's other problems because they believed the "unresolved loss issue" was at the root of them.

I gave the parents ample space to talk about this issue. However, I was at a loss for coming up with potential solutions, particularly with getting a child this young to understand the abstract concept of death and to mourn this loss. Besides offering the parents some parenting skills, normalizing Lance's regressive behaviors, and drawing with him, I had no idea where I was going with this family until our third session together.

Lance, with a little help from his mother, had put together a number of drawings of Tony and himself in book form. Once Lance created the book, his behavioral difficulties spontaneously began to improve. He stopped the ritual of searching throughout the house for Tony and calling out his name. It was as if Lance had naturally externalized his thoughts and feelings about missing Tony onto paper. He and his mother had found their own high-quality unique solution to the loss issue by creating a book about Tony.

I ended up seeing Lance and his parents seven more times over the next year. An important part of the treatment process was actively collaborating with Lance's teacher. The teacher was quite burned out; she had "four other boys" in her class who "were major behavior problems." It was not until the time of our eighth family session that the teacher noticed that Lance had changed dramatically. The parents wanted to keep Lance in treatment over the school year as a result of pressure from the teacher and her superiors to keep him in therapy because of the pathology-laden psychological evaluation results that identified Lance as exhibiting ADHD. Lance was never placed on Ritalin. By our last session together, he was symptom-free, speaking more clearly, and sporting a sunny, happy face. As a reward for being a "big boy who was taking big steps," I gave Lance one of my favorite Nerf balls. The mother also took a picture of Lance hugging me as a way for him always to remember me, a similar strategy to that of creating a "Tony Memory Book."

This was clearly a highly resilient and resourceful family. What I found most interesting about this case was that throughout the course of therapy I discovered the power of "not doing." I gave family members plenty of space to tell their painful stories and they not only provided me with what they perceived as the real problem but generated their own unique solution, which was far better than anything I could have ever possibly come up with.

The next case example concerned a Caucasian 10-year-old girl, Audrey, who had been described in past treatment summaries and psychological evaluations as "deeply depressed," "a hopeless case," "a damaged child," "ADHD," "behavior-disordered," and "severely learning-disabled." Audrey had had four inpatient psychiatric admissions for "clinical depression" and was chronically "tearing up her clothes." Audrey had had a total of 12 outpatient therapy experiences. Her father had been psychiatrically hospitalized for "clinical depression" and had had several unsuccessful and "bad therapy" experiences. Her biological mother used to beat Audrey until she was reported to child protective services; at that point, Audrey went to live with her stepmother, Emily, and father, Jim. Audrey had one biological sister, Theresa, who was 17. Emily and Jim had four children together, ranging in ages from 15 months to 8 years old.

In our first session together, only Emily and Audrey showed up. Although Emily appeared very committed to trying to help Audrey, she was highly pessimistic that Audrey would "ever change." Audrey was now having "difficulties getting along with" peers at her therapeutic day school, was still "destroying her clothes with her hands," and was stealing from her older sister, Theresa. Audrey was tall for her age and very fidgety and squirmy in her chair. She appeared to be extremely nervous and had little to say to me.

I decided to meet alone with Audrey to see if I could join with her over a checkers game. It was interesting to note that Audrey went out of her way to help me beat her in the game. Audrey did, however, disclose that she wished she had a closer relationship with her father, who was never around. I met alone with Emily to clarify what she perceived as the "real" or main problem, which turned out to be Audrey's "destroying her clothes with her hands." According to Emily, this was proving to be an "expensive bad habit" for her and Jim.

As I had discovered that Audrey "loved art" earlier in the session, I recommended that the mother buy some clay and find a quiet place in the house for Audrey to use her hands daily to make sculptures. Emily thought this was a novel idea and said she would implement this strategy immediately. In exploring past successes, I discovered that "going for long walks with Audrey" after dinner seemed to be helpful in curtailing some of her mischief-making behaviors. The mother had to stop these walks because of other parenting responsibilities. Jim "did very little" to assist her "with the kids."

After four sessions with Emily and Audrey, we successfully resolved the tearing up clothes problem. I also got a look at some of Audrey's "best" animal sculptures, which were quite good. Another important change occurred in the context of our checkers matches, namely, Audrey was showing signs of wanting to win the games, no longer setting herself up to lose. She also appeared to be happier and more self-confident. Emily was very pleased with Audrey's progress both at home and at school. In fact, the special school that Audrey attended wanted to gradually start mainstreaming her back into a regular school in her district because of her "academic and behavioral progress."

I ended up seeing Emily, Audrey, and some of the other children eight more times over a 2-year period. I actively collaborated with Audrey's school throughout the 2-year period we worked together. Another big change was that Audrey beat me in checkers three times! Audrey also excelled in her classes in the regular school.

Throughout the course of therapy, I oscillated between feeling pessimistic and being hopeful that Audrey would change. My therapeutic optimism greatly increased once we resolved the tearing up clothes problem.

Mary, a highly depressed Kenyan woman, sought therapy for feeling like a "failure as a parent," wanting help in learning how to "better manage" her "difficult" and chronically oppositional 6-year-old daughter, Tomika, and having difficulties coping with her marital separation of 3 months. Another major stressor for Mary was the separation from her older daughter, Keisha, who was living with Mary's mother in Kenya. Mary did not have a green card, and she could not freely leave and return to the United States after visiting her daughter. She had not seen Keisha for 5 years and felt "very guilty" about "abandoning" her.

When Mary first came to see me, she was severely depressed and had fleeting thoughts of wanting to kill herself. She was also presenting with a wide range of vegetative symptoms. Although Mary did not have a suicide plan, I made sure that she had some semblance of a support system. Mary and Tomika had been living with her "caring" and "supportive brother," Walter, for the past 3 months after Mary separated from her abusive husband, Winston, who was also Kenyan. According to Mary, Winston used to "yell at" her all the time and found it "unacceptable" for her to "work." Whenever Mary challenged Winston, he would "scream at" her or "slap" her. As another way of exercising his power and control over Mary, Winston would not try to help her get a green card or brainstorm ways to secure a "visa for Keisha to come visit" them. Winston used to call Mary "a whore" because Keisha was the product of an out-of-wedlock relationship. Culturally, Winston was a traditional African man. He believed strongly that Mary should adopt a subordinate position to him in regard to all decision making.

After Mary secured a secretarial position for a small company, Mary and Tomika moved out and went to live with Walter. Throughout the session, I provided Mary with plenty of support, empathy, and room to tell her painful story. She spent a lot of time complaining about Tomika's oppositional behavior. Mary was also quite pessimistic about "ever being able to see Keisha again" and having the ability to change Tomika's behavior. Mary had been yelling a lot at Tomika, which seemed to make the situation worse. I gave Mary an observation task of keeping track on a daily basis of any encouraging steps on Tomika's behalf and anything she was doing to promote these prosocial behaviors. I also hooked Mary up with a psychiatrist to see whether an antidepressant medication was necessary. By our second session together, Mary had observed that her daughter was being less oppositional. However, Mary still felt quite hopeless about the future. In exploring her feelings of hopelessness, Mary disclosed that she went back and forth with the idea of "moving back to Kenya" so that she could be "reunited with Keisha." Mary also "felt like a prisoner" in her marriage in that, because of her strong religious beliefs and in her culture, divorce was considered a "sinful act."

Tomika accompanied Mary to our second session. She appeared to be a very loving child who worried about her mother. Tomika disclosed that she "missed not playing games" with her mother like they used to. I decided to have Tomika and Mary make a family mural drawing of how they wanted the family situation to look. Both Tomika and Mary seemed to have a lot of fun making the family mural together. Tomika drew her mother holding hands with her, with a smile on her mother's face. She also added a big bright sun and colorful houses. Neither Mary nor Tomika added Winston to the picture. When asked about this, Tomika said she was "scared of" her dad and that he had done "bad things" to her mother. Mary disclosed that a strong part of her wanted to "start a new life" with Tomika either in the United States or back in Kenya.

I ended up seeing Mary and Tomika six more times. Mary was placed on Zoloft, which successfully stabilized her vegetative symptoms. By our last session, Mary had courageously decided to leave Winston permanently. Tomika was no longer oppositional, and the two of them were getting along much better. Mary had been saving up her money to get her own apartment. She had gotten a raise at her job. Finally, Mary had discovered that playing and drawing with Tomika tended to promote Tomika's prosocial behavior.

Covering the Back Door: Constructive Strategies for Managing Family Slips and Setbacks

Many families, while on vacation from therapy, experience some slippage backward in the goal area or with their progress. Initially, family members may think that they are back to square one when this happens. Rather than perpetuating this unhelpful way of perceiving a slip or setback, I like to normalize such occurrences as being quite common and a critical part of the change process, and I share with the family the following types of comments:

- "We could not have made headway if we did not have a slip or setback."
- "When families change, it is similar to getting the hiccups: they come and then they pass."
- "Having a slip provides us with the opportunity for comeback practice" (Tomm & White, 1987).
- "Slips are like teachers and offer us valuable wisdom. What did all of you learn from that slip on Thursday that you can put to good use the next time you find yourselves in a similar stressful situation?"

After normalizing with families the inevitability of slips while they continue to change, I explore with them the steps they have already taken to get back on track prior to coming back from their counseling vacation for a tune-up session following the slip or setback. When the family still feels derailed by their recent slip or setback, we brainstorm to come up with steps that they can take to get back on track. I inquire about past successes prior to the slip or setback. Here I ask specifically what the parents and other family members were doing that worked prior to the slip or setback. I may have family members gaze into my trusty imaginary crystal ball to visually capture the future steps they will be taking to stay on track.

As part of the goal maintenance and relapse prevention process, I conduct four activities to help my clients stay on track and make further progress: (1) structure building; (2) identifying early warning signs; (3) family constructive response scenario planning; and (4) using peers and key members from the client's social network as a natural relapse prevention support system (Selekman, 2009). With the structure-building process, it is important to fill the child's leisure time with a combination of solo hobbies and engaging in flow state activities, playtime and positive activities with friends, and quality time with family members. Having this kind of structure is particularly helpful with children that have been diagnosed with ADD and are prone to get into trouble because they cannot handle situations that are too loose.

Often clients experience major derailments, prolonged relapse situations, and crises when their therapists have failed, session by session, to "cover the back door" and address any concerns of family members. We have to find a balance between amplifying, consolidating, and cheerleading for clients when they make gains while also making room for any new concerns or pieces of the original problem situation that have not been resolved.

It is critical to observe carefully and be alert for any early warning signs of a budding crisis or things starting to unravel in the family's goal areas.

Another way that we can help cover the back door with our clients is to have family members identify a few worst-case scenarios that might lead to a major setback or crisis situation for them and then have them put their heads together and come up with constructive steps they would take to stabilize the situation. By having family members anticipate and be clear in their minds what concrete steps they plan to take if any of these worse-case scenarios materializes, they will be well equipped to constructively manage adverse developments and quickly get back on track.

Finally, covering the back door is not just a family concern but should also include interested members from the collective social network as well. These key people, which can include the child's closest friends, adult inspirational others, extended family members, the family's spiritual mentors, and even involved helping professionals from larger systems can serve as a natural relapse prevention support system for the child and his or her family. It is helpful for these concerned and caring others to know what the child's key behavioral triggers are, where there needs to be more structure and support for both the child and his or her parents, and how they individually can be most helpful.

Conclusion

In this chapter, I presented numerous guidelines for optimizing therapist–family member cooperation and promoting change with families in the second and subsequent sessions. It is important to remember that each session is a unique experience; therefore, how family members present themselves in the second and subsequent sessions will guide the therapist in terms of deciding what types of questions to ask or what types of therapeutic experiments to design and select for the family between sessions. Thus, every move the therapist makes in any given session needs to be purposive and accommodative to each family member's unique cooperative response patterns.

8

Co-Constructing Change

*Hosting Collaborative Meetings
with Allies from Larger Systems*

Out beyond ideas of wrongdoing and right doing there is a field. I'll
meet you there.

—RUMI

Once upon a time a North-Going Zax and a South-Going Zax met
in the prairie of Prax. Much to their surprise, the two Zaxes came to a
place where they ran into one another face to face. "Look here, now!" the
North-Going Zax said. "I say! You are blocking my path. You are right in
my way. I'm a North-Going Zax and I always go north!" "Who is in whose
way?" retorted the South-Going Zax. "I always go south, making south-
going tracks, so you're in My way!" This proved to be unacceptable to the
North-Going Zax, who refused to budge and get out of the South-Going
Zax's way. The North-Going Zax proclaimed that he would not move for
"fifty-nine days!" The South-Going Zax countered with "I can stand here
in the prairie of Prax for fifty-nine years! I'll stay here, not budging! I can
and I will if it makes you and me and the whole world stand still!" (Seuss,
1961b, pp. 27–31).

Dr. Seuss's *The Zax* is a nice metaphor for the kinds of interactions
that can occur in collaborative meetings with those representatives from
larger systems who are involved with our cases. Often we and the helping
professionals with whom we collaborate are not as forthright and assertive
with one another about our opinions, assumptions, thoughts, and feelings

as are the Zaxes. Instead, we tend to keep our private beliefs, assumptions, and opinions about cases to ourselves, which defeats the whole purpose of working together as a group to co-create possibilities for complex and challenging cases. Senge, Kleiner, Roberts, Ross, and Smith (1994, p. 242) have identified four ways our self-generated beliefs and overly convinced selves can get us into trouble in collaborative meetings:

1. Our beliefs are the truth.
2. The truth is obvious.
3. Our beliefs are based on real data.
4. The data we select are the real data.

To help prevent us from succumbing to the mental traps that can open wide during such meetings and in our sessions with families, we can do the following: become more perceptive about our own thinking and reasoning, make our thinking and reasoning more explicit to the helpers with whom we collaborate, and more actively into what their thinking and reasoning are during our collaborative conversations with them (Senge et al., 1994).

Not only is collaborating with helpers from larger systems a powerful and effective approach to empowering families, but also it is highly cost-effective and therefore supported by most managed care companies. Any treatment method that contributes to the rapid stabilization of the child's symptoms, helps prevent legal complications, curtails problems at school, and reduces the likelihood of psychiatric admissions gets the "*Good Housekeeping* seal of approval" from managed care companies! Active and constructive collaboration with involved helping professionals delivers all of this—and more. When collaborative meetings are productive, the therapist working with the family and hosting the meetings is empowered as well. Doherty (1995) put it best when he said, "Collaboration among professionals is the most clinician-friendly thing to do because it reduces professional isolation, enhances the knowledge and skills of all providers, and reduces the crushing sense of overresponsibility given the fact of one's own limited resources" (p. 276). By applying the right attitudes and approaches, we professionals can become a "shared mind," providing fertile ground for the generation of multiple high-quality solutions to resolve the child's and family's difficulties rapidly.

In this chapter, I discuss the role of the solution-determined system, the role of the hosting therapist in family–multiple helper collaborative meetings, and the key elements of successful collaborative relationships as well as providing examples of useful collaborative questions that can be asked of such meetings. I follow with two case examples that illustrate the power of collaboration among professionals.

The Solution-Determined System

During the initial family assessment session, one key objective of mine is to find out from family members all the persons who constitute the *solution-determined system* (Selekman, 2009). In addition to the client, attending family members, the referring person, and myself, concerned absent family members, extended family members, the key members of their social networks—including adult inspirational others and close friends—and other involved helping professionals from larger systems are all members of the solution-determined system. Like family members, these important individuals are creative, resourceful people who possess certain strengths, talents, life experiences, and wisdom that can be tapped in the solution construction process. Ideally, I like to arrange with the family for as many members of the solution-determined system to attend the very first family session or have a joint meeting before the next session. There are many advantages to doing this as early in the treatment process as possible—most importantly, finding out from everyone seriously concerned about the problem what their specific concerns are, what their theories of change are, the best hopes and outcome goals for the child and family in their view, and what creative ideas they have for the problem's resolution. Having the family present affords all members of the solution-determined system the opportunity to hear what their current needs are and how specifically they can be most helpful to the family. Finally, the members of the solution-determined system can help activate and support the family's changes and serve as an ultimate relapse prevention team, if needed, across multiple settings.

The Role of the Hosting Therapist

Like all friendly and gracious hosts, we therapists should make visiting helpers feel warmly welcomed at the key initial meeting, and we must display good manners at all times. For some helping professionals, this type of demeanor and way of relating may come as a pleasant surprise, especially if in the past therapists treated them as if they were the "enemy" or a "villain" meddling in their clients' lives and maintaining and further exacerbating their clients' difficulties. Personally, I strongly believe that each involved helping professional is a potential *ally* who possesses strengths and resources that can help generate creative ideas for empowering the family. When we convey this much friendlier therapeutic attitude to helping professionals, it greatly enhances cooperation and is the catalyst for building trust. The hosting therapist must demonstrate a deep respect for each helper's expertise, knowledge, skills, and unique perspective on the case. According to McDaniel, Campbell, and Seaburn (1995), "Such behavior is like an engraved invitation that says, 'You may enter safely into my culture'" (p. 296).

Following the introductions, each helping professional is invited to share his or her story of involvement with the child and family. Family members are free to comment on or provide feedback on any of the helpers' concerns or descriptions of them with which they disagree. For the family, this experience might be the first time in their long history of involvement with larger systems' representatives that they feel like they have a "voice" in their treatment. The hosting therapist's main job in the collaborative process with the helpers and the family is to be competent at keeping conversations going as long as possible, which can help generate new meanings about the problem story. He or she needs to operate from the Buddhist perspective of "Don't know mind," utilizing the therapeutic tool of *multipartiality* (Anderson, 1997; Anderson & Goolishian, 1988b), that is, siding simultaneously with both the family member's and helper's perspectives and not permitting his or her own personal views to take precedence over others' opinions.

If the hosting therapist in any way conveys a strong allegiance to a particular view or explanation, the flow of conversation can be shut down or quite possibly alienate certain helpers attending the meeting. When we start indulging our own therapeutic views in this way or behave with missionary zeal during such a meeting, we should immediately reflect on what was said that made us so anxious or put us on the defensive, ask open-ended conversational questions (Anderson, 1997; Anderson & Goolishian, 1988a, 1988b, 1991a, 1991b), and try to determine what each participant is thinking or feeling about what was being discussed (McDaniel et al., 1995). The bottom line is that if we expect family members and involved helping professionals to be open to changing their problem-saturated views, we need to be equally ready and willing to change our own views and behaviors. Hosting therapists can model this kind of flexibility by inviting helpers in their meetings to reflect on one another's views and by welcoming alternative viewpoints. We cannot escape from the reality that we are very much a part of the problem situation and the developing solution-determined system. What we think and do can greatly influence the outcome of each family–multiple helper meeting.

Another useful collaborative tool we can use when we find ourselves having a strong emotional reaction to more pessimistic and pathology-minded helpers' negative views regarding the clients' abilities or resistance to change is called *suspension* (Selekman, 2005; Isaacs, 1993). Like comic strip characters, we need to create over our heads an imaginary bubble and fill it with our voices of judgment and emotional reaction, self-reflect, and use curiosity to invite these helpers with radically different views to help us to understand how they arrived at their conclusions about the clients. Our voices of judgment, cynicism, and fear of taking risks all serve to block us from having an *open mind* and *open heart,* which is the pathway to true collaboration (Scharmer, 2007; Senge, Scharmer, Jaworski, & Flowers, 2005).

As hosting therapists, we need to be sensitive to cultural differences

(McDaniel et al., 1995) among the helping professionals participating in our meetings. For example, a psychiatrist speaks a much different language from a child protective worker. Any two professionals may have very different responsibilities and practice styles. We need to be respectful of the various helpers' cultural differences and the role of context in determining what they can hear and see. It is also helpful for hosting therapists to be conversant with the helpers' terminology, but, when confused by certain words and their meaning, to ask the helper to explain what he or she means.

Finally, as Peek and Heinrich (1995) emphasize, hosting therapists should "watch the team score, not just your own scores" (p. 338). When a case is in crisis, all the helpers are implicated, even those doing a great job in their therapeutic area. It is crucial to be proactive and go the extra mile—with more challenging or "stickier" cases, in particular—to prevent "case fractures and misunderstandings." This type of regimen includes making phone calls and engaging in advocacy work between scheduled family–multiple helper collaborative meetings, for example.

Out of respect for the family and the involved helpers' work schedules, we mutually decide the frequency of collaborative meetings and when they are scheduled. For absent helpers who were invited but could not attend, the family and I prepare a summary statement of what was discussed in a particular meeting, and we fax it or mail it to absent helpers so they are kept abreast of important new developments. I also make myself available to meet with these helpers to discuss the case in their respective offices. The physical presence of all involved helping professionals in collaborative meetings is not necessary to create possibilities. (In point of fact, some of Einstein's most successful collaborations were by written correspondence with other scientists and scholars.) Sometimes, I put helpers who could not attend scheduled family–multiple helper meetings on the speaker phone so that they can participate from their car phone or offices. In every way possible, I try to accommodate absent helpers, including scheduling future collaborative meetings at their offices so that they can attend.

Finally, as the host of these collaborative meetings, we need to create opportunities for the outside participants and family members to share with one another what they have appreciated in their work together (Cooper-rider, Whitney, & Stavros, 2003). The participating helping professionals and the key members from social networks can learn from family members what specifically they have done that has been most meaningful and helpful to them. The hosting therapist should also seize any ready opportunity to share credit for the family's successes not only with family members but the extended helper network as well. This creates a reservoir of good feeling among all the participants and underscores synergistic benefits of their joint teamwork.

Key Elements of Successful Collaborative Relationships

Throughout history and across professional disciplines, one can find many examples of successful collaborative relationships. One of the greatest presidents of all time, Abraham Lincoln, was a master at establishing successful collaborative relationships with fellow politicians, even if—as in his case—they counted themselves among his sworn political foes. Lincoln actively recruited political antagonists Salmon Chase, Edwin Stanton, and William Seward to serve as key members of his cabinet. Able to look beyond their ambivalent or ill feelings toward him and to appreciate their strengths and aptitude for the positions to which he appointed them, Lincoln deftly converted would-be enemies into useful functionaries of his administration while neutralizing their venom through the antidote of goodwill (Kearns-Goodwin, 2005).

One study found that the majority of Nobel Prize winners had collaborated with an important colleague (e.g., Crick and Watson, the co-discoverers of the double helix theory of genetics). The famous Cubist painters Georges Braque and Pablo Picasso frequently advised each other as to when, precisely, their paintings were "finished" (Schrage, 1990). In the arts, one highly successful collaborative relationship was that of lyricist Lorenz Hart and songwriter Richard Rodgers. Rodgers recalled:

> When the immovable object of his unwillingness to change came up against the irresistible force of my own drive for perfection ... the noise could be heard all over the city. Our fights over words were furious, blasphemous, and frequent, but even in the hottest moments we both knew that we were arguing academically and not personally. (in Schrage, 1990, p. 41)

There are six key elements of successful collaboration as it applies to family–multiple helper meetings:

1. There is a climate of respect, tolerance, and trust.
2. The communications flow is free-form and spontaneous.
3. A context is provided that facilitates the cross-fertilization of multiple viewpoints.
4. A context is created that plays with multiple viewpoints, treating uncertainty as an opportunity for further exploration.
5. Consensus is not necessary; it is irrelevant to the act of creation or discovery.
6. There are no restrictive boundaries regarding who does what.

Let us discuss each element in turn.

There Is a Climate of Respect, Tolerance, and Trust

Every member of the family–multiple helper collaborative meeting must have a "voice" and be shown the utmost respect. The hosting therapist can model for collaborators' *generative listening*, that is, not only listening to the participant's words but to the very essence of his or her thinking, "the art of developing deeper silences in yourself" (Senge et al., 1994, p. 377). The hosting therapist also needs to model the importance of being nonjudgmental and suspending one's feelings (Scharmer, 2007; Senge et al., 2005; Isaacs, 1993). Each participant is treated as an equal and is given ample floor time to share stories of concern about the family. Concurrently, family members are encouraged to be coauthors of their new evolving story, without any participants serving unduly as narrative editors or blocking them from having a "voice" in their own destiny and with treatment planning.

The Communications Flow Is Free-Form and Spontaneous

As noted earlier, the hosting therapist avoids providing excessive structure for the collaborative meetings. After he or she initiates the meeting with introductions and an invitation to helpers to share their stories of involvement with the family in turn, participants are given free rein to chime in at any point during the meeting's conversations. During periods of silence the host may usefully solicit contributions from participants who have not yet spoken or make explicit his or her thoughts or reactions to what somebody has said. Again, when sharing thoughts, the host must do so from a position of curiosity and suspension of belief, not coming across as wedded to only one way of looking at the problem(s). At some point, the conversation should shift from what is not working and how to fix it to the subject of what is working and how to *leverage* it. This shift can help create a "generative field" of mutual trust and appreciation, in which the assembled helpers and family will feel encouraged to brainstorm in earnest and share their creative ideas and potential solutions (Scharmer, 2007; Brown & Isaacs, 1997, 2005; Cooperrider et al., 2003; Cooperrider & Srivastva, 1987).

A Context Is Provided That Facilitates the Cross-Fertilization of Multiple Viewpoints

Ideally, the hosting therapist needs to create an atmosphere in which multiple views of the problem situation can be productively shared. In such an environment, helpers and family members begin to entertain new ways of looking at the client's problem-saturated story and are emboldened to coauthor new problem-free narratives. Physicist David Bohm refers to this process as a "stream of meaning" flowing through us and among us (Bohm, 1985). Over time, once involved helpers are able to feel less alarmed and concerned about the child and his or her situation because new understandings about the problem situation have emerged and been internalized and their views have changed, they will feel progressively less compelled to have regular involvement with the problem's solution and will, in some cases, eventually disengage.

A Context Is Created That Plays with Multiple Viewpoints, Treating Uncertainty as an Opportunity for Further Exploration

When the hosting therapist brings together a roomful of helping providers with diverse health care and professional cultural backgrounds and a family entangled in the professional web, anything can happen. Sometimes our collaborations occur at the top of our lungs. Sometimes there may be long silences and a strong sense of cautiousness in the air. In one meeting, several high-quality solutions may be generated by the group, or a family member may self-disclose the "not yet said" (Anderson, 1997; Anderson & Goolishian, 1988b), which may be the missing piece of the family puzzle and may prove to be newsworthy to all participants. One never knows what shape or form these collaborative meetings will take. Einstein once said, "The most beautiful experience we can have is the mysterious. It is the fundamental emotion which stands at the cradle of true art and true science" (in Wujec, 1995, p. 27). The mysterious and uncertain elements of these collaborative meetings are a constant reminder that knowledge is always in the making.

Consensus Is Not Necessary; It Is Irrelevant to the Act of Creation or Discovery

That consensus should not be the overriding criterion for judging success in collaborative relationships is suggested by the bond between Francis Crick and James Watson, co-developers of the double helix theory of genetics. According to Crick, "Politeness is the poison of all good collaboration in science" (in Schrage, 1990, p. 42). In describing his collaborative relationship with Watson, he noted that "our advantage was that we had evolved unstated but fruitful methods of collaboration. ... If either of us suggested a new idea, the other, while taking it seriously, would attempt to demolish it in a candid nonhostile manner" (in Schrage, 1990, p. 42). I am not suggesting or trying to convey that hosting therapists should behave this way with helpers in collaborative meetings, but it does demonstrate that we do not have to have group consensus to make important discoveries. Through maximum input from concerned professionals and family members alike, we want to project a kaleidoscopic view of the problem story into a view that is more likely to open portals to new possibilities. Also, by avoiding the push for group consensus, we are modeling for family members that there are many ways to look at their problem situation, none necessarily more "correct" than the others. This tolerance for diverse viewpoints can help loosen up fixed beliefs that family members may have about the client and the helpers who have been involved in their lives.

There Are No Restrictive Boundaries Regarding Who Does What

One of the most touching and yet common occurrences in the day-to-day grind of collaborative meetings is the spontaneous offer by a participating professional to advocate for and assist family members in the social realms where they had been experiencing the greatest difficulty. For just one example, a school social worker spontaneously offered to advocate for and help the child client resolve a long-standing conflict with a particular teacher who was known to be "difficult." I had not suggested in any way that she intervene on the child's behalf—she came up with the idea on her own. As a result of her efforts, the child began to view her as a "caring" ally in the school who was available to him, and she became instrumental in helping him resolve outstanding issues with the teacher. This example demonstrates that the hosting therapist need not assign tasks or responsibilities to participants in the meetings. Once collaborating helpers begin to appreciate that their knowledge and expertise are respected and potentially critical to success, they begin to take more positive risks, such as offering to go the extra mile for the child and/or family members.

Collaborative Interviewing

The hosting therapist has to be a good diplomat, translator, and master conversationalist. As a key meaning maker in the collaborative process, he or she models the importance of being curious about the second and third possible explanation for the problem story and asks questions from the vantage point of "not knowing" rather than "pre-knowing" (Anderson & Goolishian, 1988b). Lao-tzu, author of the *Tao Te Ching*, offered the following words of wisdom about the dangers of adopting a pre-knowing stance: "The more you know, the less you understand" (in Mitchell, 1988, p. 47). Therefore, the hosting therapist needs to ask open-ended conversational questions (Andersen, 1991, 1995; Anderson, 1997; Anderson & Goolishian, 1988a, 1988b) that help enlarge meaning about the continually evolving problem story. At the same time, the hosting therapist should not hesitate to make his or her thinking and reasoning known to all participants in the meeting, taking special care not to offend anyone and "honoring the passion" that underlies their varying viewpoints (Senge et al., 1994).

I now present some examples of the types of collaborative questions I may ask family members and helpers in the context of our meetings together, followed by a brief discussion on the importance of the therapist's use of self-reflexive questions.

Collaborative Questions

Collaborative questions are open-ended and the hosting therapist's primary tool in the meaning-making process. Such questions contribute to the restorying process, which ultimately leads to the authoring of new and more preferred family narratives. Examples of collaborative questions include the following:

To the family:

- "Let's say that this group of providers, including myself, proved to be most helpful to you [the family]; what sorts of things would we have done that benefited you the most?"
- "What leads you to that way of seeing things?"
- "What do you mean by that view?"
- "You may be right, but I'd like to understand more. What leads you to believe … ?"
- "If you [the family] were conducting this meeting, what do you think all of us providers really need to know about this problem situation and your family?"
- "What are your thoughts about why this problem exists?"

To the helpers:

- "How did you first get involved with this family?"
- "What is your present role in this family's life?"
- "What ideas do you have about this problem situation?"
- "What are you most concerned about?"
- "What question, if answered, could make the greatest difference to the future of this difficulty we're discussing right now?"
- "When you said that, what did you mean?"
- "Is there something that needs to be talked about that we have not touched on yet?"
- "What has kept that issue from not being talked about?"
- "What question would you like to ask now?"
- "If our success were completely guaranteed in resolving this problem, what bold steps might we choose to take?"

Self-Reflexive Questions

Self-reflexive questions (Kegan & Lahey, 2009; Scharmer, 2007; Bohm, 1996; Schon, 1983; Senge et al., 1994, 2005) can aid hosting therapists in paying closer attention to how their own emotional reactions, beliefs, and opinions block them from being totally open to all possible viewpoints that are generated in the context of family–multiple helper meetings. All hosting therapists and participating helpers bring to collaborative meetings assumptions about the cases with which they are mutually involved. Our assumptions can block us from truly hearing what others are saying and from entertaining new ways of looking at a case. According to Bohm (1996), we need to "suspend our assumptions, so that we neither act on them nor suppress them. Suspension is helpful in that it creates a mirror so that you can see the results of your thought" (p. 25). We can ask ourselves these questions as a form of private dialogue during the meeting or when reflecting to ourselves immediately after the meeting. Examples of self-reflexive questions include the following:

- "What has really led me to think and feel this way?"
- "How might my comments have contributed to the difficulties in our meeting?"
- "What unhelpful assumptions am I making about [a particular helper]?"
- "How has my voice of judgment and cynicism prevented me from listening respectfully and deeply to what certain helpers are saying?"
- "What were my intentions in this meeting?"
- "What prevented me from behaving differently?"
- "By having this meeting, did I achieve the results I was intending?"
- "What differences did this meeting make for the family?"
- "As a result of this meeting, did the family appear to leave feeling empowered, or did it not seem to make much of a difference to them?"
- "If I had an opportunity to replay this whole meeting over again, what would I have done differently as the host facilitator?"

Case Examples

A Case of the LD Blues

Victoria Smith brought her 11-year-old son, Sebastian, in for therapy for his "aggressive behavior" toward peers, "poor grades," and "low self-esteem" because of his "learning disability" problem. The Catholic school that Sebastian attended had threatened to kick him out because of his "aggressive tendencies," "mischievous ways," and "failing grades." The Smiths had been to "five therapists" prior to seeing me. Victoria was convinced that Sebastian's behavioral difficulties were "at the root" of his "feelings of inadequacy," caused by his alleged "visual-perceptual processing deficit," which had been "identified through testing by the district psychologist" when Sebastian was in the third grade. Victoria's key question for years had been: "Has the visual-perceptual processing deficit caused Sebastian's low self-esteem?" When I explored past treatment experiences with Victoria, she made it quite clear to me that none of the former therapists could "provide answers" to her question, nor could they develop a "relationship with Sebastian." In some ways the latter problem became a negative self-fulfilling prophecy that had been perpetuated with every new therapist. I, too, experienced great difficulty connecting with Sebastian. He refused to say a word to me, even when I met with him alone. The use of humor and the miracle question (de Shazer, 1988) proved to be fruitless with Sebastian. By the end of the session, the best I could do was ask Victoria to experiment by "not mentioning a word about school to Sebastian for a whole week." She had agreed that "hounding him daily about doing his homework" tended to lead to "arguments" and made matters worse. After our collaborative strengths-based family assessment session, Victoria was eager for me to talk with Sebastian's teachers, the school principal, and their pediatrician, who was also concerned about Sebastian's situation. Victoria and Sebastian signed the consent forms so that I could collaborate with the school personnel and the pediatrician.

As my office was not too far away from the school, the art, gym, and homeroom teachers agreed to come there for our first collaborative meeting with Victoria and Sebastian. Because of scheduling problems, neither the school principal nor the pediatrician could attend this first meeting in person but were available to be put on the speaker phone at various times. After brief introductions, I invited each of the helpers to share his or her story of involvement and concerns about Sebastian. In the school context, only the homeroom teacher had some positive things to say. Despite Sebastian's "testy" behavior at times, the homeroom teacher shared that she thought Sebastian possessed "excellent assertiveness skills" and was a "natural-born leader." I noticed that a slight smile appeared on Sebastian's face after his homeroom teacher acknowledged his strengths.

In responding to Sebastian's nonverbal response, I asked him whether he thought his homeroom teacher wanted to "join his fan club." For the first time, I got Sebastian to laugh and respond. He pointed out that he liked his homeroom teacher the most. Suddenly, the art teacher voiced a strong desire to "join Sebastian's fan club" as well. Sebastian appeared very surprised by his art teacher's response. He asked her, "Why would you want to join? I'm getting an 'F' in your class." The art teacher responded by complimenting Sebastian on his "artistic abilities when he applies himself." She also pointed out some ways that Sebastian could "pick up" his grade. Despite the positive interactions between Sebastian and two of his teachers, this was not newsworthy to the gym teacher or the principal. Although the gym teacher began by complimenting Sebastian on his "athletic abilities," he switched gears to tell how Sebastian was a "big troublemaker" and often "does not follow the rules." The principal chimed in that there is "no other child" he "sees more" in his office than Sebastian. Sebastian cried out, "You never have anything good to say about me!" Victoria defended her son and put the principal on the spot by asking him to give her son "a chance" and "stop beating his self-esteem down all of the time." The principal was silent for a few minutes and made it clear that he didn't like "playing the heavy" and "would love" to see a reduction in Sebastian's visits to his office. Sebastian pointed out that he didn't like to have to visit the principal either. Finally, the pediatrician had nothing but praise for Sebastian's talents and good qualities.

We scheduled a follow-up meeting 4 weeks later. The mother hugged and kissed Sebastian at the end of the meeting and told him how proud she was of him. Both the art and homeroom teachers patted Sebastian on the back and said they would help him in any way they could. The Smiths and I decided not to meet until our next collaborative meeting.

Four weeks later, we met as a group at the school. The pediatrician could not attend because of his hectic schedule. Across the board, the multiple helpers had only glowing reports about Sebastian's behavior. The district psychologist had retested Sebastian, as a new attendee, and reported in our meeting that he could not find any signs of learning deficits or problem areas for concern. All the teachers reported that Sebastian was "well behaved," "cooperative," and "showed good self-control" when provoked by peers. Both the gym teacher and the principal were astonished by Sebastian's complete behavioral turnaround. Victoria pointed out that his behavior had improved at home and he seemed "much happier these days." We all agreed that we could hold off on scheduling another group meeting because Sebastian had made such tremendous progress behaviorally and academically. I ended up seeing the family two more times, and therapy was successfully concluded.

As a result of the family–multiple helper meetings, new narratives were generated about Sebastian's alleged learning disability handicap and being perceived as the big troublemaker at school. An alternative preferred story was coauthored in our first collaborative meeting that described Sebastian as being a natural-born leader, being artistic, possessing excellent assertiveness skills, and having good athletic abilities. Sebastian was empowered by our meetings and did a nice job of asserting himself, which challenged his mother's long-standing belief that her son was "paralyzed emotionally" by his "low self-esteem." It was also a newsworthy experience for me to witness the spontaneous and assertive dimensions of Sebastian.

A Little Daredevil

Cedric, a 10-year-old African American boy, was court-referred for treatment because of his long history of "shoplifting" from "toy stores" and such school behavioral problems as "mouthing-off" to teachers and other school personnel and "stealing from students." Cedric had been adopted by the Hineses when he was 3 years old. The adoptive parents knew very little about Cedric's biological parents. Because they were unable to bear their own children, they were thrilled to get Cedric. However, they described Cedric as being "difficult to raise since day one" and as always being "a little daredevil." Cedric was constantly testing their limits and engaging in "temper tantrums," and he began stealing from them at the age of 8. "Yelling at him" and "taking his toys away" proved to be ineffectual in curtailing those behaviors, which continued to the present day. In school, he was constantly in the principal's office, which eventually led to his being placed in a behavior-disordered (BD) program in the school district. According to the parents, Cedric associated with "older" peers in the neighborhood who were "up to no good." One time, the mother came home after work and found Cedric and these "older boys" on the roof of their house. Finally, Cedric had been caught a few times by store security guards trying to steal "Game Boy" computer toys. The last time Cedric got caught, the store owner pressed charges.

Cedric was tough and very precocious. He acted more like a 16-year-old. He appeared to be very street smart and shared with me when I met with him alone that he mainly hung out with older kids in their midteens. I asked Cedric how I could be helpful to him. Cedric's main complaints were that his parents always went through his "bedroom drawers looking for things" and his probation officer made "surprise visits" to his house and school. I played Columbo with Cedric and asked, "What could your parents possibly be looking for in your bedroom?" He responded with, "Oh … Game Boys." I shared with Cedric how confused I was about what he did with all the Game Boys he had taken. I asked him if he stole them for friends or sold them for money. Cedric was quite open with me and reported that he did both. We related well to each other, talking about how much each of us liked Michael Jordan and the Chicago Bulls basketball team.

After reconvening with the family, I explored their thoughts on whom I needed to collaborate with. The parents suggested the probation officer, the school social worker, the principal, and their church pastor, who was very concerned about Cedric's behavioral problems. Family members signed the appropriate consent forms. The initial treatment goals were for the parents to experiment with "not going through Cedric's bedroom drawers for a week." Cedric agreed to reconnect with a friend his own age and "stay away" from the "older friends" with whom he tended to get into trouble. I also shared with Cedric that I would help get his "probation officer off his back." Cedric was happy that I was willing to help him out with the probation officer. Because I had a good working relationship with the probation officer, I could easily negotiate with him to help my clients.

Present at our first collaborative meeting were Cedric, his parents, the school social worker, the probation officer, and the pastor. The principal made it quite clear to me on the telephone that he had already "wiped his hands clean of Cedric" and had no time to attend after-school meetings. After everyone shared his or her story of involvement with this case, the pastor began with a minisermon about how worried he was about Cedric's "ending up in a street gang" if he didn't change. The parents chimed in that they thought it might already be "too late by the looks of some of the older boys Cedric runs with." Cedric took a risk with the group and disclosed that he used to run with "Anthony and Leon," who were both members of the "Disciples" street gang. He had cut off contact with them because they used "drugs" and "beat up" kids in the neighborhood. Out of curiosity, I asked Cedric if Anthony and Leon had anything to do with his stealing Game Boys. Again, Cedric took a risk with me and the group and disclosed that they had threatened to "kick" his "ass" if he didn't steal for them. This information proved to be quite newsworthy to all the participants in our meeting. They had no idea that Cedric was being "bullied to steal for the gang members." Out of concern, the probation officer offered to intervene on Cedric's behalf with the two gang members. He also shared his plan to "let the judge know the truth" about Cedric's "shoplifting" situation at the next court date. Cedric thanked the probation officer and shared with the whole group how "scared" he had been about "getting caught stealing" and the gang's coming after him if he "quit doing this" for them. The school social worker and the parents offered to help out with support and protection. For added protection, the pastor offered to hook Cedric up with an African American community leader who was respected by the street gangs. He also pointed out to the group that Jesse, the community leader, "coached a basketball team" for kids around Cedric's age. Cedric got excited about this and left our meeting more hopeful and in good spirits. The next scheduled collaborative meeting was for 6 weeks later.

During the interval break, I saw Cedric and his family twice. The parents reported that Cedric was being a "good boy" and "following" their "rules" and had "stopped stealing." Another important change was that the parents "did not receive one call from the school" about Cedric's problem behavior. Cedric also met Jesse and began attending his basketball practices to help "keep him off the streets."

Six weeks later, I met with all of the helpers, the Hines family, and Jesse. Across the board, all the helpers and Jesse had glowing reports to give about Cedric's progress. The parents also shared in front of the whole group how pleased they were with Cedric's progress. Mrs. Hines brought a large cake that she had baked for the group as a token of her appreciation for all of their "kindness" and "help" with Cedric. Even the school principal, who was originally so skeptical and pessimistic about Cedric's ability to change, became a true believer that the "new responsible Cedric" was here to stay. We mutually agreed to meet one more time as a group in 3 months.

I ended up seeing Cedric and his family four more times over a 6-month period. Cedric's behavior continued to improve both at home and at school. His mother no longer referred to him as a little daredevil; instead, she used the words "responsible young man" to describe him. Cedric had become one of Jesse's "star" basketball players. Cedric also got let off of court supervision 3 months earlier than the judge originally ordered because of his tremendous progress.

As readers can clearly see, by actively collaborating with the involved helpers in the child's social network, rapid and quite dramatic changes can occur in one or more group meetings. Doing and thinking collaboratively can make treatment much more efficient and effective. Margaret Mead summed it up best when she said: "Never doubt that a small group of committed citizens can change the world; indeed, it is the only thing that ever does" (in Vandenberg, 1993, p. 91).

9

Collaborating Successfully with School Professionals

In the long history of humankind (and animal kind, too) those who learned to collaborate and improvise most effectively have prevailed.
—CHARLES DARWIN

Normally both the problem- and solution-maintaining patterns of interaction that occur at home also extend to the child's interactions with fellow students, teachers, and other school personnel. However, what is first brought to the parents' attention by teachers and school officials are the child's negative and disruptive behaviors, often labeled as "ADD," "attitude problems," "bipolar tendencies," "autism spectrum disorders," and the like. Once these narratives begin to serve as the dominant story or central explanation for the child's behavior in school, any encouraging, responsible, or positive steps that he or she takes that counter or contradict these descriptions often go unnoticed because they do not accord with the emerging consensus at school. As a way to help introduce qualifiers or counterplots to the dominant story and provide a more complete picture of how the child actually functions, parents are well advised to keep open the lines of communication and to actively collaborate with their child's teachers and other concerned school personnel. Some parents have no difficulty in calling or meeting with teachers and other concerned school personnel when necessary, while others may feel uncomfortable doing this and would prefer that their therapist serve as the bridge builders from the home to the school. The bottom line is that when parents have strong cooperative and positive relationships with their children's teachers and other involved school personnel, behavioral and serious academic difficulties are least likely to occur. Once contacted by a parent, school social worker, psychologist, or school counselor about a particular child, I find it advisable to schedule a family–school collaborative meeting at the school either prior to the initial family assessment or the week following it—whichever the family prefers. That approach affords me with a wide-angle perspective on the child's behavioral difficulties in both settings, enabling me to learn from the teacher and other involved school personnel their overall assessment of the problem situation. Bringing the family and school personnel together early on also conveys to all participants the importance of collaborating on a common solution since it may be newsworthy to the school personnel to learn that the child's problematic behavior is occurring not only at school but also at home.

In this chapter, I describe ways of promoting teamwork among the client and his or her parents, teachers, and other involved school staff members to co-construct solutions together. I first describe some guidelines for how therapists can foster cooperative relationships with teachers and other school personnel and tap their expertise in the solution construction efforts, and present some highly effective family–school team tasks or exercises that directly or indirectly involve the child. I then present a solution-oriented family–school team meeting format that can be used in the context of either individual meetings or teacher team meetings. Finally, two case examples of successful family–school helper collaboration are detailed at length.

Guidelines for Fostering Cooperative Relationships with Teachers and Other School Personnel

I present four practical guidelines on how therapists and school professionals can establish a strong partnership in their work with challenging at-risk children and their parents. Once cooperative relationships are in place with the teachers and other involved school personnel, positive results can occur quite rapidly with at-risk children, largely resolving their problematic behaviors at school as well as their difficult interactions with parents and other family members.

1. *Familiarize yourself with schools in the vicinity of your practice by having informal lunch meetings with teachers, school psychologists, social workers, counselors, principals, and the heads of parent–teacher associations.* One highly effective way to begin fostering collaborative and cooperative relationships with teachers and other school professionals is by arranging with the head of the school social work or counseling department or the school principal a lunch meeting at a time when many members of the school staff are available to meet. In this informal setting professional rapport can be established, and the therapist can explore with school personnel some of

the challenging student behaviors or difficulties they have experienced with parents that they might like some help with. The therapist should share with the school professionals his or her own training background and specialty areas and cite the overriding importance of active collaboration in the event of any referrals.

As part of this dialogue, it is instructive to first find out what has worked best in previous collaborations with therapists in the community and the school professionals' expectations of outside therapists, that is, the frequency of meetings and telephone contacts. Finding out about prior worst-case scenarios (i.e., where there was minimal to no collaboration or open lines of communication, or where a split had occurred, with the therapist and family opposing the school) is also useful. Two common pet peeves that school professionals report are therapists who leave referring school staff members totally in the dark about their subsequent disposition of referred cases and therapists who conspire with parents against school officials, exacerbating differences unnecessarily. The therapist should end his or her get-acquainted session by inviting more such meetings in the future and by addressing any concerns school staff members might have. I also offer to make free presentations on managing disruptive behaviors or any other behavioral difficulties they would like help with.

I have also found it beneficial to offer free presentations to parent–teacher associations and have informal lunch meetings with PTA officials as well. The parents can specify what parenting and child topics they would like to learn more about; in return I learn about some of the challenges and concerns they struggle with daily.

2. *When beginning the family–school collaborative process, take a one-down "not knowing" position and use curiosity.* As therapists, we need to avoid at all costs coming across as privileged experts parading our esoteric knowledge before the teachers and other involved school personnel. Instead, we must adopt a one-down "not knowing" position and be truly curious (Selekman, 2005; Anderson, 1997; Fisch et al., 1982). It is helpful to first listen to the teacher's and other involved school staff members' stories about how they view the child's behavior and their theories of change (Murphy & Duncan, 2007; Selekman, 2005; Hubble et al., 1999). The parents are then invited to share their views, concerns, and needs. Next, map out on a flip chart or blackboard how the teacher and other school professionals typically respond when the child acts up and track the whole circular sequence of events. Not only may this be the same problem-maintaining pattern of interaction that occurs at home with the parents, but also all the participants involved see how their attempted solutions are inadvertently exacerbating the very behaviors they want to see changed. Furthermore, this exercise offers the family–school collaboration team several focal points

around the problem life-support circle to disrupt the problem-maintaining pattern. Since those enumerated may not be their only attempted solutions, I want to elicit from the teacher and other involved school staff officials everything they have tried to do to resolve the child's challenging behaviors, including in particular problem-solving strategies that seemed to help a little bit as well as what they were doing even before the objectionable behavior began. This important information can be used in the co-construction of solutions together.

3. *View teachers and other involved school professionals as the experts and allies in the solution construction process.* When I collaborate with teachers and other school personnel, I want to know not only what they are currently doing to prevent the child's behavior from getting much worse but what seems to be helping even a little bit that we may want to increase. In addition, I want to find out about their past successes at resolving similar students' behavioral difficulties, as this may serve as a blueprint for resolving the student's current behavioral difficulties. In addition, if I have implemented with the family a ritual or change strategy to resolve similar behavioral difficulties at home, I will recommend to the school professionals that we also use it at school. By doing so, we are able to effectuate change in both settings simultaneously and usually more rapidly than otherwise.

4. *Identify and utilize the services of the child client's adult inspirational other(s) in the school to the maximum extent possible.* When working with children and adolescents, I ask them the following question: "Are there any adults outside the home that you turn to for advice or support when you are stressed out or worried about anything?" More often than not, the child identifies a teacher or other school staff member with whom they have established a meaningful relationship and who cares about him or her. It is this or these *adult inspirational other(s)* that can help co-create a solution that enables the child to overcome his or her presenting problem(s) (Selekman, 2005, 2009; Anthony, 1984). Once identified, the adult inspirational other(s) can join the family–school collaboration team if not already involved. With the parents' and child's approval and written consent, I regularly involve adult inspirational others also in my family therapy sessions.

Occasionally, the child client is unable to identify an adult inspirational other in their life, and I will involve another child's adult inspirational other to fill this void in his or her life. This is particularly helpful when, for whatever reason, they are very emotionally disconnected from one or both of their parents and desperately need some caring adult in his or her life to have a strong and meaningful emotional bond with.

Family–School Team Interventions

In order to co-create long-lasting changes across multiple systems, it is advantageous to encourage family–school team tasks. There are a number of therapeutic experiments that are typically employed in individual and family therapy sessions with the child and his or her family that can also be implemented in schools. By making the solution construction process truly collaborative, the whole helping team eliminates outmoded views and abandons unsuccessful problem-maintaining actions. I present below 10 highly effective therapeutic tasks that can be extended to classroom and school settings.

The Teacher as a Supersleuth Detective

Most teachers who have challenging at-risk children in their classes get so stuck and frustrated about how to manage these children's difficult behaviors that they become completely oblivious to the times when they are behaving better, even if only for short periods of time. *The teacher as a supersleuth detective* experiment helps the teacher to view all of the child's behaviors, good and bad, with a wide-angle lens. The therapist can share with the teacher the following:

> "I have learned a lot from you today about _____'s difficult behaviors that you would like some help with changing. Now, in order for me to have a more complete picture and better understand the patterns of these behaviors, I would like you to do an experiment for me over the next week. I would like you to pretend to be like the supersleuth detective Miss Marple [for female teachers]/Sherlock Holmes [for male teachers] and pull out your imaginary magnifying glass and carefully observe daily in class for any positive, encouraging, and/or responsible steps you see _____ take and what you are specifically doing during those times that may be promoting those behaviors when he or she is behaving *better*. Please write down all of your important observations, clues, and hunches about what works, and we can review them when we get together next week."

Not only do stuck and frustrated teachers discover that their difficult students are not always having problems but that they are already using certain strategies or have generated some new ones that are promoting the kinds of positive behaviors they want to see more of. Their narrow and outmoded original views of the children shift, which leads to a change in their interactions with them. Once we identify what the teacher is doing that works, we want to have him or her increase these constructive ways of responding.

Pretend the Miracle Happened, or Being Zapped by a Magic Wand

In the initial family–school collaborative meeting, as part of the goal-setting process and a way to co-create possibilities together, it is helpful to ask the *miracle question* (de Shazer, 1988, 1991). How the school professionals benefit from this miracle inquiry is that they bear witness to the child's testament regarding how he or she sees him- or herself changing and also offers them guidance about how they should be doing things differently to help the child resolve past behavioral difficulties. Just talking about the kind of future reality all parties involved would like to have often triggers positive emotions, laughter, and playfulness among the helper group. The added bonus is that when the child, teachers, or others involved are asked "Are any pieces of the miracle already happening a little bit now?," often they will remember recent glimmers of progress when the child was behaving better or performing better academically, or liked the way he or she was being treated, or said or did something encouraging. In such cases, the therapist facilitator of the meeting should immediately inquire what the teacher or other school professional specifically had done to elicit the better behavior. The parents should also share their positive observations of miracle-like behavior from their child and what they might have done to contribute to its emergence. There may be certain parental actions on the home front that work quite well that the teachers could usefully implement in the classroom with the child.

As one of the proposed family–school team tasks, the child, parents, teachers, and other involved school personnel can pick 2–3 days over the next week to engage in each other's "miracle" behaviors without letting the other(s) know that they are doing so (Selekman, 2005, 2009; de Shazer, 1991). They are instructed to carefully notice how the others respond to them on those days. If they find that their miracle-like actions are producing really positive responses from others, they should increase the time that they engage in these new actions.

With younger children, I use an imaginary or toy magic wand and have them zap themselves, the parents, teachers, and other involved school personnel to find out what kinds of changes they want to see for themselves and everyone else involved. In a similar fashion but with simpler language, I tell the child and all other parties to pretend as though they have been magically zapped over the next week and individually to monitor closely the changes in their behavior and how it helps them improve their relationships and resolve the presenting problem(s).

The Secret Surprise

The *secret surprise* (Selekman, 2005, 2009) tasks (discussed earlier, in Chapter 6), is very similar to "pretend the miracle happened." During the family–school collaborative meeting, I have the child step away momentarily so I can meet alone with the adults. I then invite the parents and school professionals to come up with two surprises they can spring on the child that will shock him or her in a positive way over the next week. These need to be surprises that the child will really notice and appreciate. Furthermore, they are not to tell the child what the surprises are—he or she will have to play detective and figure them out. The results of this experiment will be discussed in the next family therapy session, family–school collaborative meeting, or via telephone conversations with the teachers or other involved school personnel. Prior to concluding the meeting, the child is brought back in and told that there are going to be some positive surprises happening over the next week both at home and at school and he or she will have to play detective and try to figure them out. The child is also told that everyone involved will be eager to discover what a great detective he or she makes. This is a fun and playful experiment that often triggers positive emotions, generates solution-building interactions in key relationships, and promotes better behavior from the child.

This format can also be reversed, with the child creating the positive surprises in his or her relationship to parents, in the classroom with the teacher, or out of class in his or her relationship to other involved school professionals. The adults involved end up playing detective and trying to figure out what the surprises were. I have consistently gotten good results using either format.

Do Something Different

The *do something different* experiment (de Shazer, 1988, 1991; Selekman, 2005, 2006, 2009), introduced earlier (in Chapter 4), is incredibly effective in disrupting the child's rigid and entrenched problem-maintaining patterns of behavior both at home and at school. Common traps that parents, teachers, and school authorities fall into in their interactions with the child are: being "superresponsible," thereby relieving the child of responsibility for his or her actions; engaging in threats or lectures; pleading with the child to cooperate and change; viewing the child's negative behaviors as being "manipulative" and therefore inconsistently intervening; and on the home front using bribery (awarding the child with material items) to get him or her to do homework, get better grades, or behave better in school.

I have successfully used the "do something different" strategy in family therapy, and it can also be equally effective in the classroom, particularly after the teacher has tried more conservative and straightforward approaches and is stuck doing *more of the same* in his or her attempts to eliminate behavioral problems. In a meeting with the parents, the teacher, and/or the assistant principal, the therapist can explore whether the parents have experienced similar challenging behaviors with their child at home. If so, both the parents and the teacher can experiment with the "do something different" experiment both at home and at school. They are told that they are too predictable in their typical responses to the child when he or she acts up. Accordingly, the next time the child breaks home or school rules, does not cooperate with directives, fails to complete tasks in class or bothers other students, or fails to complete homework assignments, they are to respond differently than their usual course of action—no matter how absurd or off-the-wall their responses are, so long as they are different from anything the child has ever experienced from them before. Not only does this dramatic experiment disrupt long-standing problem-maintaining patterns and strengthen parents' and teachers' reflective skills in sizing up the problem and determining what options to pursue, but also it can confuse the child and promote more positive behaviors from him or her.

Sometimes I reverse this strategy and have the child experiment with doing something different in response to the teacher that will "blow his or her mind" in a positive way. Usually I discuss possible options with the child in session prior to his or her implementing creative ways of acting differently in response to negative teacher behaviors he or she has been complaining about to parents or to me in our family sessions.

The Imaginary Time Machine

The *imaginary time machine* (Selekman, 2005, 2009) is one of the most versatile therapeutic tools that can be used with virtually any presenting problem, at any stage of treatment, and in any setting. As the case examples in Chapter 5 demonstrate, the other bonus with this experiment is the child's exhibiting for the parents and interested others his or her inventiveness or creativity in using the time machine to generate solutions for the current difficulties. Some children go back in history and connect with such historic figures as Ben Franklin, Pocahontas, Martin Luther King, Abraham Lincoln, and the like, presumably seeking to access important words of wisdom and ideas to help them resolve their current difficulties. In fact, I often have the child invite their historic figure to join us in our family–school collaborative meeting. Using an empty chair, I have the child pretend that his or her historic figure is there as an adviser or guest consultant to offer us some fresh ideas. Through this fun and imaginative process, the child is able to generate some additional practical strategies for resolving his or her problem situation.

Another way to use the imaginary time machine strategy is to have the child hop into the time machine and take it to the future, where he or she is now a senior in high school or a first-year college student. He or she has come by the school to visit the former fifth- or sixth-grade teacher to let him or her know how well he or she is doing academically and in his or her life. This use of the time machine is particularly effective with chronic situations where the child has a long history of behavioral difficulties and the current situation has been very negative for the child, parents, teacher, and assistant principal. Having the assembled adults experience the child's envisioning a bright future for him- or herself gives everyone pause momentarily, enabling everyone to summon up fresh hope that together they can co-create a context for change. The therapist can invite the child to try to identify the steps he or she took to be successful in school. One or more of these steps can serve as initial treatment goals in helping him or her get on that road to success, "starting today."

We also can have the teacher hop into the time machine and go back to a time earlier in the school year when the child was not only behaving better but academically doing better as well. The teacher is asked to reflect on what the child was doing differently back then that helped him or her behave and perform better academically—and also what the teacher was doing differently to promote this positive behavior. We can then dialogue with the parent(s), child, teacher, and interested others about what useful practices or remedies from the past can be reinstated to try to ameliorate current difficulties.

Invisible Inventions

Similar to the imaginary time machine, *invisible inventions* (Selekman, 2005, 2009) can tap the inventiveness and imagination powers of the child to generate creative solutions to his or her presenting problems, as illustrated in the case examples cited in Chapter 5. The child is asked to use his or her imagination to invent a machine or gadget that would benefit other children. Once the child comes up with his or her invention, he or she is asked to draw it on paper and describe specifically how it would benefit other children—or even adults, like his or her own parents or teachers. Often both the teachers and parents are amazed not only by the child's creativity but also by the practical uses of the inventions, some of which can be put into action with the child's current school difficulties. An added bonus and fun part of performing this experiment is that the children like to go home and try to build their inventions with their parents. Another positive outcome of this playful experiment is that it showcases the child's competencies and the desire to improve his or her behavior and/or academic performance, which can challenge the parents', teachers', and assistant principal's outmoded beliefs that he or she does not want to change.

The Habit Control Ritual

The *habit control ritual* (Selekman, 2005; Epston, 1998; Durrant & Coles, 1991) can be quite useful for children being pushed around by "attitude problems," ADD, stealing issues, anger problems, and other school disruptive behaviors, as illustrated by the case example in Chapter 5. This exercise is quite effective with chronic and oppressive behavioral difficulties that seemingly have a life of their own. What is most important when externalizing the child's problem is that it is co-constructed from the language used by the child, parents, teacher, and assistant principal in describing the problem and their beliefs about why they think it exists. As part of the family–school team and with written consent from the client's parents and the friends' parents, the child is invited to include his or her closest pals to serve as members of the family–school team as well. The child's pals often come up with some very creative ideas for frustrating and outwitting the client's oppressive problem. Next, the therapist has to summon up from the members of the family–school team sufficient emotionality to get them fired up to work together as a team to conquer the problem. A chart can be developed to keep track of the family–school team's victories over the problem and the problem's victories over them. The members of the family–school team can identify criteria that would indicate that the problem is lurking about or starting to push the child around. They are to keep track of what specifically they do (useful self-talk and effective problem-solving strategies) to stand up to the problem and achieve victories over it. Conversely, they also need to keep track of the problem's victories over them and how it still outsmarts them at times. Strategy meetings are scheduled both at home and at school to determine where they need to tighten up with the structure and what they need to increase doing to weaken and achieve more victories over the problem. On the home front, I have the child and parents work out together to get themselves in better shape to contend with the challenges— both mental and physical—that the problem presents to them. Usually, after a few weeks of using the habit control ritual, dramatic changes occur in the child's behavior and in school officials' conceptions of that behavior.

Pattern Intervention

Another effective way to disrupt problem-maintaining patterns at school is to invite the teacher to track for you the whole circular chain of responses, beginning with his or her response to the child's acting up, then the child's response to the teacher's actions, then what the assistant principal does, how the child responds to that, how the parents respond once contacted, and then how the child responds to the parents' involvement. Mapping this procession of responses out on a flip chart enables all the parties involved to see graphically his or her part in keeping the circular problem life-support system intact. It may be newsworthy for parents, teachers, and interested others to see visually how, despite their best efforts to resolve the child's difficulties, the very same problematic behavior they want to see eliminated is not only maintained but often made worse. In this context, the child can no longer be viewed in isolation as the problem; rather, everyone's attempted solution also figures in the mix (Watzlawick et al., 1974).

Once we have the circular map diagramed, *pattern intervention* strategies (Selekman, 2005, 2009; O'Hanlon & Weiner-Davis, 1989; O'Hanlon, 1987) can be used to disrupt the problem-maintaining pattern that the child's behavior is embedded in. We can do the following: change the order of various persons' involvement; add something new to the context in which the problem occurs; prescribe and "schedule" the child's problematic behavior to occur at different times, for different durations of time, or in different locations; or in other ways make it an ordeal for the child to engage in his or her problematic behavior.

Splitting the Team

Another type of pattern intervention that can be used with oppositional defiant children is to *split the team* (Selekman, 2005; Papp, 1983). The therapist and/or the teacher take the side of the child, while the assistant principal and other involved school staff can predict that the child will have behavioral difficulties on specific days or times during the coming week. Sometimes parents will divide themselves up, one forecasting a better school week for the child and the other being skeptical and predicting some bumps in the road over the following week. Oppositional defiant children love proving skeptical adult authority figures wrong, which can consciously motivate them to engage in more positive and prosocial behaviors in response to this challenge. Predicting slips in general is great for relapse prevention—for two reasons. First, it helps keep clients on their toes, making better choices and doing more of what works to stay on track. Second, if the therapist or skeptical parents or school professionals were accurate in predicting slips, it would indicate that the child needs to make better choices. It also is important to reassure the child, parents, teacher, and other involved school professionals that occasional setbacks go with the territory. Armed with such assurances, members of the family–school team will not view slips or setbacks as being disastrous occurrences or an indication that we are back to square one.

Writing Letters

One powerful way to generate change and help foster cooperative relationships among parents, children, teachers, and interested others is by writing selective letters. As the old adage goes, *there is nothing more powerful than the written word.* Children's parents can play an integral role in resolving teacher–child conflicts and improve the quality of their personal communications by taking the time to write the teacher a caring and thoughtful letter about their commitment to remedying their children's challenging behaviors and academic difficulties through mutual teamwork.

In the letter, the parent conveys empathy and support for the teacher in an admittedly tough job, one made not any easier by the subject child's difficult behaviors. The parent points out that even at home the child engages in objectionable behavior that is unacceptable. Finally, the parent shares in the letter that the parent has given the child a special assignment to do in the teacher's class today, namely, to play detective and carefully notice two to three things that the teacher does that he or she really likes and come home and tell the parent what the positive things were that the teacher did. The letter is then signed by the parent after acknowledging his or her best wishes to the teacher, put in an envelope and sealed, and hand-delivered by the child to the teacher. Not only does this letter channel positive emotion into the conflicted teacher–child relationship but both the child's and the teacher's views of one another can dramatically change, which will help them to communicate with each other in a more positive way. In addition, the teacher really appreciates the parent's backing him or her up and expressing the need to work together in remedying the child's behavioral and academic difficulties.

Letters in the opposite direction are just as useful and welcome. In clinical and school situations where the parents are very negative and the child is living in the shadow of an older sibling whose success story at school or in extracurricular activities is well known, occasional letters from the teacher regarding the younger child's academic and behavioral strivings can have a positive affect on the parents and help them see him or her in a new light. Teachers that I collaborate with in these clinical situations quickly pick up on the angelic–devil divide between the scapegoated younger child experiencing behavioral problems and the star sibling to which he or she is constantly compared. Such teachers see the value of using letters to acknowledge the child's behavioral and academic improvements as an effective way to inject positive information into the parents' minds and challenge their negative and unhelpful beliefs about the child. Some teachers have gone the extra mile by inviting parents in to see some of their children's high-quality classroom work and even provided parties after school for the parents and their children to celebrate (in some cases, along with selected pals) their gains or achievements.

Solution-Determined School Team Meetings

Although most schools go to great lengths to try to involve parents more in important decision making regarding curriculum development and planning activities at the school, and strive to create school climates that are healthy and intellectually stimulating for their children, there are still some important planning meetings and conversations among teachers and school officials from which parents and children are deliberately excluded. Two such meetings are *teacher team meetings* and *individualized education planning meetings*.

Teacher Team Meetings

When teachers have their team meetings, they rarely invite parents or children to sit in—even though the latter are being talked about and important decisions are being made regarding what the teachers think is best for a particular child. The focus in these meetings is usually exclusively on the child's behavioral difficulties and learning issues rather than what is *right* and working with the child. If these meetings sought to empower children, teachers would spend more time talking about what they are specifically doing that brings out the best in a child and how they could increase these solution-building patterns of behavior. For teachers who feel stuck about how best to manage a particular child's challenging behaviors, peer teachers who had similar students in the past could share their problem-solving strategies that worked.

Ideally, a family representative should be invited to relevant teacher team meetings to share knowledge about what works best with the child at home, to consider the ideas and concerns that the teachers express, and to be involved in the action planning process. Having a parent participate in relevant teacher team meetings would help keep the lines of communication open from the school to the home, and if difficulties were to arise at school, the parent would be actively involved in the problem-solving effort.

Individualized Education Planning Meetings

Throughout my professional career, I have sat in on numerous individualized education planning meetings (IEPs) where neither the parents nor the child had any real input into the goal formulation process and choice making in terms of what services they thought could best meet their needs.

Typically, parents are never asked such questions as "Do you think your child can achieve that goal? What do you think would be a smaller but more realistic goal? What do you think of the overall plan? Are there any specific support or remedial services that you think your child could benefit from?" The professionals sitting around the table ultimately decide what *they* think is best for the child. In many cases, the goals that are established in the IEP are too lofty and vague to be realistically achievable. Thus, children are thereby set up to fail.

In contrast, a *solution-determined* individualized education planning meeting would look very different. The parents and child would be invited to determine their goals and share their expectations about how the teachers and other school personnel could help them best in achieving their goals. The parents and child could indicate how they would know when they achieve their goals and specify the indicators for teachers and other school personnel to look for. They should have the lead voice in determining which special school services and programming options they would like to pursue. Finally, if anyone anticipated any obstacles to achieving these goals or implementing the change strategies successfully, the teachers and other involved school staff should join forces with the family to remove these barriers to help ensure the child's ultimate success.

Case Examples

In this section, two case examples are presented that illustrate how to establish successful collaborative relationships with teachers and other school personnel. In both examples it was the close and strong family–school teamwork that made the critical difference in the treatment outcomes.

Is It Symbiosis, or Is He Just an Emotionally Sensitive Boy?

TELEPHONE INTAKE CONVERSATION WITH THE SCHOOL SOCIAL WORKER

Haim, a bright and precocious 11-year-old boy, was referred to me by Ellen, the social worker at his private elementary school, for problems with anxiety, somatic complaints that included upset stomachaches, and frequent visits to the nurse's and principal's offices to get them to call his mother to come pick him up when he was not feeling well or in the midst of conflicts with some of his teachers. According to Ellen, "this pattern of Haim's behavior and his mother, Barbara, coming up to the school to rescue him and fight his battles started a few weeks after the new school year began." She described Haim's relationship with his mother as being "symbiotic," and she thought that he might be experiencing "separation anxiety."

In my efforts to learn more about Ellen's school and Haim's teachers, I asked her to fill me in. Ellen explained to me that at her school the children are team taught to help provide them with a well-rounded Jewish educational experience. The two teachers that Haim had the most trouble with were Mrs. Goldberg, his Hebrew teacher, and Mr. Weinberg, the gym teacher, who both had been teaching at the school for close to 25 years. Ellen pointed out to me that she was constantly putting out fires between these two teachers and Haim and Barbara. Barbara would call them up to complain about their teaching styles and mistreatment of her son and then call Rabbi Schwartz, the principal, to complain about the teachers as well. He, in turn, would ask Ellen to try to mediate the conflict. Ellen shared with me that this was "one of the biggest stressors and headaches" of her job at the school.

In regards to the teachers' complaints, Mrs. Goldberg contended that at times Haim was disruptive in class, talking to fellow students when she was giving a lesson, and he tended to complain about stomachaches whenever he did not understand the classroom material. One day she decided to move Haim into the front row of the class to try and stop him from talking, and he immediately objected that he did not think that was fair. Attempting to discipline him, she was unsuccessful in gaining his cooperation and soon had to send him to the principal's office. His mother, Barbara, was contacted and came to the school fuming; in this instance, the principal got Haim to go back to Mrs. Goldberg's class and take his new seat for now. Barbara then demanded that the principal talk to Mrs. Goldberg about trying to handle Haim in a better way, noting that he was an "emotionally sensitive" boy.

In Mr. Weinberg's gym class, Haim would often display his stubborn side by either refusing to participate in certain activities he did not wish to engage in or going through the motions but not putting forth his best efforts. These actions caused Mr. Weinberg to yell at him, and his fellow students also would get mad at him for not trying and causing them to lose team games. In one gym class, after Mr. Weinberg yelled at him loudly, Haim walked out of the class crying and went to the principal's office to complain. Haim succeeded in getting the principal to call his mother, who, in turn, came to the school fuming about "Mr. Weinberg's abusive behavior" toward her son. Haim continued to cry and asked his mother to take him home. Later that day, the principal confronted Mr. Weinberg about this incident and requested that he talk with Ellen to learn some new methods of working with challenging children like Haim. Ellen shared with me that not only did she feel stuck with the management of this situation but so did Rabbi Schwartz. This is what led to her referring Haim and his family to me with the hope that I could also offer consultation to the school professionals involved with him.

FIRST FAMILY THERAPY SESSION

Although Ellen had offered us some potential dates to have a collaborative meeting at the school with her, Haim's teachers, and the principal, Barbara wanted to have a family therapy session first before meeting at the school. Present at the first family interview were Haim, Barbara, and her husband, Noah. Zeva, the 18-year-old daughter, could not attend because she was away at college. Haim was very close to Zeva and missed her. In addition to this family life cycle transition and loss, Barbara had shared that she lost her mother to cancer right around the same time Zeva was moving out to go to college. Her mother was a cigarette smoker who, even after being diagnosed with lung cancer, continued to smoke. This had been a major stressor and worry for Barbara. Haim also was close to his grandmother and was saddened by her death. When asked if Ellen and Haim's teachers were aware of these two significant losses, Barbara shared with me that she had not told them.

Barbara shifted the conversation to the problems with Mrs. Goldberg and Mr. Weinberg, complaining that she felt at times that Ellen and Rabbi Schwartz would take the teachers' sides and not support her or Haim. Barbara went on to say that Haim was a "very emotionally sensitive boy," and if the school staff would "take the time to get to know him better and treat him in a more gentle way," they would bring out the best in him. Noah interjected that he agreed with his wife that the teachers should be kinder to Haim, but in his opinion it did him more harm than good for her to come to the school and confront the teachers and take their son out of school. He noted that Barbara and Haim were very close and that Haim had been a big support to his mother in trying to cope with his grandmother's smoking, death, and Zeva's moving out, adding "He's a good Mama's boy." Barbara started to cry and said that she felt a real emptiness in her life after losing both her mother and Zeva. Haim got out of his seat and went over to hug and comfort his mother. She shared that her father had died from a stroke 5 years earlier. In fact, after these two losses, Barbara became a "homebody" and put both her social life and working on the "back burner." I shared with the couple that it might be helpful, in eliciting more compassion and support from Haim's teachers and the other school officials, if they were aware of the emotional pain and sadness she and her son were experiencing. Both parents agreed that sharing this information might help them to establish a more collaborative partnership with the school staff. Finally, Barbara mentioned that it had also been especially hard over the past few months with having Noah out of town because of his business. Both parents and Haim agreed that I should arrange a school meeting with Ellen during the following week. I recommended that we arrange for some of Haim's other teachers to join us for the meeting to hear their perspectives on the situation, as well.

Haim had been very quiet and respectful while his parents shared their stories. I asked him how he had been experiencing the school situation, particularly his interactions with Mrs. Goldberg and Mr. Weinberg. He described Mrs. Weinberg as being "very stern and mean." I asked him what specifically he would call "mean." Haim shared that she told him to move up to the front row of the class without any explanation; he found this to be "very embarrassing," and a few of the male students had "teased" him about it. She also would yell at him "loudly" when he would be "talking in class." He further added that she was a "hard teacher" and she expected students to "learn Hebrew at a fast pace." When asked if there was anything he did like about Mrs. Goldberg, Haim did say that it was interesting to hear all of her stories about having lived in Israel for a long time and all of her unique experiences there. In fact, hearing all of these interesting stories about Israel contributed to his own strong desire to visit Israel in the future. I asked him if he had ever shared these sentiments with Mrs. Goldberg, and he said he had not. I made a mental note to encourage him to share this important information with her before or after class one day.

The two things that Haim disliked about Mr. Weinberg was his "yelling" and "making students do hard workouts and activities" that Haim found to be "too challenging." Haim admitted that Mr. Weinberg's yelling scared him—even when he yelled at *other* students. Apparently, Mr. Weinberg was a tall and muscular man. Haim shared how sometimes he got stomachaches in class when he was feeling nervous around Mr. Weinberg. I asked him if his stomach had a voice and could talk during those times, what would it say? Haim said, "Mr. Weinberg is so angry—what if he hits me or another student?!" Although the parents were alarmed to hear that, they never had any concerns that Mr. Weinberg would ever hurt a student. During this discussion, Noah admitted that sometimes when his own temper flared up at home and he yelled at Barbara in front of Haim, it really scared him. Although there were no reports of family violence, Haim did share that sometimes he worried that his father might get so mad that he would go on a work trip and then never return. Barbara interjected at this point that, while she and Noah did sometimes have heated arguments, she nonetheless felt that they were happily married. She also reassured Haim that there was "nothing to worry about losing Dad." Haim smiled and hugged his mother. At the end of our meeting, I told everyone that I would get back in touch with them as soon as I was able to schedule a school meeting.

FIRST FAMILY–SCHOOL COLLABORATIVE MEETING

Present at the first family–school meeting were Ellen, Rabbi Schwartz, Mrs. Goldberg, Mr. Weinberg, Mrs. Goldblatt (the science teacher), Mr. Rubin (the history teacher), Barbara, and Haim. Noah could not attend because he was out of town on business. We began the meeting with introductions, which I found to be very instructive. Haim's two favorite teachers, Mrs. Goldblatt and Mr. Rubin, began the meeting by sharing what a "bright and outstanding student" he was—a "real delight" to have in their classes. Haim naturally had a big grin on his face. Barbara thanked the teachers for saying such nice things about her son. Urging the teachers to share their expertise in bringing out the best in Haim in their classes, I invited them to share what specifically they did that enabled him to do so well in their classes. They related that they just interacted with him in a relaxed way, using humor and inviting him to share his thoughts and to ask as many questions as he wished to about the course material. This approach appeared to keep him engaged and enabled them to build a positive relationship with him. They both asked Haim about what they had just shared to get his feedback. Haim agreed with what the teachers had said and added that he really appreciated not only how they made their subject matter interesting but also how they had treated him in a "nice and kind way." Mrs. Goldberg asked both Mrs. Goldblatt and Mr. Rubin if they had experienced any problems with Haim's talking in class, not being cooperative, or asking to go see Rabbi Schwartz. Neither Mrs. Goldblatt nor Mr. Rubin could think of even one time in their experience when they had observed those behaviors. Mr. Weinberg wondered if they had ever had any problems with Haim's complaining of stomachaches. Again, neither teacher had had this problem in their classes.

I took a risk in the collaborative meeting and decided to tap Haim's expertise about what he thought might help him and Mrs. Goldberg and Mr. Weinberg to have a more positive working relationship in the future. Barbara blurted out, "Treat him nicer and be gentle with him!" I asked Barbara to hold off for a moment until we had heard from Haim. I decided to ask Haim a hypothetical question for each teacher. First, I asked him, "If we were to pretend that you were Mrs. Goldberg, how would you try to work with a student like Haim?" Haim shared with Mrs. Goldberg that "I would try to refrain from yelling at him, help him if he was having trouble with learning Hebrew, and share more of my wonderful and interesting stories about Israel with him and the class." Mrs. Goldberg turned to Haim with a surprised look on her face and shared that she did not know that Haim liked to hear her stories about Israel so much. Haim told her that her stories were what he liked most about her class. Next, I asked Haim, "If we were to pretend that you were Mr. Weinberg, how would you try to work with a student like Haim?" Haim shared with the group that if he were Mr. Weinberg he would be more aware that the student was nervous and scared around him—which gave the student stomachaches, especially since Mr. Weinberg was so large and prone to yelling. Also, Haim said that he would notice that the student was not that great at sports and try not to put so much pressure on him to perform well in sports activities. Mr. Weinberg shared with

Haim and the group that he had no idea that he had been scaring Haim, and he felt really bad about it. He shared with Haim that he really would try to lighten up on the pressure and work on his habit of yelling in class. He also requested that Haim pull him aside either in or after class and let him know if he was doing anything that was upsetting to him. Mr. Weinberg added that there were a few kids in Haim's class who acted up and were not good listeners and that sometimes he had to yell at them to get them to stop misbehaving. Barbara, taken aback by Mr. Weinberg's graciousness, gushed that she was pleased to hear him offer to help make gym class a much more positive experience for Haim.

Both Rabbi Schwartz and Ellen shared how frustrating it had been trying to resolve the conflicts and difficulties occurring with Haim, his mother, and the two teachers at hand. They conveyed their hope that, thanks to this meeting, there would be more teamwork among all the parties and that if problems did recur they would be positively and constructively resolved immediately. I pointed out that often how conflicts and difficulties worsen is that the parties involved fail to communicate what their needs are, share specific action steps to remedy the situation, and genuinely listen to one another, preferring instead to listen to their own thoughts or to cling to their narrow assumptions about the other parties involved. Everyone around the table agreed that communications had really broken down in the past and the attempted solutions employed had only added more fuel to the fire; everyone also agreed that, going forward, they would try to work together as a team to resolve Haim's difficulties. We scheduled our next family–school collaborative meeting for 1 month later.

SECOND FAMILY–SCHOOL COLLABORATIVE MEETING

Present at our second family–school collaborative meeting were Ellen, Rabbi Schwartz, Mrs. Goldberg, Mr. Weinberg, Mrs. Goldblatt, Mr. Rubin, Barbara, Noah, and Haim. In 1 month's time considerable progress had been made. Mrs. Goldberg and Mr. Weinberg both acknowledged that Haim was doing extremely well in their classes. According to Mrs. Goldberg, Haim was no longer talking in class, he had been much more cooperative, had not asked to leave the class even once, and his grasp of the Hebrew language had greatly improved as well. Haim agreed that he and Mrs. Goldberg were getting along much better. In fact, she had loaned him a beautiful photography book on Israel that she thought he would enjoy looking at. Haim shared with her that he really appreciated that and thanked her again. Noah chimed in, "Thanks to you, he is putting pressure on us to take him to Israel!" Everyone laughed. Mrs. Goldberg shared with the group that she really missed not living there because it is such a special place.

Next, Mr. Weinberg shared with the group that he was impressed with how hard Haim had been working in gym class to master sports fundamentals and was even evolving as a leader. Apparently, he did a stellar job as the captain of his dodge ball team, leading them to victory. Haim shared that he was discovering that he was not such a bad athlete, after all. Mr. Weinberg asked Haim if he had noticed that he had cut back on his yelling in class. Haim complimented Mr. Weinberg on toning down the yelling and treating him nicer. Barbara shared how pleased she was to hear that things were so much better all around. In fact, Noah mentioned that Haim had confided to him the other day, "Mr. Weinberg is not such a bad guy!" Mr. Weinberg smiled and voiced his hope that Haim might discover *other* positive qualities about him in the future. Both Rabbi Schwartz and Ellen reported that, although they missed not putting out fires with Haim, Barbara, Mrs. Goldberg, and Mr. Weinberg, they appreciated that everyone was working together so well as a team. Mrs. Goldblatt and Mr. Rubin chimed in that Haim continued to be one of their top students. I complimented the school staff for all of their great efforts in working with the family and myself in rapidly turning this situation around. We all mutually agreed to continue the close teamwork and to schedule a future meeting only if there was a need for it.

LAST FAMILY THERAPY SESSION

I ended up seeing Haim and his family one more time 1 month later to amplify and consolidate their gains. Barbara opened up the session by saying that she had finally resumed working out at the health club regularly and getting together with friends for lunch and shopping most days. Noah had been around a lot more, and he and Barbara shared a few "nice dates" together. He also took Haim to his first Chicago Bulls basketball game. They had a great time together. In fact, Haim was wearing his Chicago Bulls hat at the meeting! According to Barbara, things were going great at school for Haim. He reported that he was getting along much better with both Mrs. Goldberg and Mr. Weinberg. We mutually agreed to terminate the therapy.

A Resilient Child Breaks Free from the Aftershocks of Family Violence

Benny, a 7-year-old biracial only child, was referred to me by a former client who attended the same Narcotics' Anonymous (NA) group as his mother, Cassandra, who was a recovering heroin addict. Benny was having difficulties at school and at home. On the telephone prior to my setting up the first family therapy session, Cassandra shared with me that her ex-husband was in jail for drug dealing and repeated domestic battery charges. Apparently, Benny had witnessed his father, Lonnie (both when intoxicated on cocaine and/or alcohol and even when sober), batter Cassandra. Child protection authorities had gotten involved after the local police had contacted them after the first domestic disturbance. Once Lonnie was incarcerated and Cassandra had stopped using heroin and gone through drug rehabilitation, the child protection caseworker closed their case. However, the aftershocks of the past family violence continued to haunt Benny. He was having night terrors and experiencing grave difficulty in sleeping alone, leaving his toys all over the house, acting "very clingy" with Cassandra, and at school experiencing learning difficulties with math, spelling, and reading. Additionally at school, he was having difficulty both staying on task and sitting still for extended periods of time, and was allowing a fellow student, Winston, to bully him. Apparently, Benny began having more difficulty with his learning issues after Winston started bullying him. His main classroom teacher, Miss Terry, recommended to the mother that he be assessed for ADD with hyperactivity. Miss Luce, Benny's special resource teacher, was not totally convinced that Benny had ADD. Cassandra took him for a comprehensive evaluation at a clinic that specialized in ADD, and the psychologist made a positive diagnosis. Despite this conclusion, Cassandra still felt that Benny did not totally meet the criteria for this diagnosis. Because of this, Cassandra decided not to pursue treatment for Benny with this psychologist, and she contacted me for another opinion. In ending our initial telephone conversation, I shared with Cassandra that it might be helpful for the teachers to know what she and Benny had been through to help them better understand him and his behavior. She agreed with me that it was better to bring this up without Benny present during our first school meeting.

FIRST FAMILY SESSION

I began the first family interview getting to know Cassandra and Benny by their strengths and talents. Cassandra, now a librarian in a public library, regularly attended NA meetings, had been abstinent for 5 years, was very close to her older sister and parents who lived out of state, was a devout Christian who regularly attended church, and enjoyed spending quality time with Benny. As I watched her interact with Benny, Cassandra struck me as a very loving, caring, and committed parent.

Benny was a very handsome, energetic, and loving boy. Cassandra shared that he was a very fast runner and excellent athlete for a boy his age. She also shared that he had a great sense of humor and could be a big helper around the house. Benny and I connected while swiveling around in circles together in my swivel office chairs. We also bonded while playing together on the floor with toy cars and small figurines of people and animals. He laughed when I would have animals driving cars.

The main areas of concern that Cassandra wanted help with were to reduce Benny's clingy behavior so she could have a little more space and time to take care of herself and cook dinner after work and for Benny to be able to stay in bed at nighttime. I reviewed with Cassandra all of her prior attempted solutions. When frustrated and tired after work, Cassandra tended to react by yelling and pleading with Benny to give her space, sometimes even locking herself in her bedroom; she also would place him in front of the TV for long periods of time, and at bedtime she would need to lie with him until he fell asleep. On the school front, Cassandra had had numerous telephone conversations and meetings with both of Benny's teachers, and she greatly resented that they were unable to stop Winston from bullying her son. In fact, Cassandra complained to the assistant principal, Mrs. Grant, about the Winston situation, but she felt emphatically that nothing had been done to remedy the situation.

Although Cassandra could not identify any pretreatment changes after I had asked her the miracle question, she was able to assure me that reducing Benny's "clingy behavior" and enabling him to stay in his own bed would definitely result in her yelling a lot less and being much more relaxed. With Benny, I handed him an imaginary wand, and he zapped his mother with it so she would yell less and play board games and go to the playground more often with him. At school, he would zap Winston with the magic wand so he would stop trying to hurt and tease him and be nicer to him. When asked about how that would make a difference for him at school, Benny shared that he would be less scared and he would learn better in class.

I asked Cassandra if she had instituted any reward system or bedtime ritual for Benny. Cassandra had put into place a star chart system that had worked for a few weeks, and then Benny returned to his clingy behavior, making messes with his toys throughout the house, and not staying in bed at nighttime. When asked if she had made any changes or deviated from the system in any way, Cassandra said that she had been very consistent. As far as bedtime rituals went, she would turn off the TV well before Benny's 8 o'clock bedtime and have him brush his teeth, wash up, and put his pajamas on, escort him to bed, and kiss him goodnight. I shared with Cassandra that other parents that I had worked with usually had their child take a warm bath and then would read to the child right before saying goodnight. Cassandra thought these suggestions sounded good and said she would try to implement them. I also told her that, in helping children to wind down in the evenings at the end of the day, it paid to reduce the amount of TV viewing and video game play as well as sweets and caffeinated beverages like soda pop. Cassandra admitted that sometimes, out of just needing a break, she allowed Benny to have too much time in front of the TV and playing with his Game Boy in the evenings. She also acknowledged that she never thought about how sweets like chocolates and soda had a lot of caffeine in them, which could also contribute to Benny's being too wired before bed-time.

Over the next week, Cassandra was asked to play the role of detective and keep track of what she did whenever Benny was less clingy, put his toys away, and stayed in bed at nighttime, and to celebrate those sparkling moments with him when he was more self-sufficient and capable of tolerat-ing being apart from her. She also agreed to eliminate evening sweets like chocolate and soda pop altogether from his diet, substituting natural fruit drinks when necessary. Cassandra also planned to try the warm evening baths and the daily ritual of reading to him in bed right before saying good-night. Prior to ending the session, I made a fun game out of turning my back to Benny and slowly moving clockwise while he surprised me by putting my office toys in the box that were strewn all over the floor. This was a great opportunity to model for Cassandra how to make taking responsibility a fun activity and that she could use this strategy at home with Benny. Benny set a land speed record of putting all of the toys back in the box faster than any other kid I had ever worked with! I made a big deal about this, and Cassandra hugged and kissed Benny. We ended the session with Cassandra signing a consent form so I could collaborate with the teachers and Mrs. Grant.

FIRST FAMILY–SCHOOL COLLABORATIVE MEETING

Present at the first family–school collaborative meeting were Cassandra, Benny, Miss Terry, Miss Luce, and Mrs. Grant. Introductions were made and the purpose of the meeting was discussed. Cassandra shared what her best hopes were that would come out of the meeting. At the top of her list were putting a stop to Winston's bullying and teasing of Benny, getting the teachers more familiar with Benny's strengths, and helping him overcome his learning difficulties. In response to Cassandra's concerns about Win-ston, Miss Terry had spoken to both Winston and his mother about his behavior and felt stuck about what to do. Mrs. Grant asked, "Why did you not come to me about this?" Miss Terry had felt that she could handle the situation. Cassandra shared that she had mentioned this problem once before to Mrs. Grant, but nothing had happened. Mrs. Grant replied that she must have gotten in touch with Winston's mother, but then possibly forgot to follow up. She made a commitment to resolve this problem by speaking to both Winston and his mother together soon after our meeting. Cassandra emphasized that it seemed to her that Benny's behavioral and academic difficulties had worsened considerably since Winston had begun harassing Benny; both Miss Terry and Miss Luce agreed with this obser-vation. Miss Terry shared her thoughts about Benny having ADD, with hyperactivity as well. At this point, I thought it might be helpful to have

Benny step out of the meeting while labels were being bandied about and to make it more comfortable for Cassandra to share some of her and Benny's past painful story with the school staff. As Cassandra began to share her story she started to cry; she voiced her strong desire to provide Benny with a better life and the opportunity to be successful in school. Miss Terry brought a box of Kleenex over to Cassandra and she, Miss Luce, and Mrs. Grant provided support and complimented her on her courage to share her story and persevere with Benny. I pointed out that having worked with other children who had lived in violent households, I knew that the aftershocks could be long-lasting and affect the child's behavior and learning abilities. I added that, considering what Cassandra and Benny had been through, they seemed very resilient and things could be a lot worse for Benny. Both the teachers and Mrs. Grant agreed and thanked Cassandra for helping them to better understand what Benny had been through and to make better sense of his academic struggles in school. The school staff could see how Winston's bullying behavior was reactivating Benny's worst nightmares about not feeling safe and getting hurt.

At this point in the meeting, Mrs. Grant and Miss Terry wanted Benny back in the room to share with them the specific times during the school day when Winston had tried to hurt and tease him. According to Benny, Winston tended to bully him the most both "on the playground" and in the "gym locker room." Mrs. Grant said that she would talk to Mr. Cooper, the gym teacher, so that he could more tightly monitor the locker room times. Miss Terry shared that she would be more vigilant on the playground for any difficulties with Winston. Mrs. Grant assured Cassandra and Benny that she would not stand for any violence occurring at her school and would take care of this problem with Winston immediately. We all agreed to meet in 1 month's time to assess progress with the school situation.

SECOND FAMILY–SCHOOL MEETING

The participants attending our second family–school collaborative meeting were Miss Terry, Miss Luce, Mr. Cooper, Mrs. Grant, Cassandra, and Benny. Across the board, all of the teachers had glowing reports about Benny's behavioral and academic progress. According to Miss Terry and Miss Luce, Benny was much more focused, able to stay on task, less fidgety, and better able to sit still for longer periods of time over the preceding 3 weeks. Miss Terry shared with the group that she was now questioning her original theory about ADD being the problem. Miss Luce pointed out that Benny had made considerable progress in the academic areas he had been struggling with. Benny was beaming from all of the praise he was receiving. Mrs. Grant shared with the group that she had resolved the Winston bullying situation with him and his mother by threatening possible suspension if he did not get his act together. Since her meeting with Winston and his mother, she had not heard of any further bullying or teasing episodes. Both Miss Terry and Mr. Cooper also indicated that Winston had not been observed on the playground, the boys' locker room, or anywhere else in the school bullying or teasing Benny or any other students. Benny shared that—much to his surprise—Winston even apologized to him. Benny and his mother both thanked the teachers and Mrs. Grant for resolving the bullying problem. Because of Benny's great progress and because no other concerns were raised, the group unanimously agreed that we no longer had to meet, subject to change.

FUTURE FAMILY THERAPY SESSIONS

I ended up seeing the family two more times, with 4-week intervals between the sessions. Cassandra found that the combination of eliminating candy and desserts and soda pop from Benny's diet, reducing TV and Game Boy time in the evenings, and giving Benny a warm bath and reading to him each night right before bedtime helped him to settle down a lot and to sleep through the night without visiting her. According to Cassandra, Benny was less clingy, more self-sufficient, and better able to respect her private time and space when she needed it. Benny also had made two new friends and was having more play dates, which offered Cassandra more break time after work to take care of herself. He also was now participating on a park district soccer team. Cassandra proudly shared that Benny was now reducing his time with his special resource teacher, Miss Luce, because he was making such great progress in math, spelling, and reading. Also, there were no further reports from Benny or his teachers about Winston bullying him anymore.

10

Establishing Successful Family-Oriented Primary Care Partnerships with Pediatricians

The wisest mind has something yet to learn.
—GEORGE SANTAYANA

Since the inception of health maintenance organizations (HMOs) and managed health care, pediatricians have been experiencing increased demands on their productivity, reflecting much more time required to fill out paperwork and to deal with insurance reimbursement issues, which in turn limits the amount of time they can spend with their patients. To compound the problem, the Surgeon General's Office has indicated that 20% of the children seen in pediatricians' offices typically have mental health problems with 11% of total patients evidencing significant functional impairment and 5% extreme functional impairment at home and in school and that there has been a 7–19% increase in children presenting with psychosocial problems over the past 20 years (Taras, Frankowski, McGrath, & Mears, 2004; U.S. Public Health Service, 2000; Briggs-Gowan, Horwitz, Schwab-Stone, Leventhal, & Leaf, 2000). Not only do many pediatricians feel ill equipped to make an accurate DSM-IV-TR diagnosis and treat these troubled children in their practices, but even in those situations where they felt qualified to make accurate diagnoses they often lack the time to provide high-quality treatment for the patients and counseling for their parents (Stein et al., 2008; Heneghan et al., 2008; Brunk, 2008; Viswanathan, Brucia, & Daymont, 2006; Brunk, 2008; McDaniel, Campbell, Hepworth, & Lorenz, 2005; Williams, Palmes, Klinepeter, Pulley, & Meschan, 2005; Hacker, Weidner, & McBride, 2004; Jellinek et al., 1999; Jellinek & Murphy, 1988).

Other dilemmas pediatricians grapple with is knowing where and to whom to refer their patients within the community and being able to keep the lines of communication open and maintain an ongoing collaborative relationship with the mental health providers they eventually select. Many pediatricians do not have access to human services directories of places in the community to refer their patients to or know of private practitioners in the community they service, particularly mental health providers who specialize in specific DSM-IV-TR childhood disorders or psychosocial problems. In some cases, pediatricians may have successfully referred their patients to the appropriate mental health provider but never heard back from the provider and wanted to establish an ongoing collaborative relationship with him or her. In other cases, it proved to be an arduous task just to talk on the telephone with the mental health provider because of conflicting schedules or having to go through several other staff people to reach him or her. Finally, some pediatricians have reported that the only way they were ever able to communicate with the mental health provider was via occasional faxed, if they were lucky, assessments or treatment updates (Viswanathan, Brucia, & Daymont, 2006; Williams et al., 2005).

Another stressor pediatricians grapple with today is the push from the American Academy of Pediatrics (AAP) to secure more knowledge and training in the assessment and treatment of childhood mental health disorders and behavioral health issues other than ADD/ADHD (Stein et al., 2008). Thanks to training opportunities sponsored by the AAP, pediatricians have and continue to receive empirically validated training in the assessment and treatment of ADD/ADHD. Both pediatricians and child psychiatrists agree that childhood ADD/ADHD can be successfully managed in pediatric settings (Stein et al., 2008; Viswanathan et al., 2006). Because of many pediatricians' lack of medical school and residency training in family therapy or in the assessment and treatment of childhood mental health disorders other than ADD/ADHD, Tolan and Dodge (2005) contend that pediatricians miss opportunities to prevent and intervene early in behavioral health issues that place children at risk for later and more serious problems.

Glenn (1987) has identified 10 types of situations in which collaboration with and referral to a therapist can greatly aid pediatricians (and other physicians) in establishing cooperative relationships with highly challenging patients and their families:

1. The patient's symptoms are not explained by medical findings.
2. The problem involves other family members.
3. The patient is noncompliant with medical treatment recommendations and/or with taking medication.

4. The physician is feeling overwhelmed by the emotional and relationship difficulties of the patient.
5. The physician is being triangulated into family relationship conflicts.
6. The physician is constantly in conflict with the patient over diagnostic and treatment issues.
7. The patient's problem coincides with a transitional event in the family's life cycle.
8. The patient's problem leads to the discovery of cancer, sudden changes in physical health, or in some other terminal disease.
9. There appear to be family secrets that are affecting the patient's functioning.
10. The patient exhibits emotional difficulties during the course of medical treatment.

Clearly, all of these clinical situations can be adequately addressed by therapy. It may also be beneficial to have the pediatrician (or physician) participate in the initial family therapy session to receive his or her input and expressions of support for the patient. Ongoing interest and involvement in the course of therapy is also to be welcomed. Throughout the course of family treatment, I strive to combine meeting with the pediatrician alone, having him or her join us when available or when a crisis or special concern with the patient occurs, and updating him or her on the telephone periodically about both the patient's and the family's progress.

In this chapter, I discuss several *unhelpful* assumptions that, if made by therapists, can prevent true collaborative partnerships from developing with pediatricians, and I present several good reasons why therapists and pediatricians should collaborate in behalf of referred patients or patients held in common. Finally, two case examples are provided that illustrate how collaborative teamwork with pediatricians can greatly benefit the therapist and contribute to positive treatment outcomes.

Why Do Therapists Avoid Collaborating with Their Clients' Pediatricians?: Some Common Reasons and Unhelpful Assumptions

In consulting with clinicians and mental health organizations worldwide, I often hear purported reasons why mental health professionals should supposedly avoid collaborating with their clients' pediatricians. I will discuss six common ones at length in turn, namely:

1. Confidentiality concerns.
2. Assuming pediatricians lack the knowledge and clinical skills to understand and treat contemporary childhood mental health disorders and behavioral health issues.
3. Assuming pediatricians will look down on therapists or not be interested in their clinical opinions.
4. Assuming pediatricians are too busy to collaborate (so why bother?).
5. Operating from a Cartesian–Lockean mindset in which there is a clear separation between the body and the mind: separate problems, separate treatments.
6. Assuming that seeing clients in pediatricians' offices will be too disruptive to the treatment process.

Confidentiality Concerns

Many therapists are concerned that, even with the requisite consent forms signed and privacy guidelines well understood by all, pediatricians may end up sharing client-divulged information with other patients, which could rupture the therapeutic alliance by diminishing clients' trust in their therapists. Therapists need to inform any new clients in their first family assessment session that the therapist will be collaborating with the client's pediatrician to ensure comprehensive high-quality care and support for them throughout the course of treatment. Therapists should also discuss in detail with their clients specifically what can and should not be shared with their pediatricians. They should also be upfront with their clients about what they find helpful to share and discuss with pediatricians, such as notes on diagnosis for insurance purposes, the effects of any medical condition or illness on the child's psychosocial functioning, the treatment plan and goals, case progress updates, and how they can work effectively as a team to benefit the client to the maximum extent possible.

Conversely, pediatricians are naturally concerned about sharing their patient information with therapists, largely because they fear that important medical disclosures made only to the parent(s) and not the child patient might inadvertently or prematurely be divulged to the child by the therapist. Such disclosure could damage the child, impair or even destroy the pediatrician–family relationship, and most likely lead to the end of any collaboration with the pediatrician. Just as in the initial family assessment, the therapist must know clearly from the point of referral from the pediatrician what medical information can or cannot be shared with the child patient and his or her parents. When and if the time comes to share privileged medical information more widely, the pediatrician should be present in the session and take the lead in this discussion.

Pediatricians' Lack of Knowledge and Skills to Treat Mental Health Discorders

Many therapists assume that pediatricians lack the clinical skills to accurately diagnose and effectively treat child mental health disorders and behavioral health issues. Some therapists may think that, apart from thanking the pediatricians for their referrals, it is a waste of time to have ongoing collaborative relationships with persons less experienced than themselves in addressing child mental health and/or family problems. First, therapists who adopt this attitude need to ask themselves, "How do I know that this highly concerned and involved pediatrician does not possess good assessment and treatment skills and couldn't aid me greatly in resolving this child's difficulties?" Second, therapists need to realize that pediatricians can be valuable resource people and allies to them; after all, they have known the child and parents much longer, may have important background information to impart, and may well have powerful leverage with the family, potentially facilitating the therapists' engagement process with the clients. Third, therapists need to view pediatricians as part of the solution-determined family–multiple helper system in not only addressing clients' concerns but also in co-generating solutions to their problems.

Pediatricians' Attitude toward Therapists and Their Clinical Opinions

Many therapists assume that most pediatricians and psychiatrists are so arrogant as to think themselves gods. Often, this erroneous and highly destructive assumption originates with past negative experiences therapists may have had with certain doctors throughout their professional careers. The truth of the matter is that there are just as many arrogant and know-it-all therapists as physicians. Clearly, research indicates that not only would pediatricians like to collaborate with therapists more but would also welcome the opportunity to have them join their staff and work in their practices (Clark, Linville, & Rosen, 2009; Viswanathan et al., 2006; Brazeau, Rovi, Yick, & Johnson, 2005). Clark and her colleagues (2009) found that 48% of their sample of 153 family physicians would refer to marital and family therapists to resolve their patients' psychosocial difficulties. Moreover, increasing numbers of pediatricians are recognizing nowadays that child mental health problems and behavioral health issues are on the rise and that—time-constrained as they are—referring these child patients and their families to a trustworthy and skilled in-house therapist or one in their community is a necessity that also best meets their patients' needs.

Pediatricians' Busy Schedules

While pediatricians are doubtless busier than ever these days with heavier patient loads and overwhelming demands on their time, they nonetheless have an abiding interest in both referred patients and patients held in common with preferred therapists, and, given a choice, they welcome continued collaboration and being kept "in the loop" of communications. They recognize they have much to contribute and much to learn from well-planned face-to-face collaboration in determining therapeutic outcomes for patients held in common with selected therapists.

A Cartesian–Lockean Mindset of Clear Separation between the Mind and the Body

Some therapists (and pediatricians, for that matter) operate in their own separate world with a Cartesian–Lockean mindset that has pervaded Western thought since the Enlightenment, one emphasizing a clear separation between the body and the mind. These practitioners fail to see the relationship between the increased incidence of stress and the proliferation of both mental health and physical health problems or even how high levels of family stress can exacerbate existing medical conditions in children and in some cases lead to life-threatening crisis situations. Prescriptively, Jeffrey Brosco put it best:

> In the future, integration of pediatric and behavioral health will require that systems of care do not perpetuate myths about the distinction between [the] two fields. ... It is clear at both a biological and psychological level that distinctions between physical and behavioral health are specious at best and generally impede attempts to maximize child health and well-being. (2003, p. 3)

Engel (1980) was the first to argue that to understand a patient's illness the therapist needed to attend to the interrelationships among biological contributions, the patient, patient and family interactions, the social contexts they interface with, and how all affected the development of symptoms and illnesses. He calls his model a *biopsychosocial* treatment approach. I would further expand Engel's biopsychosocial framework to include the interactions among family members, the therapist, and all of the involved helping professionals from larger systems.

In the family therapy field, Salvador Minuchin and his colleagues at the Philadelphia Guidance Center and Philadelphia Children's Hospital were the first family researchers to show the intimate relationship between family functioning and physiological processes. They called these families *psychosomatic families*. They found in their research that parental conflict is detoured, or defocused, through the chronically ill child, be it with diabetes, asthma, or anorexia nervosa (Minuchin, Rosman, & Baker, 1978). Campbell and Patterson (1995) found in their study that chronic family conflict, lack of parental teamwork, and low family cohesion have all been associated with poor diabetic management issues and crises with children.

Rolland (1998) has established a useful categorization of illness dimensions to help determine the impact of a particular medical condition on a particular family. The major dimensions include onset (whether acute or gradual), course of illness (progressive, constant, or relapsing), outcome (fatal or nonfatal), and degree of incapacitation. Each one of these dimensions and their many combinations put a particular kind of intensity and pattern of demands on the child patient and his or her family. According to Rolland, a careful assessment of these illness features helps to organize our clinical understanding of the psychosocial impact of a child's illness and the levels of adaptability, problem solving, role responsibilities, and family cohesion resulting from the illness.

Disruption to the Treatment Process

Depending on where in the pediatrician's office suite therapists typically see the pediatrician's referred patients, interfering noises may or may not be a problem. If the designated therapist's office is next to patient examination rooms, it may be very noisy. If the office is down the hall away from the examination rooms, and happens to be a conference room, it may be sound-proofed or at least the noise level is more manageable. Therapists should not get too hung up on the noise level because most clients tend to not be bothered by it and the engagement process is not hindered by it. There are three good reasons why therapists should choose to spend some or all of their clinical practice time working in pediatric settings. First, there will be a steady stream of referrals. Second, the shaman effect will be fully operative, in that clients generally trust their doctor and by extension his or her judgment in referring them to you. Thus, their expectation levels are elevated that the therapist will be able to help them to resolve their difficulties. Finally, these clients will be less likely to drop out of treatment, knowing that you are actively collaborating with their own trustworthy doctor.

Partnering Successfully with Pediatricians

Many pediatricians today not only welcome the opportunity to collaborate with mental health providers but also are open to adding, or have already added, psychologists and social workers as part of their practice team. Viswanathan et al. (2006) found in their survey sample of pediatricians that 88% believed that close collaboration was necessary with patients they shared with mental health providers in the community. Similarly, Brazeau et al. (2005) found that 60% of the physicians surveyed valued collaborative care and would consider having an in-house therapist in their practice. Ruddy, Borreson, and Gunn (2008) argue that physicians want to make referrals to mental health providers they know and who are committed to actively collaborating with them in providing quality care. However, many pediatricians as well as therapists do not think systemically enough and would not consider partnering, in part owing to some of the false assumptions outlined earlier.

Several advantages result from combining both professionals' knowledge bases and skill sets. For pediatricians, close collaboration with both in-house and community-based therapists offers them the opportunity to get valuable clinical experience and further develop their skills in treating mental health disorders and assessing family parenting issues. Research indicates that many physicians have not had coursework or specialized training in medical school or in their residency specifically devoted to diagnosing and treating children with mental health disorders (Stein et al., 2008; Heneghan et al., 2008; Viswanathan et al., 2006; Williams et al., 2005). Since pediatricians' severe time constraints make it onerous if not impossible for them to carry out comprehensive child mental health assessments and provide ongoing treatment, having on-site mental health providers as part of the pediatric team can successfully meet this need. Moreover, it may be a unique service offering in the community that helps attract referral sources and the public.

Mental health providers working in-house in pediatric practices enjoy such advantages as having a steady stream of referrals, patients' and their parents' trust and faith in their pediatricians can speed up the engagement process with them, and close case collaboration and teamwork with the pediatricians can make for high-quality comprehensive treatment for children and their families. Other bonuses include greater opportunities to learn much more about human physiology, disease processes, pharmacology, and the latest research on serious and life-threatening illnesses afflicting children.

Such brief therapy approaches as the collaborative strengths-based brief therapy (Selekman, 2009), solution-focused brief therapy (de Shazer et al., 2007; de Shazer, 1988, 1991), and the MRI (Mental Research Institute) brief problem-focused therapy (Fisch & Schlanger, 1999; Fisch et al., 1982) are the key therapeutic approaches most suited for use in fast-paced pediatric practices where large numbers of children are regularly seen. Since the main emphasis of these approaches is on nonsymptomatic periods—that is, when behavioral difficulties *are not* occurring—increasing clients' positive emotions and hope levels and building on *what works* for the clients to co-construct solutions can greatly reduce the length of treatment (when required), thus allowing for high volumes of clients (Selekman, 2009; Unwin, 2005; Park, 1997; Mauksch & Leahy, 1993). In addition, once they are well versed in using either the collaborative strengths-based brief therapy or the solution-focused brief therapy approaches, clients do not need to be seen for a full hour, but only for 30–40 minutes, making these approaches especially appropriate for pediatric practice settings. Furthermore, when using either approach, the therapist does not have to have everyone in the family present and actively participating in every session. In fact, what is most crucial to success is to have the most involved and concerned parent—that is, the true *customer*—working most closely with the therapist in implementing change strategies at home. The child client, of course, is perhaps the best agent of change for key relationships in the whole family.

Unwin (2005), a primary care practitioner in England, contends that solution-focused thinking and therapeutic strategies are the most ideal ones for his practice setting. He adopts the point of view that his office waiting room is filled with a *room full of heroes* rather than people with problems. He finds it to be much more empowering to his patients to focus on the present and future rather than the past and avoids at all costs inviting his patients to share any toxic or negative memories associated with their presenting problems.

Such family therapy approaches as strategic family therapy (Madanes, 1981, 1984; Haley, 1986, 1987) and structural family therapy (Minuchin & Fishman, 1981; Minuchin et al., 1978; Minuchin, 1974) also are ideal treatment models for pediatric settings in that they are short-term (12–15 sessions) and are efficient approaches for stabilizing children's symptoms and behavioral difficulties related to family and other psychosocial stressors. One of the main challenges in using either one of these family therapy approaches, however, is that it may be difficult to schedule all family members during the day for sessions if pediatric clinic evening hours are limited. Another option, of course, would be to see families on Saturdays.

Case Examples

In this section, I present two challenging case examples where the client child had a chronic illness that could become life-threatening unless constructively managed. Both cases illustrate that the child's physical health problems, which can be exacerbated by psychosocial stressors, are a powerful force in shaping family dynamics.

Seth's Dilemma

Seth, a Caucasian 10-year-old only child, was referred to me by his pediatrician, Dr. Stein, for family therapy. Dr. Stein had been Seth's doctor since he was a toddler and treated him for asthma. According to Dr. Stein, ever since Seth's parents divorced when he was 8, there had been intense conflicts and continued arguing between them. He felt that "Seth's dilemma" was that he was getting caught in the middle of the postdivorce parental battles and being forced to take sides, and as a result it was worsening his asthmatic condition. In fact, four times during the past year Seth had had to be taken to the emergency room of a local hospital after severe attacks. Seth had opened up to Dr. Stein a few times about how it upset him that "Mommy and Daddy could not be friends." He also shared with Dr. Stein that both parents had frequently said mean things to him about the other. Another problem reported to me by Dr. Stein was that at times Seth would fail to use his inhaler or even lose it; his breathing would immediately become labored, and the mother would rush him in for an emergency appointment. Finally, Seth's school grades were slipping as well. Dr. Stein had described Seth to me as being a very bright boy who was getting A grades in school up until the parents' divorce.

Typically, when starting up with families where there has been a divorce and I know there has been a lot of conflict, I explore with both parents if they think they can be civil and meet with me in the same room together. If they feel there is too much bitterness and conflict between them, I offer to see each parent separately and alone with the children. It is unproductive and not good for the children to watch their parents verbally attack each other in front of them. However, sometimes both parents will agree to meet with me together and be civil in front of their children, and they end up setting each other off and the session gets out of hand. In these situations, I carefully observe how the children react to their parents' bickering, whether they take sides, look and listen to their emotional and nonverbal responses, and take note of other physical responses. Next, I ask one of the parents to step out of the session and see him or her later either individually or together with the children.

FIRST FAMILY THERAPY SESSION

After contacting Seth's parents, Barbara and Mark, and exploring whether they could handle being in the same room with each other, they both agreed to maintain their composure, be civil, and try out a family session. When discussing the parents' concerns about Seth's challenging asthmatic condition and his academic decline, they started blaming each other. As the conflict and blaming intensified, I could see that physically Seth was laboring to breathe, and then when both parents observed what was happening with their son, they focused all of their attention on him and stopped their all-out verbal assaults on each other. Once Barbara reminded Seth to use his inhaler and he complied, he was able to breathe better and became more relaxed. At this point in the session, I said to Seth, "You did a heroic and courageous thing there to help your parents to stop hurting each other." I told him that I would now take over and help his parents out and that he no longer had to be the hero in this family story. Seth was asked to step out and wait in the lobby while I met alone with his parents.

I first shared with the parents that it might sound crazy to them, but children are benevolent by nature and they will go to great lengths, including placing themselves in life-threatening situations, to help their parents out. Barbara pointed out that Seth was an emotionally sensitive and loving boy. Mark agreed and asked me what he could do to help Seth out. I shared with Mark that it is just not "I" but "we"—meaning "you and Barbara as a team." I shared with the couple that research has demonstrated with children of divorce that when parents work together as a team, are civil and respectful toward each other in front of the children, share similar household rules and expectations for the children, and avoid forcing the children to take sides, the children adjust well and cope better with this stressful and difficult family change (Wallerstein & Lewis, 1998; Ahrons, 1994).

Next, I discussed with the couple their past successes with parental teamwork, both before and after the divorce. Both parents were able to identify a number of times prior to the divorce when they were able to discuss their disagreements peacefully and constructively manage Seth's asthmatic condition when there were problems. When asked about specifics regarding what made it possible to work together as a team in these situations, Barbara indicated that Mark would "listen to me" while "I made my points" and "not interrupt me." Mark shared that Barbara would "not put me on the defensive" by "blaming me for being out of town on business" and not being able to take Seth to "doctors' appointments" or "meet with his teachers at school." Barbara brought up a recent postdivorce severe asthma attack when Mark had just dropped Seth off after a weekend visitation, and a few hours later not only could Seth not find his inhaler, but also he was starting to turn blue because he was laboring to breathe. Barbara called 911 and Mark immediately. After Mark rushed over to the home and comforted Barbara, who was hysterical, he drove her over to the hospital—right after the paramedics arrived with Seth at the emergency room. Apparently the couple did not blame each other or argue even once about it after this life-threatening crisis situation with Seth. I complimented Mark and Barbara on working together so well amid the frenzy of crisis and underscored how this was teamwork at its best! Barbara thanked Mark for "being there and being so supportive." Rehashing this past successful event triggered positive emotions for both of them. Barbara added that, after Seth was stable and hospitalized for observation, "he seemed so happy to see both of us right by his bedside." According to the parents, there was absolutely "no tension or conflict," and it was "totally peaceful" in Seth's hospital room. I shared with the couple that this might be the recipe for success as a team, that is, by co-creating together in Seth's company an emotional climate that was healing and comforting. The parents agreed that they needed to establish a permanent truce—to lay aside their verbal arms and to re-create the kind of soothing emotional atmosphere that was possible when they were together for Seth. The parents asked me if I would be willing to continue to work with them to strengthen their cooperation and help them address other post-divorce issues, and we agreed to do this. Prior to the intersession break, I told the parents that I wanted to bring Seth back in and share with him that they had agreed to continue working with me to be better friends and a better team as parents. Seth, in response, not only looked greatly relieved but sported a big smile on his face. Seth shared with his parents that he had been "wishing for a long time" that they could "be friends."

After a 10-minute intersession break, I shared my editorial reflection with the family. I complimented the parents on their 180-degree turnaround during the session and for recognizing that they could be civil, respectful, and work together as a team. In fact, they had already found the recipe for success in co-creating the kind of emotional climate that most benefited Seth: no tension, conflict, or arguing, and providing a peaceful atmosphere when they were all together. I complimented Seth on his emotional sensitivity and for being such a fine, caring son that he would do anything to help his parents not argue and hurt each other, as in the past. I thanked him for agreeing to let me take over helping out his parents and said that he could now devote his time and energy to spending more time with friends and being the smart and great student that he was capable of being. In closing, I offered the family some experiments or tasks to try out between sessions: the parents were to continue to practice their teamwork and use their recipe for success with Seth; if one parent was having a bad day and started to blame or pick an argument with the other in Seth's company or on the telephone, they were immediately to pay close attention instead to how to void the blame game and keep track of what works; and I predicted to Seth that he might want to put on his cape again and be the family superhero if his parents slipped up and started arguing in his company. The family asked to meet again in 2 weeks. I had the family members sign consent forms so that I could work with Dr. Stein and Seth's teacher, Miss Brown, as all agreed that it would be helpful to involve these concerned helping professionals in our joint collaboration. They all felt quite comfortable in letting Dr. Stein and Miss Brown know more about their family dynamics and how they were all committed to taking steps to remedy Seth's difficulties.

INDIVIDUAL MEETINGS WITH DR. STEIN AND MISS BROWN

During the 2-week interval between therapy sessions, I met with Dr. Stein and Miss Brown separately. Dr. Stein was delighted to hear that Seth's parents were finally committed to working on their postdivorce conflicts and lack of teamwork in the parenting department. As Dr. Stein had detected earlier, Seth's asthma attacks often coincided with his parents' arguing or trying to involve him in their hostilities toward each other. I told Dr. Stein that I had gotten the parents' firm commitment to deal directly with each other in resolving their conflicts *without* involving Seth. Dr. Stein liked my strong emphasis on parental teamwork and keeping Seth out of the middle.

Miss Brown also was pleased that Seth and his parents were finally in family therapy. Seth had shared with Miss Brown on more than one occasion that it upset him that his parents "fought a lot" and were "not friends." She had noticed that he worried a lot, seemed preoccupied with family problems, and as a consequence was having difficulty staying on task and performing well on homework assignments and tests. I told her about my working closely with the parents to improve their teamwork and change the emotional climate in the family so that Seth could function better physically and at school. Miss Brown offered to personally provide additional support and reassurance if Seth needed anyone else to talk to. I was very impressed with Miss Brown's nurturing style and investment in her students' well-being.

SECOND FAMILY SESSION

I began the second family session by asking all three family members what further progress they had made. According to Barbara and Mark, not only did they refrain from having even one argument or from berating each other in Seth's company, but as a family they had gone "out to dinner twice" and everyone enjoyed one another's company. Seth enthused that he was really happy about the "fun family times" and his parents "being friends." I reacted with obvious amazement that the parents were able to pull this off. I asked them if they were aware of how they were able to take such a big step as a team. Both Mark and Barbara agreed to give their new parental teamwork additional test runs but to focus more of their efforts on maintaining Seth's happiness and physical health. I asked Seth what effects the two fun family dinners had had on him. He said he was feeling happier and more hopeful about his parents becoming better friends. Next, I asked everyone what else was better. Seth shouted out that he got an A on a science test. I asked him if Miss Brown had fainted after she discovered how well he had done on the test. Seth and his parents laughed. Seth said that he was able to pay better attention in class and overall do better. Both parents shared with Seth how proud of him they were that he was back on track at school.

I spent a short amount of time with the parents amplifying and consolidating their gains. I also wanted to cover the back door with the parents to keep them on their toes, so I asked them, "What would you have to do to go backward at this point?" They were clearly able to spell out what they used to do to upset each other and inadvertently place Seth in medical jeopardy. I then shared with them that slips "go with the territory of change" and are inevitable. I asked both parents, "What steps will you take individually if one of you caves into blaming or pushing the other's buttons to not allow the situation to get out of hand?" Both agreed that whoever was being attacked had to remain calm, not personalize what the other said, and not fight back. I agreed with them that whenever you don't have a sparring partner it is very difficult to do battle or keep a fight going.

I met alone with Seth to personally commend him on all of his great accomplishments. I also emphasized to Seth that I appreciated his faith in his parents' ability to be a team and to participate in going out to dinner as a family without feeling the need to be the family superhero again and do something dramatic either during the meal or beforehand. Seth shared with me that he could tell that his parents had really changed and that he was really happy about that. I brought the parents in before my intersession break to ask them where they would rate their progress on a scale from 1 to 10, with 10 being the situation is "better enough" and 1 that there is further work to be done. Both Mark and Barbara rated the situation at "a 7." To set a goal between now and the next family session, I asked the parents, "What are you going to do between now and our next session to get up one point higher, to an 8?" The parents agreed that they were committed to avoid arguing with each other, keeping the emotional climate positive around Seth, and would try more family outings.

During the editorial reflection portion of the family session, I underscored all of the family's changes and offered them a month-long vacation from counseling as a vote of confidence for their great work as a family team. I shared with them if they wished to do any work while on vacation that I wanted them to keep track of what they did that they would rate as an 8 or better. Just to keep the family on their toes, I shared with them that change can be a funny thing—it can be three steps forward and one step backward, but "that last step never means that we are back to square one." I reiterated that slipups do not have to be disastrous, and we can learn from them. I also shared with the parents that I was confident that they knew what to do if a slipup should occur. I wished them all a fun vacation and to continue to do what works.

TELEPHONE CONVERSATIONS WITH DR. STEIN AND MISS BROWN

During the family's vacation break from counseling, I updated both Dr. Stein and Miss Brown about the family's great progress. Both helpers were thrilled to hear how well everything was going. I shared with them that if the family came back from the counseling vacation break with a glowing progress report I might well explore with them the possibility of terminating if they felt okay with that. I let both of the helpers know that I have an open door policy and my clients could always contact me in the future for a tuneup or further work together if they needed it. I did not pick up on any hesitations or concerns from either Dr. Stein or Miss Brown about ending the counseling.

LAST FAMILY SESSION, WITH DR. STEIN ALSO PRESENT

The family came back from their counseling vacation reporting excellent progress. Dr. Stein also attended our third family therapy session. Barbara and Mark had not had even one argument. Seth's grades in school had continued to soar, and he was socializing more outside the home with friends. Barbara and Mark reported that they not only went out to dinner a few times as a family but also saw a Cirque du Soleil show together. Seth proclaimed that the show was "awesome!" I shared with the family how much I loved going to Cirque du Soleil shows as well. When asked what level on the scale they would rate their situation at this point, all family members shouted out "a 10!" Dr. Stein was delighted to hear about the family's great progress and remarked that they visibly looked happier as a family. He did a nice job of reflecting on how Seth and the family looked before family treatment had begun and how things were dramatically different now. After amplifying and consolidating all of the family's gains, we mutually agreed to terminate family therapy with the understanding that I had an open door policy if they should need a future tuneup.

Wrestling Back Control from "Worrying"

Chase, a precocious 8-year-old hemophiliac boy, was referred to me by his pediatrician, Dr. Walters, for family therapy due to concerns about his mother's "rigid pattern of overprotectiveness." According to Dr. Walters, Sylvia, Chase's mother, was constantly calling friends' parents and his teacher to make sure he was not placing himself in risky situations; she also maintained a watchful eye on him around the house. This rigid pattern of overprotectiveness had intensified after Chase fell off some monkey bars at a park while Sylvia was talking to another parent and briefly had her back to him. She called 911 immediately and accompanied him to the hospital. Ever since this calamity had occurred, Sylvia felt guilty and intensified her overprotectiveness with him. Dr. Walters was concerned about Sylvia—but even more about Chase's having his autonomy totally squelched. In fact, some of his friends had begun teasing him about his mother's treating him like a baby. Sylvia also sought to greatly limit Chase's participation in sports and certain play activities. Chase "pushed his mother's buttons" by rebelling against her wishes by playing certain forbidden sports and engaging in other activities she would not allow (e.g., skateboarding at a friend's house).

Sylvia had sacrificed her social life to be around more to supervise Chase. In spite of her constant worries about him, she had been able to maintain her administrative assistant position at a small business. His biological father had been out of the family's life since Chase was a toddler. Chase had a 15-year-old sister, Paula, whom he bickered with occasionally.

FIRST FAMILY SESSION

In the first family session, after getting to know all the family members by learning about their strengths and personal passions, I inquired what they all wished to change today. Sylvia loved cooking Italian food. I had discovered that Chase really loved to watch professional wrestling on TV. Paula shared that she liked to swim and got into Emo music.

When it came to discussing the problem situation, Sylvia took the floor first and stated that she wished that Chase would stop upsetting her and making her worry so much about him all of the time. I asked, "What specifically does Chase do that makes you worry the most?" She said, "He puts his life on the line by playing contact sports and engaging in other risky activities that I have outlawed!" Chase chimed in that he felt like his mom did not allow him to do anything fun. Paula confronted Chase by saying loudly, "You really need to be more careful and stop stressing out Mom!" Chase told Paula to "shut up!"

I shifted gears at this point in the session and decided to ask the miracle question. Chase said he would not have hemophilia, and he would get to do all of the fun things that his friends get to do. I shared with Chase I would wish for that too for him. I then asked him, "What else would you like in your perfect miracle picture?" Chase responded with "Mommy would not worry so much about me all of the time." I then asked him, "How would that make things better for you if she did not worry so much about you?" Chase shared that "he would be happy" and also "not worry about and get so mad at her." Sylvia responded with "If I stopped worrying so much, would you stop doing things that make me worry, like skateboarding and playing football with friends?" Paula interjected, "Yeah, you keep doing things to make Mom upset, and then I have to worry about her!" I asked Sylvia, "When you are worrying less about Chase's choice making and he is taking better care of himself, what effects would those changes have on you individually and in your relationship with him?" Sylvia shared that she would be "more relaxed" and would "stop calling his friends' parents and his teacher all of the time." I asked Chase what it would be like for him if Mom were more relaxed and did not have to worry so much. He said, "It would really make me happy, and we would get along much better." Paula shared that she would also like to see her mom "more chilled." I asked Paula to describe to me what a "more chilled" mother would look like. Paula said, "Less nervous and constantly checking up on Chase's well-being and, yes, maybe she would take more of an interest in me and my life for once!" Sylvia looked shocked to hear this from Paula. According to Sylvia, she had no idea that Paula had felt "short-changed" by her. Paula then said to her mother, "Yeah, that's right, Mother. It's always about what Chase is doing and, oh, I got to stop Chase from doing ... and Chase this and Chase that ... Well, what about me?!" When asked about any times lately or in the past when she felt that her mother was more available to her and there was more of a balance in her mother's relationships with Chase and her, she could not think of even one time in the past few years. In other words, she could not think of even one time when her mother checked in with her about her life and how she was feeling about things.

I decided at this point in the session to take a risk and address this mother–daughter conflict alone with the two of them. Sylvia told Paula that she was really surprised to hear this outburst from her. Paula disclosed that she had been keeping quiet about feeling this way because she did not want to further stress her out or have her worry about her too. Sylvia went over to hug Paula and tell her how much she loved her and to please let her know whenever she feels sad or neglected. I was curious to hear from Paula how keeping a lid on all of this emotion was affecting her mental outlook. She quickly replied that she had been feeling mad and depressed about it. Paula alarmed her mother by sharing that she had cut herself a few times to try to make herself feel better. She also said that sometimes she would deliberately go out of her way to torment Chase. Sylvia urged Paula to stop cutting herself and start talking to her more. She also asked Paula what she could do to improve their relationship. Paula replied, "Ask me how I am doing sometimes ... Let's go out for coffee ... or go shopping. You and I have not gone out together in a long time." Sylvia assured Paula that she would be delighted to do those things with her and again declared emphatically that she must stop cutting herself.

Next, after Sylvia and Paula did some great work together in opening up the lines of communication in their relationship, I brought Chase back in to continue the goal-setting process. I asked them how they all would know that they succeeded in our counseling work together. Sylvia said that she would "worry less." Paula chimed in with "Mom would worry less" and "Mom and I would spend more time together." Chase said his mom would "worry less" and would "stop calling my friends' moms and my teacher all of the time checking up on me."

I shared with the family that it sounded like "worrying" was getting the best of all of them, including friends' moms and Chase's teachers. I pointed out how it is quite common in families oppressed by an illness for "worrying" to prey on them and take on a life of its own, brainwashing family members to fight with one another, to not spend enough high-quality time together, and to engage in unhelpful and risky behaviors in an attempt to cope with it. In an effort to unite the family's efforts to take charge of this out-of-control "worrying problem," I explored with them as a family team what percentage of the time were they in charge of "worrying," versus "worrying" being in charge of them at three intervals—1 month before seeing me, 2 weeks before seeing me, and their current rating of the situation. They said that a month before seeing me "worrying" was 90% in charge; 2 weeks ago, they were at the same place; presently, however, they thought that "worrying" was now 70% in charge. I asked them to try to account for the change. Sylvia said that, by keeping busy lately, she had not made as many calls to Chase's friends' mothers and to his teacher. Paula also noticed that lately her mother had been coming to her somewhat less frequently sharing her worries about Chase. We discussed what specifically Sylvia and other family members were going to do as a team over the next week to get to 40% or better in charge of worrying, from the 30% level currently. Sylvia committed to drastically reducing her inquisitive telephone calls. Paula was going to stop annoying Chase and encourage her mother to do more things with her over the next week. Chase said he would be a better listener with his mom and try to stay away from doing things that would upset her.

After my intersession break, I presented my editorial reflection to the family. I complimented the whole family on working so hard in our meeting to improve their relationships with one another by letting each other know what upsets them and what specific steps each of them could take to get along better: Sylvia could be more relaxed, keep busy, stop making so many phone calls, and try to find more time in her life for Paula; Paula could open up more to her mom, avoid doing anything to harm herself, and stop annoying Chase; and Chase could be a better listener and not do anything that would lead "worrying" to getting the best of his mother. I shared with them that it would be hard work and a big challenge for the family to wrestle back control of their lives from the clutches of "worrying." I offered the family a few tasks or experiments to try out over the following 2 weeks.

As a family team they were to implement a "worrying" taming ritual that consisted of creating a large chart on poster board with two columns, the family team victory column and the "worrying" victory column. Daily, they were to keep track of the various things they did and told themselves to stand up to "worrying" and not allow it to get the best of them. They also had to keep track of the times when "worrying" achieved victories over them. I encouraged them to have regular family meetings to discuss what was working and where they needed to tighten up individually and in their relationships so that "worrying" did not get the best of them. I also suggested that they might want to work out together to be in great shape to wrestle with "worrying" when they needed to. Everyone smiled and Chase proclaimed loudly, "We will win this match!"

There were two other experiments I offered. Sylvia was asked to pay close attention to what she did daily to avoid caving in to "worrying's" attempts to make her pick up the phone to call Chase's friends' moms and his teacher. Paula was to pick one to two times over the following week to approach her mom to talk about anything she wished to share with her or to do something fun together. I recommended that the family try out the experiments over a 2-week period. I got the family to sign consent forms so I could collaborate with Dr. Walters and Miss Fine, Chase's teacher. Our next appointment was scheduled for 2 weeks later.

COLLABORATING WITH DR. WALTERS AND MISS FINE

I spoke to Dr. Walters on the telephone, sharing with her the results of our highly productive first family session. She was very pleased to hear that there was a breakthrough in the mother–daughter relationship. Dr. Walters had picked up on some conflict in their relationship and thought that Paula was upset about all of the attention Chase was getting from Sylvia. I shared with Dr. Walters what the family goals were and what therapeutic tasks had been assigned. She felt that these sounded right on target. For her, hearing and witnessing Sylvia's being less overprotective would be the key indication that change was really taking place. We agreed to continue collaborating throughout the treatment process.

Miss Fine was pleased to meet with me and share her concerns about Sylvia's frequent and troubling calls. Her biggest complaint was having to watch Chase so closely on the playground, which would prevent her from intervening early with other student difficulties. At times, Miss Fine felt a bit overburdened by having to field Sylvia's constant phone calls and comfort her. She felt relieved that Sylvia and her family were now in treatment. I shared with her what our therapeutic experiments were and that I would be checking in with her to see if there had been a reduction in telephone calls from Sylvia. Miss Fine agreed to assist me in any way that she could.

SECOND FAMILY SESSION

Two weeks later, the family brought in their chart to show me how, on 12 out of 14 days, they had successfully pinned "worrying" to the mat and achieved victories over it. After hearing about their great success as a family team, I gave them all high-fives and had them share with me all of the details regarding how they were able to beat "worrying" 12 of the 14 days. Although "worrying" successfully infiltrated Sylvia's mind on two of the days, she was able to do a reversal mid-day and limit her telephone calling to only two calls rather than five or six on those days. I asked her what she told herself to get out of "worrying's" clutches, and Sylvia replied that she repeated to herself, "I have got to stop myself and get out of the house and run an errand." This strategy worked well for her twice, and going to the health club also was helpful. Paula related that three times she and her mother went out for coffee and talked about what was going on in her life, and they went shopping without Chase once. Chase, in turn, reported that he tried hard to be a better listener and to steer clear of activities that would make his mother vulnerable prey for a "worrying" attack; only on two occasions did he engage in forbidden activities. Another pleasant surprise was that Chase and Paula were getting along better and played some computer games together amicably. Sylvia identified this as a big change. I asked the family what percentage of the time they were now in charge of "worrying." They unanimously agreed that they were now 80% in charge of "worrying!"

After amplifying and consolidating all of the family's gains, I took my intersession break. When we reconvened, I shared my editorial reflection with the family. Again, I gave them all high-fives for being such an awesome and formidable team. Although I shared with them that "worrying" might now think twice about trying to wrestle with and push them around, I also warned that "worrying" was a sneaky character who might strike when they least expected it and that they needed to be constantly on guard and alert for sneak attacks. I predicted that they might feel as though they were walking on egg shells, and it might be a little bit tense for a while when they are together because they are not used to having "worrying" *not* being so central to their lives. I also pointed out to Chase that "worrying" might try to prey on him at school by tempting him to try to impress his friends by doing something risky on the playground that he was supposed to avoid trying in order to maintain good health. Chase confidently stated that "we are a tough family and can handle it!" I recommended that the family continue the "worrying" taming ritual and keep track of what they do to be 90% or better in charge of "worrying." When I asked them when they wished to come back, Sylvia checked with the kids and they agreed to come back with her in 1 month.

COLLABORATIVE TELEPHONE UPDATE CONVERSATIONS
WITH DR. WALTERS AND MISS FINE

During the month-long break from counseling, I updated Dr. Walters about Sylvia and the family's progress in defeating the "worrying" problem and the other improvements they had made. She was pleased to hear the gains that Sylvia and the family were making. I asked Dr. Walters if she had any other concerns she would like me to take up with Sylvia and her family, and she could not think of anything else. I shared that we might be terminating in one or two sessions if the family was feeling satisfied and did not feel that there was anything further to work on. Dr. Walters was okay with this plan. I asked her if she would like to attend our next family therapy session. Because of her hectic work schedule and one of her colleagues being on vacation, she asked if I could arrange for the meeting to be held at her office. I told her I would contact Sylvia and see if we could work that out and then get back in touch with her to arrange an appointment time.

When I spoke with Miss Fine, she reported that she had received only one phone call from Sylvia during the past month, which was clearly an indication that Sylvia was changing. She also noticed that Chase was being much more careful with his choice of play activities and steering clear of some of the rougher kids in his class. I shared with her all of the changes Sylvia and her kids were making. Miss Fine thanked me for helping make her life less stressful, at least with one of the more challenging parents she had to deal with regularly.

THIRD FAMILY SESSION, AT DR. WALTERS'S OFFICE

One month later at Dr. Walters's office the family came in and proudly reported that they were now 100% in charge of "worrying!" Sylvia reported that she had made only one call to Miss Fine or Chase's friends' moms in nearly one whole month! Sylvia also noticed that Chase was being much more careful in his play activities and involvement with sports. Some of Chase's friends' mothers also shared with Sylvia when picking up Chase from play dates that they had noticed that he was changing his play activities with their sons and not being as much of a risk taker any more. Paula felt that she and her mother were now closer than ever before. I inquired about sneak attacks by "worrying" over the break period. No family members could remember any time when "worrying" was in the picture. I asked if they thought "worrying" had packed its bags and left town to find another family to prey on. Paula stated that "We ended 'worrying's' wrestling career!" Dr. Walters was thrilled to hear how well Chase and his family were doing. She thought it was wonderful to witness how they had really grown together as a family.

To test the waters, I asked the family what would have to happen for them to go backward at this point. All family members confidently stated that they could not see themselves going backward. I asked them to entertain some worst-case scenarios, like Sylvia's making telephone calls again or Chase choosing to take too many risks and hurting himself in the process. In looking back, both Sylvia and the kids wished to close the door on what was and open the door for new and exciting possibilities for the family. Sylvia was now socializing more with her friends and finally having a life outside the home. Paula was applying to become an exchange student in France, since she was good in French. Chase joined his school chess team.

After I amplified and consolidated all of the family's gains, we mutually agreed to terminate. I complimented each family member on his or her individual gains. Before they left, I asked them what their consultation fee would be if I needed to call them in the future to help me with another family being pushed around by "worrying." Paula said, "$1000 per hour!" Chase interjected, "No, we will do it for free!" Dr. Walters added that if they did it for free she might consider having them come in as expert consultants to help other families plagued by "worrying" difficulties in her pediatric practice. I wished the family the best of luck with their future endeavors, and we mutually agreed to terminate.

11

From Therapeutic Black Holes to Possibilities

Resolving Complex Child Treatment Dilemmas

When one door closes, another opens; but often we look so long upon the closed door that we do not see the one which opened for us.
—ALEXANDER GRAHAM BELL

$\mathbf{A}$t times in our professional careers, all of us have been faced with clinical situations in which we were intimidated by, or experienced therapeutic paralysis in reaction to, our clients' overwhelming problems. Some clients presented with such extensive treatment histories that their file folders almost had to be forklifted into the office! Other clients presented with chronic and seemingly intractable problems, some featuring families with multiple symptom bearers, including parents with serious mental health and substance abuse issues and severe marital or postdivorce conflicts; children as young as 10 years old self-harming, abusing substances, and already involved with street gangs; clients—in sum, all too often who had not responded well to seemingly well-conceived constructions of their problem situations and/or therapeutic experiments that seemed appropriate. In many such cases, we ultimately experienced a strong sense of pessimism that we would be able to co-create workable realities with these clients, particularly those whose presenting problems appeared to be impervious to our chosen therapeutic methods, despite their many successes in the past. All of these clinical dilemmas I prefer to label as *therapeutic black holes*. Stellar black holes, which are created by the collapse of supersized stars, generate such intense gravitational force that once objects come within their

265

gravitational field there is no possibility of return. Despite having invisible interiors, black holes reveal their presence by interacting with other matter (Hawking, 1998). When caught in the irresistible vortex of a therapeutic black hole, initially we may feel as though our clients' problems are impossibly difficult to resolve and as though we are therapeutically paralyzed.

In this chapter, I describe several ways we can enter and seemingly get stuck in therapeutic black holes in exiting the black hole's force field. Next, I present practical guidelines for looking for and capitalizing on open doors or entry points for co-constructing possibilities with our clients. Finally, two challenging and complex child case examples are presented, accompanied by posttreatment reflections.

Therapeutic Black Holes: Pathways to Getting Stuck

In this section, I present 14 ways we can seemingly end up in therapeutic black holes with challenging children and their families. I discuss each clinical dilemma and the steps that were taken that led to getting stuck. In the next section, I discuss the ways in which we therapists can actively resist being drawn by our clients' overwhelming problems into the vortex of a therapeutic black hole.

1. *"You've got to be careful if you don't know where you are going, 'cause you might not get there!"* *The clients' treatment expectations, preferences, and theories of change have not been solicited or clearly articulated by the therapist.* The great baseball player and manager Yogi Berra's quote (1998, p. 102) is quite applicable to the world of psychotherapy. If we fail to take sufficient time at the very beginning of treatment to get our clients to share their treatment expectations, preferences, and theories of change with us, we will have no idea how best to meet their needs. With children and their families who have chronic difficulties and have already had numerous treatment experiences in many settings, it behooves us to elevate them to expert status and have them inform us what former therapists and other professionals missed and/or did to exacerbate their problem situations; what they consider as the *right* problem to work on changing first; how they think the sessions should be structured (i.e., joint vs. separate sessions for the client and parents); who they think needs to participate in our sessions (other family members, members of their social circle, and involved helping professionals from larger systems); and how the clients will know that they are truly satisfied with their treatment experiences, particularly what specific topics or issues need to be addressed and what behaviors need to be resolved.

2. *The details regarding the referral process as well as past and present parental attempted solutions—including past treatment experiences—have not been explored. Thus, failed "solutions" are inevitably repeated.* When we fail to secure the specific details about both the parents' and former treatment providers' attempted solutions, we run the strong risk of largely replicating past unsuccessful attempted solutions and further exacerbating the clients' problem situations. This danger is most common with clients who have had multiple treatment experiences. When therapists automatically adopt a privileged expert attitude toward their clients and/or their own preferred treatment models and modalities, rather than allowing the clients' needs and preferences to drive the therapeutic process, the outcome predictably is a dead-end street.

3. *The treatment goals are vague, poorly formulated, or too ambitious.* Vague or poorly formulated goals lead to inconclusive, pointless therapy. Not knowing where you are going with your clients is like trying to feel one's way through a maze in a dark room: the likelihood of bumping into walls and feeling hopelessly stuck is all-encompassing. Moreover, the clients also will feel frustrated and demoralized when the therapist has not taken the time to negotiate with them incremental, achievable goals that the clients *wish* to pursue. In the therapist's zeal to quickly get clients on the road to change, he or she may negotiate initial treatment goals that are much too ambitious, only setting them up for failure.

4. *The client intimidation factor and the therapist's own anxiety is blocking him or her from being truly present.* Some therapists are intimidated by their clients' DSM-IV-TR diagnoses, chronic physical health difficulties, and extensive treatment experiences, particularly so for families in which multiple members have had chronic mental health and substance abuse difficulties. They may present the new therapist with a formidable file folder of psychological evaluations and treatment summaries. Rather than carefully listening to the clients' problem stories and observing the interactions in the room, the therapist may be distracted by his or her anxiety over being able to successfully help the clients out. Whenever this internal dialogue drowns out the external dialogue, the therapist is not truly present with the client, and his or her pessimism potentially sets in motion a negative self-fulfilling prophecy. As the Milan Associates aptly pointed out years ago, change cannot occur under a negative connotation (Boscolo, Cecchin, Hoffman, & Penn, 1987).

5. *There are weak therapeutic alliances with the parents and/or the child.* For most experienced therapists working with children, it is more

challenging to engage the parents than the children. When there is a weak alliance with the parents or they feel that the therapist is taking the child's side (versus theirs) or they feel blamed, he or she runs the risk of the parents abruptly ending the therapy. Our primary role needs to be serving as consultants to the parents and tapping their strengths to help them resolve their child's difficulties—not to try to reform the parent or restore the child back to better psychological well-being on our own.

In some situations, engagement with the parents is more easily accomplished than with the child. In such cases, the therapist may be talking too much rather than observing what the child likes to play with and do in the office; engaging children directly in fun and playful activities on their own level gives them a better opportunity to express themselves. However, some children are relatively unapproachable—whatever strategy or inducement is used. Some therapists interpret this behavior as resistance and something they have to figure out. The therapist may not think to involve the parents in the engagement process with the child and instead pursue a therapeutic direction that entails trying to fix what is wrong with the child that is interfering with a therapeutic alliance developing. This approach, in turn, may lead the child to feel even more uncomfortable with the therapist and therefore maintain his or her distance from the therapist. As Bohart and Tallman (1999) found in their research, clients are not passive recipients of what their therapists are trying to do with them but active participants, even when silent. We need to be patient and allow the silent child to get comfortable with us and change at his or her own pace.

6. *The therapist is not matching his or her questions or the therapeutic experiments to the family members' unique stages of readiness for change.* Many therapists do not take the time to carefully assess what stage of readiness for change family members are in when they begin treatment. In fact, only 20% of all clients that are referred to or seek treatment are in the action stage of readiness for change (Norcross, 2008; Prochaska et al., 1994). However, many therapists gear their treatment approaches and protocols to clients in the *action* stage of readiness for change rather than matching what they do to the unique stage of readiness for change each family member is presently in. For example, when family members are in the *precontemplative* stage of readiness for change and do not respond well to therapists' questions or assigned tasks offered them, therapists end up calling them "resistant" or "noncompliant." The real problem, of course, is that the therapists are being resistant, not the clients.

7. *The therapist moves* prematurely *to address the parents' mental health or substance abuse difficulties and/or severe marital or postdivorce conflict problems.* When parents bring a child in for therapy, they want help

in resolving *that child's* difficulties—not help in addressing their own mental health or substance abuse difficulties and/or severe marital or postdivorce conflict problems. However, some therapists—especially those who view the child's problems as being caused by the parents' "projections," "unresolved issues when they were the same age as their child," or "the child's being helpful to the parents by acting up and taking the focus off of their marital and postdivorce conflicts"—end up crossing the bridge too soon into the marital or postdivorce relationship system, which can lead to the parents feeling blamed or getting defensive and dropping out of treatment. The same thing happens when the referring person or therapist suspects or observes visible signs that one or both parents have mental health or substance abuse issues. In both of these clinical situations, unless the parents are in the *preparation* or *action* stages of readiness for change and can see the effects of their behavior on their child, they may not be concerned enough about or ready to commit to changing their behavior. As therapists, we need to begin first with striving to empower parents (no matter how troubling their behavior is supposed to or appears to be) to resolve their children's difficulties.

8. *The therapist has failed to build cooperative relationships with the referring person and all involved helping professionals from larger systems.* How clients are referred to us—what the referring person's and all the involved helping professionals' problem explanations, concerns, and best treatment outcome hopes are—is critical information for both our clients and us to know at the beginning of treatment. However, many therapists fail to secure this important information, keep the lines of communication open with the referring person and the involved helpers, or strive to build cooperative and regular collaborative relationships with them. They do not realize that these professionals are potential allies and key players in the solution-determined system (Selekman, 2009). Instead, they work in isolation with the child and his or her parents and are oblivious to the fact that as long as the referring person and other involved helpers are stuck viewing the child and his or her parents in a particular way or engaging in the same failed "solutions" that may have inadvertently further exacerbated the clients' problems, their *good* therapeutic work can quickly unravel.

9. *The true customer for change in the client system has not yet been recruited to participate in family sessions.* One of the most challenging clinical situations we all faced at one time or another is the *no-problem problem family* (Selekman, 2005; Eastwood et al., 1987). All family members are in the *precontemplative* stage of readiness for change, and they are in our office only because the referring person (whether a child protective worker, the principal of the child's school, or a police officer) is in a power position to enforce action. Sometimes in these situations it is the grandmother living

in the home, another relative, or the referring person or another involved helping professional that is most concerned about the child and/or family difficulties and in the action stage of readiness for change. To find out who the true customer(s) for change is, the therapist can ask the child, an older sibling, or a parent the following scaling question: "On a scale from 1 to 10, with 10 being most concerned about _____ (you [the child], your brother/sister, or your son/daughter) and 1 least concerned, what numbers would you give absent family members, relatives, close friends of the family, and other involved helpers like me?" The higher the number on the scale these concerned others are rated, the greater the need for them to participate in future family sessions. Since these individuals are in the action stage of readiness for change they will be eager to help with the solution construction process.

10. *Therapy is serious business!: The therapeutic process is boring and humdrum and lacking in spirit and energy.* When therapists work with children, the therapeutic process needs to be full of play, spontaneity, and fun. If there is too much adult talk and the experience feels like a serious science project to both the child and the parent, sessions will drag on interminably and be too humdrum, and nothing will change with the client's situation. Sometimes the reason why sessions feel stale and like they are in slow motion is because the therapist is doing most of the work and his or her agenda is driving the treatment. As the great hypnotist Milton H. Erickson once said, "It is the patient who does the therapy. The therapist only furnishes the climate, the weather. That is all. The patient has to do all of the work" (in Havens, 2003, p. 110). Given the opportunity, most parents are eager to participate in family play and art activities with their children.

11. *The therapist is inextricably wedded to his or her favorite therapy model.* Sometimes the reason we fall prey to therapeutic black hole situations with challenging clients who have extensive treatment histories is that we try to accommodate all our clients' diverse circumstances to treatment via a single-flavored therapy approach rather than tailoring our treatment to the unique needs and goals of the various clients. When we fall in love with a particular therapy model, we box ourselves into a narrow set of rigid theoretical assumptions and therapeutic experiments and strategies that greatly limits what we can see, hear, and do therapeutically. As the French existentialist philosopher Emile Chartier observed, "There is nothing more dangerous than an idea when it is the only one you have" (cited by Goolishian & Anderson, 1988). Therapists who adopt a privileged-expert attitude toward their clients ultimately meet with a high level of psychological resistance, leading clients to feel increasingly misunderstood and mismanaged, eventually terminating treatment.

12. *The child's serious physical health issues are compounding his or her behavioral difficulties, and the therapist has not actively collaborated with the pediatrician.* With some of our child clients, developments affecting their physical health can end up exacerbating their behavioral problems both at home and at school. Rather than actively collaborating with the pediatrician involved to learn more about the child's chronic medical conditions and the side effects of the medications he or she is on, some therapists gather information only from the parents, not even considering that it might be helpful to learn more about these important matters directly from the pediatrician. Some medications may produce effects resembling anxiety, depressive, and ADD-like symptoms, and, absent knowledge of his client's pharmacological regimen, the therapist involved may assume that these are underlying issues that need to be addressed. Also, if the child's teachers and other involved helping professionals are not apprised of chronic medical conditions and the side effects of the medications the client is taking, they may view troublesome behaviors as deliberate and/or pathological.

13. *Environmental stressors or obstacles may preclude change and contribute to the maintenance of the child's and the family's difficulties.* During these difficult economic times, many parents are losing their jobs, have had their hours greatly reduced, or are forced to work two jobs to help their families survive financially. In such households, the anxiety levels are often quite high, which eventually trickles down to the children. I have seen many children and adolescents in my office who are worried and upset by their family's financial struggles, which typically lead to dramatic changes in their lifestyles and family emotional climates. Other families may be living in violent communities, feature parents who have chronic physical health difficulties and possibly terminal illnesses, or be experiencing major transitions or life cycle changes that are adversely affecting all of its members. However, some therapists fail to take into consideration how both these micro- and macro-level environmental factors may be fueling and maintaining the child's emotional and behavioral difficulties. Instead, when change does not occur with the child or the parents, these therapists may view the clients as being resistant or noncompliant.

14. *The therapist has failed to cover the back door in addressing client concerns and the disadvantages of change throughout the treatment process.* Once our clients make changes, it is critical that we *cover the back door* with them and both amplify and consolidate their gains and make room for regularly addressing any concerns they may have throughout the course of treatment and afterward (Selekman, 2009). Many therapists in their zeal to constructively counsel, cheerlead, and further empower their clients, not only fail to educate them at the beginning of treatment about

the inevitability of slips but also fail to listen for any concerns on the part of family members. Budding crisis situations may be occurring that could have been prevented if addressed by the therapist early on. When a crisis does eventually occur or clients' progress in their goal areas begins to unravel, they may feel demoralized and as though they are back to square one. Norcross (2008) and Prochaska and his colleagues (1994) have demonstrated that slips "go with the territory of change," particularly during the maintenance stage of readiness for change.

Escaping into Workable Realities

Having provided an overview of the most common ways therapists end up getting stuck in therapeutic black hole situations with their most challenging clients, now I present 11 ways we can escape with our clients into more workable realities. I describe practical steps that therapists can take to liberate the treatment system from the strong gravitational pull of therapeutic black holes.

1. *Remember that we are co-pilots, not solo navigators.* No matter what models or approaches therapists use, the process needs to be collaborative. Our expertise is in eliciting *our clients'* expertise. They are the captains of the ship in determining the goals of treatment, what modalities they wish to pursue, setting each session's agenda, deciding who participates in sessions, and articulating what the ideal treatment outcome will look like to them. Research indicates that clients are much more accurate than therapists in determining what works best for them in all aspects of the treatment process (Norcross, 2008).

2. *Presence: Listen generously and observe like an eagle.* Therapists who are truly present with their clients listen closely with loving kindness and compassion to what the clients say, asking for clarification of the meaning of their key words and the themes in their problem stories (Selekman, 2009; Hoffman, 2002). Besides being skilled listeners, we have to be like eagles, viewing matters from an advantaged vantage point and carefully watching ourselves in relationship to our clients and how we interact with one another. With their keen sense of vision, eagles can follow the patterns of behavior of potential prey and determine when best to strike. In order to stay in the moment with our clients, we cannot allow our preferred therapy approach, internal voices of judgment, or even sensory perceptions to prejudice what we see and hear. When therapists are truly present with their clients, they experience the feelings felt by them. The clients feel understood,

validated, and respected by them, which are all components in creating a strong therapeutic alliance.

3. *Make maximum use of family members' key strengths, talents, passions, resources, and learning styles.* Our clients' strengths, talents, passions, resources, and unique learning styles are our key allies throughout the treatment process. All of these important natural gifts and attributes can be put to good use in designing therapeutic tasks and experiments that work to accomplish real change in clients' lives. Children naturally gravitate to therapeutic experiments and rituals that use the language and metaphors of their top skill areas. For example, a child who aspires to play soccer well also aspires to score goals with his mom: the art of therapy consists chiefly in just matching motivation to task. If one properly conceives the task, not only will the child be fired up to perform the task well, but also he or she will enjoy doing it. The more we make maximum use of our clients' likes, strengths, and resources, the shorter the road to change will be and we can greatly reduce their lengths of stay in treatment.

4. *Stop doing more of the same! Do something new and dramatically different.* One way we put ourselves into therapeutic black hole situations is by using "more-of-the-same" therapeutic tools and strategies that have not worked. Once we catch ourselves, we can shift gears and try something new and dramatically different from anything the clients have experienced from us before. No matter how challenging the client's situation may be, all we need to do is produce a small change either in the client's viewing of the situation or in family interactions, which can loosen up fixed beliefs and disrupt the patterns of interaction that are maintaining the child's presenting problem.

5. *Cirque du Soleil-infused therapy: Inject more playfulness, humor, surprises, and drama into your family sessions.* When working with children and their families, we need to create a therapeutic climate that is upbeat and filled with playfulness, lots of humor and fun, and surprises. Our therapy sessions should be conducted in the spirit of a highly entertaining Cirque du Soleil show that includes the following: at the very start, hilarious and off-the-wall clowns who capture the audience's attention and jog their funny bones; a host or guide dressed in a colorful, beautiful costume, who introduces the main story line or theme; spectacular special effects, playing on all of our senses; and lastly, death-defying acrobatics and dance numbers by well-trained gymnasts and dancers who are wearing costumes that are works of art.

Although I don't wear costumes or perform death-defying acrobatics in my office, I *do* tell jokes, share stories, sing songs, play my djembe or tabla drums, literally fall out of my chair from amazement when children and their families tell me about the big steps they have taken on their road to goal attainment, share my off-the-wall thoughts, display unashamedly the full spectrum of my emotions, sometimes climb up on my desk to conduct the session from up there and to gain a new perspective on the situation, and occasionally get up and walk out of the session without notice or idea of where I am going.

When the treatment process appears to be at a standstill, I take a risk and share with the clients the two voices I am hearing in my head, usually a confused one and a curious one. The confused voice might be asking me a question like "What am I doing or not doing that might be contributing to our standstill situation?" The curious voice might want me to ask the clients "Have we stumbled upon a topic that may be considered off-limits that is not to be talked about in this family?" or "Is there something you think I should be asking you about your family situation that we have not covered but is important for me to know?"

All of these antics can liven up the session, take the sting out of the clients' problem situations, loosen up their fixed beliefs, and open up space for possibilities. At the end of first family therapy sessions with children and adolescents, I know I have really connected with them when they share as session feedback that "That was fun!"

6. *Stop trying to be Hercules! Work with subsystems or individuals and establish separate goals and action plans for change when faced with disconnected families.* Some therapists make the mistake—or possibly have fleeting delusions of grandeur—of thinking they are like Hercules when they begin working closely with disconnected families. By "disconnected families," I mean families with multiple symptom bearers, featuring a Grand Canyon of emotional distance in family relationships, parents exhibiting chronic and severe marital and postdivorce conflict problems, and mental health or substance abuse problems galore, all of which overshadow the children's difficulties (Selekman, 2005, 2009). With challenging family dynamics like these, it truly would be a Herculean task to try to change all of these family members congregated in the same room. Therefore, it is a much more practical course of action to break them up and work with individuals and/or subsystems, establishing separate goals and work projects with each. Once individual family members' and the couple's difficulties are stabilized, we can test the waters and bring the family back together to revisit issues they wished to address and consolidate their gains.

7. *When you see daylight, seize the moment!* Like skilled running backs, we have to look for daylight—for a brief opening gap in the defense—and capitalize on that opportunity to gain a lot of yardage—even go for a

touchdown when we think we have a shot at it! In every given session, if we carefully scan the room, observing family interactions and listening carefully to what is being said, entry points and open doors for taking risks and offering new ideas or trying out therapeutic experiments with family members abound for the taking! As the great modern architect Frank Gehry put it: "Look for that slither of space. It's an opportunity. I love that first move. It's dangerous!" (in Pollack, 2005). However, in order for us to take risks, we need to feel comfortable allowing ourselves to be vulnerable, to overcome our fears of upsetting clients or worrying about our therapeutic moves not working, and to be at ease while living with uncertainty. The bottom line is that, once we create a firm therapeutic alliance with our clients, they are forgiving—even if what we try does not work or was too much too soon. We need to be able to trust our own guts and establish a base of confidence in our therapeutic decision making and risk taking. As Yogi Berra said, "When you come to a fork in the road, take it" (Berra, 1998, p. 48).

8. *Regularly solicit feedback from all family members on the quality of your therapeutic relationships and their perceptions of the change process in every session.* Since the client's perceptions and the therapeutic relationship are the most important determinants of positive treatment outcomes, it behooves us in every session to constantly solicit feedback from our clients on the quality of our relationships with them and their perceptions of the change process (Norcross, 2008; Hubble et al., 1999). We need to ask our clients about their perceptions of each session, what has not been talked about that needs to be addressed in future sessions, what concerns the clients have or changes they would like us to make so that we can strengthen our alliance with them, and their thoughts about the change process or the lack of progress. By securing this important feedback and input from our clients, we can adjust our own thinking and do things differently to better meet their needs and prevent premature dropouts from occurring.

9. *"With a little help from my friends": Engage and actively collaborate with key members of each client's social network.* In any challenging child case situation, we can make our lives less stressful by including key members of the client's social network in our family sessions. Potential helpers can include any of the child's closest friends and adult inspirational others, grandparents and other extended family members, the family's spiritual mentors, and close and concerned adult friends of the family. By reaching out to and involving these key members of the family's social network, we become less isolated and thereafter have allies working for us in social contexts to which we do not have access to help the child stay out of trouble and support the parents. These individuals can be instrumental in preventing child and/or family relapses.

10. *Conduct regular family–multiple helper collaborative meetings.* Ideally, therapists need to maximize opportunities for involved helping professionals from larger systems both to observe changes in clients' problematic behaviors and to hear their situations communicated about in new ways. Unless we do this, the helpers may be stuck viewing the clients' situations as they were when they first got involved and engaging in the same failed attempts to change them. In my clinical practice, ideally I like to alternate family sessions with family–multiple helper collaborative meetings. By conducting therapy in this way, I am able to involve all concerned parties actively in the change effort from the very beginning of treatment.

11. *Look for blips on the radar screen: Carefully listen for and promptly address clients' concerns throughout the course of treatment.* If we go back in time and dissect some of the common threads in such horrific and tragic events as the 9/11 terrorist attacks, the Columbine High School shootings, and the Virginia Tech massacre, there were two important factors that might have helped prevent these incidents from occurring, or at least lessened the human carnage involved, namely, a breakdown in communications and a failure to act more forcefully on the part of bystanders. With all three of these tragic events, there were both individuals who tried to communicate to others their concerns—but to no avail—and individuals who were alarmed but unmoved to act. When it comes to our clients' problematic situations, it is critical that we regularly provide them with session time to communicate their concerns (even if their progress is exemplary) and immediately take steps to help them to remedy these concerns. If we fail in this regard, the blips on the radar screen can grow into calamities that can derail the change process and lead to a prolonged relapse, or, at the least, have a demoralizing effect on the client.

Case Examples

I present two challenging case examples to illustrate how to escape into workable realities with clients when faced with tough therapeutic black hole situations. Posttreatment reflections are provided after each full-length case presentation.

"It's Like *Mutiny on the Bounty*—and the Pirates Have Taken Over the Ship"

REFERRAL PROCESS

Terrence, a Caucasian 10-year-old, was referred to me by his school social worker, Elizabeth, for what she believed was "ADD, oppositional defiant behavior, fighting with peers, and having a difficult time following the classroom rules." According to Elizabeth, she had had "a long history with Terrence's family at the school." She had worked with Terrence's 14- and 17-year-old brothers when they had attended her school, and they "exhibited similar behavioral difficulties." Elizabeth shared with me that "the parents were highly inconsistent with keeping meetings" with her, both presently and in the past, and "have failed to actively collaborate with their children's teachers" to try to resolve their problematic behaviors. When the parents would come, they were "very conflicted, had difficulty agreeing with each other, and Melanie [the mother] had a tendency to blame her husband, Bill, for the children's problems" because, according to Melanie, Bill was "weak and would not set limits on them when necessary." Melanie also described Bill as being "very passive-aggressive and deliberately going out of his way to frustrate" her by resisting teamwork in managing the boys' challenging behaviors. Elizabeth shared with me that she suspected that it was "super-chaotic at home," and sometimes when she would call Melanie after school she could "hear the boys fighting in the background." Finally, she reported that the family had been in family therapy four times before.

FIRST FAMILY SESSION

Prior to meeting the family in the waiting room, I could hear Melanie screaming at the boys to stop bickering and fighting. When I eventually brought them into my office, immediately the boys started going at it physically and verbally with one another, and Melanie and Bill just sat there looking overwhelmed and frustrated. Present at the session were the parents; Terrence; Stephen, who was 14; and their older brother, Mark, who was 17. While building rapport with each family member I learned that this was a basketball-loving family, and they were all big Chicago Bulls fans. I discovered that Bill had been an All State basketball star who was heavily recruited by many top college teams. However, he could not get a full ride at any of the schools that recruited him, and he was forced to drop out during his third year at a Midwestern university, owing to lack of funds to cover the rest of his education. His other major love and talent was car mechanic work, and he had landed a good-paying job with a foreign car dealership. Melanie was an English major and college graduate. When she was part of the workforce in the past, she had done secretarial work for a company and climbed the ranks to being an office manager. She was an avid reader, particularly a big fan of classic books. Since the boys were born, she had become a stay-at-home mother. I asked Mark what his favorite hobbies and interests were, and he said, "Playing computer games, shooting hoops (playing basketball), listening to classic rock tunes, and girls." Melanie interjected that "Mark is very popular with the girls," and they were "always calling" him at home or "e-mailing him." Stephen loved playing basketball and was "the top scorer" for his junior high school team. He also liked his father's "classic rock music, like Led Zeppelin, the Allman Brothers, and Grateful Dead," to name a few. According to Bill, Mark was an "incredible basketball player and made the varsity team at his high school as a freshman." However, Mark shared with me that he had injured his ankle during his sophomore year and after that decided to stop playing for the high school team because of the tremendous time commitment and due to his active social life. All the boys were die-hard Bulls fans. Mark's all-time favorite Bulls player was Michael Jordan because, like Michael, he himself liked "to mix it up with fade-away jumpers and driving the ball in and taking it to the hoop." Stephen, on the other hand, loved "going for those 3-pointers, taking field goal shots from 30–40 feet outside the hoop." His favorite Bulls player was Ben Gordon. Terrence interjected that he loved both of these players and "Curt Heinrich because he was a good dribbler and helped his team out a lot." He also liked his "PlayStation games." I asked the parents if they had any favorite Bulls players, and they both agreed with their boys that the names they had mentioned were their favorites as well. Our discussion about family members' strengths and interests seemed to temporarily quiet all of the bickering among the boys.

As soon as I asked the family what they would like to change, Stephen and Terrence started to go at it, trying to provoke each other. Michael yelled at them to stop and tried to separate them. Melanie then yelled at them to stop and be quiet. Then she yelled at Bill about just sitting there. She then proceeded to blame Bill for being "weak and not taking charge of the boys." Both Mark and Stephen, like tag team wrestlers, started yelling at their mother for putting their father down. At this point in the session, I asked the boys to go out to the waiting room and allow us to meet alone. In a nice way, I asked them to try and chill out there since other therapists' clients would be coming in and out. The parents stopped arguing after the boys left the room. They both indicated that they were worried about Terrence's difficulties in school. When asked about their theories about what was going on with Terrence, they both agreed that all of the bickering and fighting among all of them was having a negative effect on him. Melanie went off on a long monologue about how "Bill's failure to step up and take charge of the boys" forced her to have to "yell a lot and be 'the heavy' with them." Bill was quick to admit that he did not like "yelling and conflict" because he grew up in a household where his "mom yelled a lot" as well. He said he was a lot like his father, who would distance himself from his mother when she "went on the warpath" with his brothers.

Bringing us back to the here and now, Bill shared with me that his "work hours had been greatly reduced" recently, and he was "really worried about" losing his job. He went on to say that he had been "feeling really guilty and depressed about this for the past 2 months." Melanie added that she had reluctantly been forced to have to take a secretarial position with a company to try and recoup some of the income lost because of the reduction in Bill's income. However, she turned to Bill and in a loving way said to him, "Don't worry—we will make it." Melanie also shared with Bill that he was finally "opening up" to her about what was "going on inside of him." Bill thanked Melanie for being supportive. I complimented them on supporting each other and how they had come together as a team and the leaders of their family.

I explored with the couple all of their past and present attempted solutions, including past treatment experiences. As parents, they had tried "yelling, taking meaningful things away from the boys for long periods of time, sending them to their rooms as timeouts, and grounding." According to Bill and Melanie, any changes that occurred with their children ended up being only "short-lived." Given their past family treatment experiences, both admitted that they felt "blamed for their boys' problems and that the therapists would just sit there and allow the bickering and fighting to carry on throughout our meetings just like what was happening at home." All of the therapists had tried to get them to "do marital therapy" with them rather than helping them to try to resolve the boys' problems. The therapists also thought that both Mark and Stephen had ADD, which the parents did not buy into. Both Melanie and Bill felt that the boys' bickering and fighting problems had gotten progressively worse, even after all of the family counseling. Melanie shared, "It's like *Mutiny on the Bounty,* and the pirates have taken over the ship" in their home. In addition, they had "caught both Mark and Stephen recently with alcohol and small bags of marijuana." They also were concerned that Mark was beginning to run around with some rowdy types of guys lately. When asked about their past successes, the parents could not initially think of anything they had done lately or in the past to curtail their boys' challenging behaviors.

I returned the couple back to the goal-setting process. I asked the following question: "Let's say that by the end of our session today you left here completely satisfied and feeling glad that you had come. While driving home as a family, what will you notice first that will tell you that 'Wow! Our situation is better'? What will be different?" Melanie said, "The boys would not be bickering and fighting in the car." I asked them, "What effects would that change have on you individually and as their parents?" They both shared that they would be "less stressed-out," they would be "arguing less and getting along better," and it would be "more peaceful in the household."

In an effort to find out if pieces of this positive outcome scenario were already playing out a little bit, Bill shared that a week ago he had joined the boys "on Saturday afternoon for a few hours shooting hoops, and there was absolutely no fighting." In fact, "the boys showed good teamwork." I asked if the boys were less likely to argue with one another when Bill was present, and Melanie agreed they were. She felt that the boys wanted more involvement with their father. I shared with the couple a crazy idea that had popped into my head, which was "I wonder if the boys were fighting for Bill's love and attention." Both Bill and Melanie felt that my idea was not that crazy. Bill shared that there were periods of time that a combination of life disappointments and work stress were contributing to his distancing from his sons. I asked about other sparkling moments that had occurred before our meeting. A week ago, the parents had stood side by side and successfully broke up a big fight that had erupted between Mark and Stephen. Apparently, both boys stopped immediately when they experienced them as a unified team. Bill and Melanie had also discovered that cutting off "the boys' technological links to their social lives" was a very effective weapon in their arsenal—"taking away cell phones and Internet use" for periods of time had worked well in the past. However, a new challenge they faced with Mark was his "crawling out of his bedroom window and sneaking out when grounded," and also "the older boys refusing to relinquish their cell phones." Moreover, they felt that the older boys were "corrupting Terrence by not following the rules and modeling bad ways to resolve conflicts with others by bickering and fighting."

To complete the goal-setting process, I asked the parents the following scaling question: "On a scale from 10 to 1, with 10 being your leaving here today and the boys' bickering and fighting behaviors are no longer happening and 1 being there is *a lot more work* to be done on their bickering and fighting, where would you rate the situation today?" Melanie said, "At a 5," while Bill thought things were "at a 6." I asked them what specifically they had been doing to prevent the situation from being much worse and down at a 1 level. According to the parents, there were other times that they did not mention earlier when they "teamed up and nipped these behaviors in the bud before they got out of hand." Melanie shared that she had "greatly reduced" her "yelling at the boys" and had "tried to be more firm with them when dishing out consequences." Bill had the idea of trying to devote "one-on-one attention time with each boy" and that seemed to "really help." I asked each parent if they were aware of how they had come up with such creative ideas. Melanie shared with us that she had "come to the realization that yelling a lot just made the boys more out of control." Bill had been reflecting on how he had been "shortchanging the boys" with his time and thought "one-on-one attention time" with each of them would help strengthen his relationships with them. I asked the parents what they were *going to do* over the next week to further reduce the boys' bickering and fighting behaviors to bring us up to a 6 and 7 on the scale. The parents shared that they would "try to join forces more and be a unified team with the limit setting," Bill would "spend more time with the boys," and Melanie would "try to not yell at or threaten the boys with severe consequences." We discussed the importance of playing solution detectives and trying to catch them when they are good and exhibiting the 6- and 7-rated behaviors over the next week as well. I encouraged the parents to increase doing what they were doing that was working and keep track of other creative things they came up with that would also help reduce the boys' bickering and fighting behaviors.

I met alone with Terrence and his brothers and asked them which parent they worried about the most. The boys unanimously picked their father. I asked why. Both Mark and Stephen felt that their dad had been "real down over the past few months about losing his job" and used to spend a lot more time with them "building things and shooting hoops together." They were also upset about how their mother was "always on their dad's case." Terrence shared that he and his father used to "build model cars together" and he had been teaching him how to be a "better basketball player." I asked the boys if playing more basketball with their father together would help them get along better, and they all agreed that it would. Both Mark and Stephen shared with me that their father was "a great high school and college basketball star," and he taught them "his best shots."

Hearing how important basketball was to the boys and how it connected them to their father, I came up with a basketball ritual for them. I asked them what specifically each of them could do over the next week to score points with their parents, especially things that they would really notice and appreciate. Mark said he would "stop swearing as much and drop the attitude" with his mother. I asked him what he meant by "drop the attitude." He replied, "Not mouthing off to her, try to not use weed and drink, and try to stop my brothers from fighting as much." I was curious as to how he would pull off the mediation trick with his brothers. Mark said, "I would act like a big brother and try to help them to be cool with each other and remind them that this only stresses dad out more." I complimented Mark on his great ideas, saying he was right on target. I asked Stephen how he would nail his Ben Gordon fade-away three-pointers with his parents, and he said, "Not pick on Terrence, straighten up my bedroom, and not have an attitude with my mom." He said "not having an attitude" with his mom meant "not swearing at her" and doing what she would tell him to do "without arguing." Terrence said playing like Curt Heinrich over the next week would look like "being good in school," "being a better listener with Mom," and "not taking things out of Stephen's room without asking." I complimented all of the boys on coming up with such great moves to score points with their parents over the next week.

In addition to encouraging the boys to experiment with all of their great ideas with their parents, I asked them what they thought about initiating a three-on-two basketball game with their parents as well. All of the boys thought this would be a lot of fun and loved the idea of playing together as a family. I asked them what NBA team they would be, and they shouted loudly and in unison "the Bulls!" I wanted to know how they planned to cover their dad, who was much like a LeBron James, given his considerable abilities! Mark shared that he and Stephen would have to "double team" him and "try to not let him inside the lane to the basket." Stephen hoped to "get hot" with his "three-pointers" and give his team "a big lead early in the game." Terrence shared that he would "pass the ball a lot" to his brothers when "they are open." I asked the boys if they were aware that their mother was a good dunker like Michael Jordan. They all laughed. Before we ended our time together alone, I had the boys place their hands in the center and, like a coach, I said, "One, two, three—this will be your game!" Again, they all laughed.

After a short intersession break, I brought the family back for my editorial reflection. First I complimented the parents on recognizing how unified teamwork not only helps them get along better but also perform better as well. Then I complimented Melanie for cutting back on her yelling and recognizing the importance of Bill's spending more time with their sons. I complimented the boys for being so respectful toward one another and working together to come up with many meaningful ways to score buckets with their parents over the next week. The parents were asked to pretend to be play-by-play commentators and pay close attention to what each of their sons did to score these buckets with them. I asked Mark to share with his parents the other fun thing they wanted to do with their parents over the next week. He explained the three-on-two basketball game idea to them. Melanie said to her sons, "I'm not very good." Terrence responded with, "Mommy, you have to play!" Bill snorted, "No problem, we will be ready for you!" I asked if I were to place bets on this great matchup of two teams, who would win— who should I go with? Bill shouted, "Us, of course!" Stephen's rejoinder was "We'll see about that!" I told the whole family that I would be on the edge of my seat all week wondering who won. We all agreed to meet 1 week later at the same time.

Prior to wrapping up the session, I solicited from everyone what their experiences were like in our first family meeting. Bill and Melanie found the session to be really helpful. Bill shared that it gave him "hope and made us more aware as parents about what we are already doing that works and other useful things to try," like focusing more on their "sons' positive behaviors." Melanie said that she "felt really supported" by me and liked my "positive approach." Both Mark and Stephen declared that "the meeting was fun." I asked them what was "fun" about the meeting, and they both said, "We talked about what we liked to do and how we could make our family better." Terrence agreed, noting that he really liked all the "talking about basketball" and "spending more time" with his dad. Before ending the session, I secured family members' signatures on a consent form so I could collaborate with Elizabeth and Mrs. March, Terrence's teacher at the school. The parents and Terrence thought this was a good idea.

FIRST COLLABORATIVE MEETING AT THE SCHOOL

I held the first collaborative meeting with Elizabeth and Mrs. March at the school one week after my initial family session. Both parents had been invited to our meeting, but they could not get out of work to attend. Since I had a long history of working with Elizabeth and already knew her concerns, I was most interested in hearing Mrs. March's views and concerns about Terrence's behavior. Mrs. March agreed with Elizabeth that he "may be ADD because he has a hard time staying on task, is impulsive, does not follow the classroom rules, and bickers and fights with other students." Elizabeth interjected, for Mrs. March's appraisal, that Terrence's older brothers also used to have the same behavioral difficulties. I wanted to know all of Mrs. March's attempted solutions. Apparently, she had tried "prompting him, moving him away from students he did not get along with, and sending him out of class to Elizabeth whenever he refused to follow the rules or began fighting with fellow students." Although sometimes these strategies worked, Terrence would behave for a while and then "start acting up again." Mrs. March was beginning to wonder if Terrence might do "better in a self-contained BD" (a class for behavior-disordered children). Mrs. March also complained that "the parents were uncooperative," refusing to take her concerns about Terrence's behavior seriously enough. Elizabeth had planned to "talk to the parents about holding an IEP [individualized education planning meeting] and ordering a case study evaluation for Terrence."

Prior to ending our meeting, I asked Mrs. March if she would do an experiment so that I could have a more complete picture of Terrence's classroom behavior. She was to carefully notice daily the times when Terrence's behavior was *better,* what he was doing specifically during those times, and pay close attention also to what she was doing that might have contributed to Terrence's positive behavior. We all agreed to meet in 3 weeks.

SECOND FAMILY SESSION

When I greeted the family in my waiting room at the beginning of our second family session, it was in a very different atmosphere than our first meeting together. The boys were not bickering or getting physical with one another, and Melanie and Bill were sitting together in good spirits. After the family sat down in my office, Melanie began by praising her sons for having "a great week." According to Melanie, not only was there "very little bickering," but also she and Bill "did not have to break up even one fight." I asked the boys how they were able to pull that off, and Mark responded with "I said to my brothers that we need to play like the Bulls when they are playing well as a team—rather than like a bunch of individuals." Bill responded to Mark with "You put that very well. All of you *did* work better together as a team than I have ever seen before." I asked Bill to share some examples of their great teamwork. He reported that they helped him out with "yard work and with some other house projects, they straightened up their bedrooms, and Mark was a good big brother and leader in helping Stephen and Terrence not push each other's buttons." Melanie reported happily that she "did not receive a single phone call from Mrs. March or Elizabeth about Terrence getting into trouble at school." I asked Terrence how he had pulled that feat off. Terrence shared with all of us that he ignored two of the boys in his class that often teased him and made him mad and that he was trying to behave better. When asked if Mrs. March had been doing anything differently, he shared that she was letting him know that he was doing "a good job" and treating him in "a nicer way."

I shared with the family that I had been on the edge of my seat all week wondering who won the three-on-two basketball game. Stephen loudly exulted that "we beat them 58 to 35!" To my surprise, Bill admitted sheepishly that "they were too much for us. Once Stephen started hitting a string of three-pointers and Mark was dominating the boards with rebounds, there was no stopping them!" He added, "Terrence made some good shots too." Melanie piped up that "they really played well as a team—without even one squabble." Mark pointed out that "when we can hold our father to 28 points, we have done our job." Apparently, 2 years earlier Bill had "scored 50 points" against them. Stephen praised his mother for her performance. "Although she was held to 7 points, she made a few nice shots, got some rebounds, and stole the ball once from Mark, which is really hard to do!" Melanie smiled and said, "It was really fun playing together as a family." Bill recommended that as a family they try to make playing basketball together a more frequent activity. The boys agreed emphatically.

I met alone with the parents to assess their progress as a team. Melanie was quick to point out that she and Bill were "much more united as a team." She also shared that there were "two occasions when Stephen was trying to push Terrence's buttons" and she "set a firm limit on him" and refrained from yelling. When asked about her useful self-talk, Melanie told herself that "yelling just makes things worse, don't do it!" Bill was spending "daily one-on-one time with each boy." He also picked up some "extra work hours with a good friend who had his own automobile repair business." Bill shared with me that this had helped lift his spirits more. I asked the couple to rate the bickering and fighting situation at this point. Melanie felt things had "shot up to a 7." Bill rated the boys' behaviors "at an 8." When asked about the next steps they will take as parents, Melanie shared that she will try to "avoid yelling, we will stay unified as a team," and maybe "come up with one other fun family activity to do together." Bill planned to increase his "one-on-one time with each boy" and also "build something with all of them." In the past, he had thought that they may "enjoy building a motorized go-cart."

I cautioned the parents that although we were on an upswing with dramatic improvements in the boys' behaviors, that there may be days ahead where either one of you or your sons will lose it and it may feel like we are back to square one. However, I pointed out to them that slips go with the territory of change and are just an indication that we need to tighten up more with the structure and also learn from these experiences. I also encouraged them to keep the lines of communication open with Elizabeth and Mrs. March. I pointed out that the more Mrs. March felt supported by them, it will have a positive influence both on how she views and interacts with Terrence. They planned to attend our next scheduled collaborative meeting at the school.

I met briefly with the boys to praise them on their great individual and team efforts over the past week. I gave them all high-fives. Furthermore, I let them know that their parents were very proud of them and would like to see more family teamwork and playtime rather than yelling and fighting. I shared with Terrence that I was happy to hear that Mrs. March was noticing that he was doing better in her class.

After the intersession break, I reemphasized many of the significant steps family members were taking to improve their situation. I noted, in particular, how they were playing so well as a team that they could have given the *real* Chicago Bulls a tough battle! Everyone was smiling. I encouraged them to increase doing more of what was working. As a vote of confidence in the family, I offered them a vacation from counseling. They decided to come back in 2 weeks. I told them that I was looking forward to hearing what further progress they could make.

SECOND COLLABORATIVE MEETING AT THE SCHOOL

Both of the parents and Terrence attended our second collaborative meeting at the school, along with Elizabeth and Mrs. March. Mrs. March was delighted to reel off all the changes she had been observing in Terrence's behavior. Apparently, when taunted by some troublemakers in her class, "he would ignore them, walk away, or let me know if he needed my support," adding "Terrence has been more focused, staying on task, listening better, and completing his classroom work without reminders." Terrence was smiling. I reached over to give him a high-five and told him, "Good job!" Both Melanie and Bill were all smiles and voiced how proud they were of their son's tremendous improvement. I asked Mrs. March what adjustments she had made that might also be contributing to Terrence's great progress. Mrs. March shared that she was "getting better at catching Terrence at his best, praising him, and involving him more as a classroom leader." She felt that having him be a classroom leader was making his "self-esteem higher and helping him behave better." Melanie thanked Mrs. March for helping Terrence do better in class. Elizabeth shared that she had "missed not seeing Terrence more times" in her office. Although she saw him once a week as a check-in, there were some weeks when he had been sent down to her office "5 out of 5 days!" I shared with the group that it sounded as though "we have closed the door on how things used to be." Both Melanie and Bill thanked Elizabeth and Mrs. March for all of their help. We agreed to arrange a future meeting only if there were any serious concerns with Terrence's behavior and academic performance. By the end of our meeting, there was no longer any discussion of calling for a case study evaluation, an IEP, or trying to get Terrence placed in a BD self-contained class.

THIRD FAMILY SESSION

Bill kicked off our third family session by sharing that he and the boys had "built a motorized go-cart together." He got hold of "an old Briggs and Stratton lawn mower engine, purchased some wood at Home Depot," and he was able to "buy some wheels at a special hobby store." All the boys chimed in about how fun it was to build the go-cart and ride in it. Terrence shared that he and his father had never built a motorized car "so big before." Melanie was very pleased to see Bill spending more time with their sons. She also was happy to report that in their last family basketball game she had "scored 12 points!" Mark gave his mother a high-five. Bill commented that he was proud of his wife's play in their last game. I amplified other gains the family had made. The best news was that there had not been one fight among the boys! Also, the parents had not received any phone calls from Elizabeth or Mrs. March.

To test the waters with the family, I asked them a consolidating question: "What would you have to do to go backward at this point?" The parents confidently shared that they could not see that happening. The boys, on the other hand, pointed out that they would "start fighting again, not listening to" their parents, and "being disrespectful" toward their mother, such as "swearing at her." Terrence said he would have to "be bad in school" to move backward. I then asked them, "Let's say we had not seen one another for a month or so and there is a big argument or fight that erupts between all of you. What steps will each of you quickly take to get back on track?" Melanie said that she and Bill would "stay unified as a team and calmly put out the fire without yelling and losing it with them." Mark shared that he would "take some deep breaths" and then try to get his brothers "to chill out." Stephen said that he would "stop swearing and going after Terrence."

When meeting alone with the parents to assess their present ratings of the sons' bickering and fighting on the scale, they both reported that they thought the situation was "at a 9." I inquired of them: if they were to replace our Saturday meeting time with a fun family activity, what they would be doing instead? Bill said that he would "take the boys fishing, ride in the go-cart, or shoot hoops with them." Melanie shared that they would "play basketball or go to the water park together." I asked them if they were satisfied with where they were mentally and emotionally and whether they felt that we needed to meet again since they were making such great progress. Both parents felt that it would be okay to stop for now. I shared with them that I have an open door policy and if they needed a tuneup in the future they could always call me. Finally, I shared with them that I would let Elizabeth know that we were stopping for now and ask her to provide backup for Terrence if he ever needed support from her.

After the intersession break, I complimented all of the family members on their great individual efforts and outstanding teamwork. I encouraged them to keep doing more of what works, especially playing so well together as a team that the real Bulls would be intimidated by them. I let the boys know that we were going to stop for now and that I would check in with them down the road to find out what further progress they had made. I wished them well, and we parted.

TELEPHONE FOLLOW-UP

I contacted the family 6 months later and also 1 year later. Melanie answered both of my calls. In the telephone conversations she indicated that "the boys rarely bickered and fought with one another." Although Bill was working full-time, he was "still protecting" his individual and group time with his sons. Melanie was delighted to report that, as parents, they were "a unified team" and their "marital relationship was stronger." I asked Melanie both times that I spoke to her who had the edge with victories in their family-grudge basketball games, and the boys' team was in the lead.

POSTTREATMENT REFLECTIONS

What was most challenging about Terrence's family situation was that there were multiple family members with difficulties. For most therapists, it would have been tempting to adopt a problem-focused orientation and buy into the former therapist's, Elizabeth's, and Mrs. March's beliefs that Terrence and his brothers had ADD; to do "more of the same" as the former therapists in shifting the focus from the children's problems to the couple's marital difficulties; and to view the father as being clinically depressed and possibly needing antidepressants and individual therapy. As in Robert Frost's famous poem "The Road Not Taken," I chose to take the therapeutic road typically less traveled by families such as this one and to use family members' unique individual and shared family strengths to resolve their presenting difficulties and co-produce long-lasting changes at home and at school. Since basketball was the first love for this family as well as their favorite pastime and they were all Chicago Bulls fans, I used star players' names and descriptions of their best shots and other basketball language and metaphors to establish greater rapport with the boys, who ultimately wielded the power in the family. As Melanie put it, "The pirates had taken over the ship!"

Another important part of our work together was facilitating connection building by helping Bill become more present in his sons' lives and reinstating pleasurable activities they used to enjoy together; together with the parents, we even managed to come up with some new activities and present them to the boys as fun options. Bill's great strides in this area helped us to resolve the couple's conflicts regarding his lack of involvement with the boys and Melanie's feeling like a single parent. Bill's sons had a lot of respect for him, particularly his past basketball accomplishments, and were longing for him to be more available to them. I shared with the parents my crazy idea that the boys were actually fighting each other mainly for his attention. Melanie was so pleased with Bill's changed attitudes that they were able to work together as a team to put an end to the boys' chronic bickering and fighting problems.

The bickering, fighting, and breaking rules problems from home spilled over into Terrence's classroom setting. So, what looked like ADD was really the replication of learned behaviors in the home setting being played out at school. The observation experiment I offered to Mrs. March was designed to help her see the big picture, the periods of time "in between" when Terrence was behaving well, and to keep track of what she was doing during those times that contributed to these sparkling moments and prosocial behavior. Mrs. March came up with some very helpful and creative strategies that contributed to Terrence's remarkable progress in her class. Once Terrence's behavior changed dramatically, the change dissolved both Mrs. March's and Elizabeth's original problem explanations that Terrence was a child with ADD, needed a case study evaluation, and needed to be placed in a special class.

From Drug Dealer for the Street Gang to Landscaping Entrepreneur

Keyshawn, a precocious 11-year-old African American boy, was referred to me by Mr. Harris, the youth officer at the local police department, for getting "arrested on the street with two ounces of marijuana and 6 Ecstasy pills." Upon being brought to the police station and interviewed by the officers, "Keyshawn refused to tell them who he was running drugs for and cooperate with their investigation." This was not the first time he had been picked up by the police, as Mr. Harris had had to intervene with Keyshawn "three times before for curfew violations and twice for shoplifting." Keyshawn lived with his grandparents since his father had abandoned the family when he was born, and his mother was "in jail for prostitution and theft and had a serious heroin addiction problem." She had "lost custody of Keyshawn to her parents because of her past problems with physically abusing him."

Mr. Harris shared with me that "the grandfather was sickly and suffered from severe arthritis and bad asthma." Keyshawn spent most of his time with "his grandmother playing on his PlayStation, watching movies, and playing football in the park with his friends." In school, Keyshawn had a long history of "not doing well academically and getting into trouble for flashing gang signs and wearing gang colors"; nonetheless, the principal reported that "he is a very smart boy and is well liked and respected by his peers." Mr. Harris wished me good luck in trying to engage the grandparents. Apparently, they had yet to follow up with any of his referrals to therapists. Since Mr. Harris had a good relationship with Keyshawn, I asked him if he would be willing to participate in future sessions once I engaged the family. He gladly agreed to participate. After securing the grandmother's telephone number from him, I called Mrs. Heath, the grandmother, to schedule a family meeting in my office.

FIRST ATTEMPTED FAMILY MEETING

Prior to our first scheduled family meeting, Mrs. Heath called me to cancel because her husband was not feeling well. Apparently, his arthritis was acting up. Mrs. Heath also said that Keyshawn failed to come back after going out with his friends. She had no idea where he was, and he had left his cell phone at home. The grandmother went on to tell me that Keyshawn hated counseling and often refused to go. I explored with her what she thought he disliked the most about counseling and with the past counselors. Mrs. Heath said that they would lecture at him about "staying away from drugs and gangs, telling him to do better in school, and listening to his grandparents." She told me that Keyshawn was "a real independent person who does not like to be told what to do," even by her and her husband. According to Mrs. Heath, it had been "a real challenge trying to raise Keyshawn," and she felt that they had "lost control of him to the Vicelords," a street gang.

I asked Mrs. Heath about Keyshawn's key strengths, and she said, "He has lots of friends, he is good in sports, and he does a great job cutting our lawn and helping me in the garden." She felt that Keyshawn was "very intelligent and capable of doing much better in school."

I explored with her whether there were any other adults in Keyshawn's life other than Mr. Harris whom he looked up to or who had taken a liking to him. Mrs. Heath believed that Mr. Steele cared a lot about him, and Keyshawn also respected Mr. Steele. Apparently, he used to be his "football coach in the Park District football program for elementary school kids." In fact, Mr. Steele once had taken Keyshawn to "a Chicago Bears football game and introduced him to some of the players he was friendly with." He also had taken him "to the movies" a few times. Mr. Harris had once or twice come by "to talk to Keyshawn and throw the football around with him." When asked if Keyshawn was a good football player, Mrs. Heath said, "For his age, he is very fast and has great hands for catching passes." Before ending our telephone conversation, I asked Mrs. Heath if we could try doing a family meeting at their home. We scheduled the session during their typical dinner hour as the best time to have Keyshawn present. I also asked if she would feel okay if Mr. Harris joined us since both Keyshawn and I had a good relationship with him and it could help with the engagement process. She thought this was an excellent idea.

FIRST OFFICIAL FAMILY SESSION

Present at our first family meeting in the Heath home were the grandparents, Mr. Harris, and Keyshawn. I could tell by the look on Keyshawn's face that he was not too thrilled about having a family counselor in his home. Keyshawn was tall, and he looked a lot older than other 11-year-olds I had worked with in the past. I asked Mr. Harris to introduce me to Keyshawn and his grandparents and share with them our long history of collaborating together. This appeared to help Keyshawn to relax and be a bit less defensive. I shared with him that his grandmother had told me on the phone that he was an awesome football player. I asked Keyshawn who his favorite National Football League player was, and he said, "Chad Johnson of the Cincinnati Bengals." He shared with me that he liked Chad because he has "great moves and great hands." I told him that his grandmother had said that he also had "great hands." I then asked him if he was going to be the next Chad Johnson. Keyshawn smiled and said, "I wish, man!" Mr. Harris also felt that if Keyshawn would keep working on his great catching ability and stick with football, he could have a great playing career ahead of him. I asked Mr. Harris what he thought might get in the way of Keyshawn's playing junior high and high school, and he said, "Drugs and gangs." At this point, Keyshawn got up and left the room shouting, "I am sick of people telling me what to do!"

The grandparents shared with us how frustrated and stuck they felt.

Mr. Heath said he "no longer had the physical strength to chase after Keyshawn." The grandmother had tried to fill up Keyshawn's free time with sports and positive activities, but she could not always be around to monitor him because she had to work as a saleswoman at a department store. Mr. Harris pointed out that Keyshawn was too young to qualify for court supervision, and therefore Mr. Harris had no legal leverage with him. I explored with the grandparents whether they thought more actively involving Mr. Steele in Keyshawn's life could be helpful if Mr. Steele had the time. They agreed that it would be worth a try. The grandparents also wanted me to meet with Keyshawn's teacher, Mrs. Stanley, and Miss Rosen, the school social worker. I had them sign consent forms for me to collaborate with Mr. Steele, Mr. Harris, Mrs. Stanley, and Miss Rosen in the future. Prior to ending our meeting, everyone was in agreement that we had to get Keyshawn off the streets and tightly structure his free time to involve him more in sports and other positive activities.

In an attempt to better engage Keyshawn, I asked him if he would be willing to throw the football around so I could throw him some long-bomb passes. He reluctantly agreed to throw the ball around with me. I was very impressed with his speed and great hands. I asked him if I could call him "Chad" rather than Keyshawn and he said, "Okay." After working up a sweat, I asked Keyshawn if he would be willing to meet with me again. He agreed to see me again. I then asked him if he would prefer to meet at his home rather than my office and he said, "At the crib" (the house). Before leaving, I scheduled another family meeting at the home with the Heaths.

FIRST SCHOOL COLLABORATIVE MEETING

I met with both Keyshawn's teacher, Mrs. Stanley, and Miss Rosen, the school social worker. Mrs. Heath could not join us because of her job, and Keyshawn was making up an important test that he had missed when he missed school one day. According to Mrs. Stanley, Keyshawn was a bright boy and had good leadership abilities; quickly adding, however, "He rarely does his homework, and he never studies for tests." This comment explained why his grades were so poor. Mrs. Stanley felt frustrated because, when she raised these concerns with his grandmother, there appeared to be "no follow through or monitoring to make sure he completed and turned in his homework assignments and was better prepared for his tests." Apparently, she had spoken to Mrs. Heath on numerous occasions about this problem. Although Mrs. Stanley and Keyshawn got along, she said he was "very laissez-faire about doing his school work." He also "did not see any problem with wearing gang colors and flashing gang signs."

Miss Rosen also felt frustrated with Keyshawn because he was so guarded. Apparently, he "never opens up to" her about "stressors in his life, such as missing his mother or running with the gangs." When he would get into trouble for wearing gang colors and flashing gang signs, "He did not think it was a big deal and did not see the potential dangers of doing these things." We agreed to meet again in a few weeks and have Mrs. Heath and Keyshawn join us.

TELEPHONE CONVERSATION WITH MR. STEELE

When I phoned him, Mr. Steele was delighted to help out in any way with Keyshawn. He, too, was very concerned about Keyshawn's choice making and safety. I shared with him that Mr. Harris, the grandparents, and I were trying to come up with as many positive activities to fill up Keyshawn's free time that would be more inviting and meaningful than gang life. We discussed the importance of surrounding Keyshawn with strong and positive African American adult role models to look up to and empower him to flourish in life. Mr. Steele made a commitment to see Keyshawn twice a week to help further develop his football playing skills and spend some quality time with him doing something fun together. I also told him about Mr. Harris and how he was invested in helping turn Keyshawn's situation around as well. Finally, I asked Mr. Steele if he would be willing to come to our next family meeting, and he readily agreed to come.

SECOND FAMILY SESSION

Present at our next family meeting were the grandparents, Mr. Steele, Mr. Harris, and Keyshawn. I told Keyshawn that I will make sure to leave some time for us to throw the football around, and if we were lucky, Mr. Harris and Mr. Steele might decide to join us. Mrs. Heath began our meeting sharing her concerns about Keyshawn's "D and F grades in school." Mr. Steele quickly interjected, looking at Keyshawn, that in order for him to be able to play football on both the junior high and high school levels, he would have to attain at least a C grade point average. He went on to say how "incredibly talented" Keyshawn was in football, and if he "kept further developing his skills as a wide receiver," he would be able to "play college ball somewhere." Keyshawn smiled and became less defensive. I shared with the group how impressed I was with Keyshawn's athletic abilities when we threw the ball around at our last meeting.

Mrs. Heath then changed the subject, confessing emotionally that she was "praying daily" that she would not "lose Keyshawn on the streets to gang violence." She murmured quietly, "I know it makes you feel big and bad, but you got to get out of it ... I don't want to lose you!" Mrs. Heath started to cry. Mr. Heath shared with Keyshawn and all of us that their "friend's grandson in the hood was just gunned down." He went on to say that "these things happen when you least expect them." Keyshawn consoled his grandparents, "You worry too much ... I will be fine." Mr. Harris disclosed that when he was "a few years older than Keyshawn" he had "dabbled with the gangs" and thought he was "real bad" until he "witnessed his closest friend get shot and killed" right before his eyes. After that shocking and painful experience, he steered clear of any future gang involvement. Mr. Steele chimed in that he could have joined the gangs when he was Keyshawn's age but chose the right path of striving to do well in school, play football, and pursue his dream to play college ball. He ended up getting a scholarship and full-ride to play football at a Big Ten Midwestern school. Keyshawn sat there quietly listening to the men's experiences.

In an effort to get to know Keyshawn better, I met alone with him for a short while. I wanted to come to understand his involvement with the Vicelords street gang and where it fit into his life situation. Keyshawn took a risk with me and shared that he only did "some dealing for them" and was not involved with violent activities. He said that he "made a lot of money so he could buy nice threads [clothes], gym shoes, CDs, an iPhone, and new PlayStation and computer games." I asked him how I could be helpful to him. Keyshawn replied with, "I don't know." I asked him if there was anything he wanted me to change with the grandparents. He said he wished they would "stop nagging" him so much "about school, getting out of the gang, and straightening up my bedroom." I explored with him if he liked to party (use drugs) and, if so, what he used. Keyshawn shared that sometimes he "smoked a little weed" and "drank some beers" but nothing more. He pointed out that "drugs like heroin make you crazy!" I asked him what he meant by this, and he said his mother was "addicted to heroin" and "used to beat up on" him. He went on to add that he "hated" his mother. I thanked him for being so open and honest with me. At this point, Keyshawn, Mr. Steele, Mr. Harris, and I went in the backyard to toss around the football.

Prior to ending our family meeting, I met alone with the grandparents, Mr. Steele, and Mr. Harris to pull our heads together to come up with a game plan. Both Mr. Harris and Mr. Steele each agreed to devote 2 days a week to spend quality time with Keyshawn throwing the football around and doing fun activities together. I shared my idea of tapping two of Keyshawn's talents—salesmanship and being a good landscaper—to help him develop his own lawn-mowing and gardening business and earn money legally and safely. The entire group thought this would be a great idea. In fact, the grandparents offered not only to buy Keyshawn a new lawn mower but gardening tools as well. Since I knew Mr. Steele also taught computer graphics art design at his high school and served as the head football coach there, I asked him if he would be willing to help Keyshawn create an attractive and eye-catching flyer and some business cards. He agreed to start working on this project the next time they got together. Mr. Harris and the grandparents offered to call around the community and help line up some initial business for Keyshawn if he would commit to starting his own business. I had Keyshawn join us, and I asked the two men to present our idea to him and what everyone was willing to do to help launch his business. Keyshawn thought this would be a lot of work but he would be willing to try it out.

THIRD FAMILY SESSION

One week later, we all met again, and there was some exciting news to report. Not only had Mr. Steele and Keyshawn put together a beautiful landscaping business flyer and business cards, but also he already had eight customers lined up in their neighborhood and by Mr. Harris's house. The grandparents bought Keyshawn a rugged and versatile lawn mower and a variety of garden tools so he would be well prepared to launch his new business. Both Mr. Steele and Mr. Harris agreed to make themselves available to Keyshawn if he needed support with his work and while he was trying to build a regular customer base and attract some new customers. Keyshawn was very excited about the prospect of making some good money and having his very own business. To help cover the back door, I explored with him if he had any worries about taking on this very responsible job or being pulled away from it to deal for the Vicelords. Keyshawn openly admitted that he was more worried about his "homies from the gang" trying to sabotage his efforts to change and be responsible. The good news was his junior high and high school-aged fellow gang members did not live in the areas that he was working. Both Mr. Steele and Mr. Harris reiterated to him that he could always call them for support if he needed it when trying not to cave in to "gang pressure to hit the streets again." Keyshawn had a look of relief on his face, knowing that his two adult inspirational others were backing him up and cared so much about his well-being. I wanted Keyshawn to know that I was also there for him with the support as well. Mr. Heath had mentioned that when he was a teenager he had cut neighbors' lawns and made good money. I shared with Mr. Heath that you must be very proud of your grandson and happy that he is keeping a family tradition going. I also recommended that Keyshawn consult with his grandfather if he needed any helpful pointers about the lawn-mowing business. Both grandparents were very pleased that Keyshawn was willing to work to try to turn his situation around.

Keyshawn shared with the group that Mr. Steele had the junior high football coach come by and meet him while they were tossing the football around, and he had complimented him on his skill as a wide receiver. I shared with Keyshawn that Mr. Constantine (the junior high football coach) did not know that he was going to have on his future team the next Chad

Johnson. Keyshawn, Mr. Steele, and Mr. Harris all laughed. Mr. Steele speculated that maybe someday Keyshawn would be even better than Chad Johnson if he kept working at it!

Mrs. Heath reported some other good news. Keyshawn's teacher had sent her a letter informing her that he was performing better on tests and starting to complete and turn in his homework assignments. I initiated the group's applauding Keyshawn for his school progress. He smiled. I asked him if he was aware of what he was telling himself or doing differently that was helping him do better in school. Keyshawn replied that he was telling himself that he wanted to "play football in junior high—and higher grades were necessary." I told him that it sounded like the voice of Mr. Steele was like a flashing neon sign in his mind. Keyshawn emphatically agreed. He also was "sitting away from Jesse and Willie," who were two troublemakers in class that often set him off and distracted him. After school, Keyshawn was making a concerted effort to come directly home rather than "hooking up with my homies." We praised Keyshawn for his good choice making and the big steps he was taking to stay out of trouble.

I decided to tap Mr. Harris's youth officer expertise and wisdom and see what ideas he had for Keyshawn about how to avoid caving to gang pressures to deal again. One tactic that had worked for other youths that Mr. Harris had been involved with was to have them "tell their gang homies that they are being watched by the police and they need to hang low for a while so nobody gets busted." According to Mr. Harris, this strategy had worked very well, because "you are like a bad case of the flu, and nobody wants to get sick." I acknowledged that this sounded like a great idea. Mr. Steele also thought this was a wonderful idea and a great tactic Keyshawn could use. Another tactic Mr. Harris shared was that "Keyshawn could stretch the truth and tell the gang homies that some rival gang members have been following him around in cars and he is worried about being clipped [shot or killed] and robbing his drug stash." He further added that "Keyshawn becomes a real liability for the gang, who do not want to lose their drug supply or money with him." Keyshawn thanked Mr. Harris for all of his great ideas.

In keeping with past practice, all of the men went out to the backyard to toss the football around. Keyshawn wanted to show me a Chad Johnson pass pattern he liked running. Although Mr. Heath could not run, he asked to throw some passes to Keyshawn. Keyshawn thought this was really "sweet" (cool) that his grandpa was throwing passes to him and joining us. He also was smiling a lot more and appeared happier about his life situation. When we reconvened with the grandparents, I asked the family as a vote of confidence for their great progress if they would like to meet in 2 or 3 weeks. We agreed to meet in 3 weeks. I encouraged Mr. Steele and

Mr. Harris to keep doing what was working and for Keyshawn to tap his grandfather's expertise about the lawn-mowing business and to work out a transportation arrangement with his grandmother to help him take his landscaping supplies to his jobs.

SECOND SCHOOL COLLABORATIVE MEETING

Present at our second school collaborative meeting was Mr. and Mrs. Heath, Mr. Harris, Mrs. Stanley, Miss Rosen, and Keyshawn. Across the board every adult in the room had great praise for Keyshawn's 180-degree turnaround. Mrs. Stanley was happy to report that Keyshawn was "now earning mostly B grades" and his "behavior in class had greatly improved." There were no further reports of his "wearing gang colors and flashing gang signs." The lines of communications between the Heaths and Mrs. Stanley also had improved. In fact, they were now monitoring that Keyshawn studied for tests and completed his daily homework and turned it in the next day. Mr. Harris reported that Keyshawn's new landscaping business was going well and he and Mr. Steele were both very proud of him and how responsible he had been managing this challenging task. Both Mrs. Stanley and Miss Rosen were happy to hear that Mr. Harris and Mr. Steele were so actively involved in Keyshawn's life and paving the road for his success. Keyshawn let Mrs. Stanley know that he was committed to doing better in school and she shared with him that she was also proud of him and could tell that he was really growing up. Since everything was going so well at school, we all mutually agreed to discontinue our collaborative meetings.

LAST FAMILY SESSION

Present at our last family meeting were both grandparents, Mr. Steele, Mr. Harris, and Keyshawn. The grandparents kicked off the session by sharing with us that they were "very proud of Keyshawn and were lucky to have him as their grandson." Keyshawn had a big smile on his face. Mrs. Heath pointed out that he was "doing double duty with landscaping work" as he was assisting her with "planting a whole new bed of flowers" in her garden. Mr. Harris wanted the adult participants to know that Keyshawn had "already been tested by some of his Vicelord homies to get back into drug dealing again" and he "successfully used the two strategies" that he had recommended in our last family meeting. I asked Keyshawn how he was courageously able to maintain his composure, keep a straight face with his gang homies, and pull this off twice. Keyshawn confidently shared with us that "it was nothing!" He also pointed out that he could not see himself "running with his gang homies anymore." Keyshawn shared with us that he was "making more money" with his landscaping business and "besides, you don't have to worry about getting busted or killed!" Everyone laughed and Mr. Harris blurted out, "You got that straight!"

Both Mr. Harris and Mr. Steele promised to continue to keep a strong central presence in Keyshawn's life. I complimented both gentlemen on their fantastic work and great displays of compassion and commitment with Keyshawn. The grandparents also thanked Mr. Harris, Mr. Steele, and me for greatly helping their grandson. After Mr. Harris, Mr. Steele, and I amplified and consolidated all of Keyshawn's and the grandparents' gains, we mutually agreed to stop meeting. Keyshawn thanked me for my help and I asked him to let me know when his first home junior high football game was so I could cheer him on. He acknowledged that he would. In keeping with our tradition, all of the men, including Mr. Heath, tossed the football around in the backyard. Before leaving, Keyshawn wanted to show me a new pass pattern he came up with. I shared with him that I bet even the real Chad Johnson could not run that pass-pattern route better than him! Keyshawn smiled and said, "Goodbye!"

FOLLOW-UP

I spoke with Mrs. Heath at 6 months and 1 year after our termination. At 6 months, Keyshawn's landscaping business was doing so well that he had to bring aboard two of his friends to help him. Apparently, he decided to branch out and offer "fall and winter services like raking leaves and shoveling driveways." I knew Keyshawn was a starter on his junior high team because I went to his first home game with Mr. Harris. Keyshawn had scored two touchdowns. Academically, he was "earning straight Bs." There were no reports of further gang involvement.

POSTTREATMENT REFLECTIONS

In reflecting on this challenging case situation, clearly what made the difference and gave the grandparents and me powerful leverage with Keyshawn was the active involvement of his two adult inspirational others: Mr. Harris and Mr. Steele. These two men maintained a strong presence in Keyshawn's life and helped steer him away from dangerous gang involvement. They helped him strengthen his football-playing abilities, make better choices, and mature into a responsible young man. In addition, by utilizing his talent as a successful drug dealer to becoming the CEO of his own landscaping business proved to be a good therapeutic move on many fronts. It steered Keyshawn clear from gang involvement, it filled up his free time with a positive structured activity, and he could take pride and joy in his accomplishment. The added bonus was that he not only ended up making a lot more money than he had as a drug dealer, but was able to expand his services into the fall and winter seasons.

Keyshawn's grandparents were also empowered by his two adult inspirational others. Mr. Harris and Mr. Steele helped him stay on track and kept the spark going with his landscaping business and passion for playing football. Their strong relationships with Keyshawn had spilled over into having a positive effect on his relationships with his grandparents, teacher, and Miss Rosen.

12

Collaborative Strengths-Based Brief Therapy and Beyond

*Major Themes and Implications
for the Future*

Leave the beaten path occasionally and dive into the woods. Every time
you do so, you will be certain to find something that you have never seen
before.

—ALEXANDER GRAHAM BELL

Major Themes of the Book

Throughout this book, I have presented many cutting-edge theoretical ideas
and therapeutic strategies that can increase our clinical effectiveness when
working with challenging children and their families. At this point, I review
and summarize some of the major ideas discussed in the book and then follow with a brief discussion of the implications of these therapeutic ideas for
the future.

I have presented a collaborative strengths-based brief therapy approach
that continues to evolve, building in more and more flexibility and therapeutic options. Therapists can now view their clients and their presenting
problems through multiple lenses and can choose many numerous pathways
for producing therapeutic solutions even for their most chronic and challenging child cases.

One major component of my approach with children is to use family
play and art therapy experiments extensively. By incorporating family play
and art therapy techniques as one possible therapeutic pathway to pursue
with children, we can gain access to the children's inner emotional worlds
and capitalize on the natural ways children best express themselves. As

shown in the case examples presented throughout this book, the play and art activities of children can serve as the catalyst for altering their parents' unhelpful beliefs about them and problem-maintaining parent–child interactions. By using play and art techniques with children and their families, we are also breaking down the barriers that have divided child and family therapists for decades.

A good grasp of child development, particularly what a child is capable of cognitively understanding, feeling, and mastering behaviorally at any stage of development, can inform how we interview the child and what we choose to do with therapeutic experiment design and selection. By having this knowledge base, therapists can educate parents on what to expect at a given stage of development and normalize for parents child behaviors that typically occur at a particular age or in response to family life-cycle changes.

Throughout this book, I have stressed the importance of empowering children by giving them a "voice" in their own treatment and in their own lives. Too often, therapists working with children concentrate most of their therapeutic efforts on intervening through the child's parents and tend to act as the child's spokesman at collaborative meetings with school personnel or other involved helpers from larger systems. Rarely do family therapists, or brief therapists for that matter, invite their child clients to specify the goals of their therapy; nor do they normally advocate for the children to offer a rebuttal to the school psychologist's case study evaluation report or to have a say in their future school planning. Much too often, mental health professionals and parents seem to forget that children are people too and should be given the respect and freedom to be active advisers on their own lives.

The research on resilient children has identified several key protective factors that clinicians should attempt to identify and fully exploit in their problem-solving efforts in behalf of their child clients and their families. Many findings from recent research studies have challenged the traditional wisdom of social scientists and mental health professionals that children with mentally ill, substance abuse-impaired, or abusive parents will necessarily grow up to be emotionally and socially handicapped. The results of several longitudinal studies with resilient children indicate that they can and will grow up to become well-adjusted, optimistic, and in most cases fully productive adults.

Implications for the Future

As client indemnity insurance plans are increasingly being replaced by the health plans of health maintenance organizations and preferred provider organizations, private practitioners and agency staff will need therapeutic tools and strategies to survive and thrive in our rapidly changing health care environment. With today's economic crisis, clients are increasingly relying on their insurance plans to cover their treatment and are scrupulously avoiding paying out of pocket for services. I have heard from many private practitioners that they have had to take on more managed care clients because there has been a major reduction in their fee-for-service business due to the current economic hard times. The collaborative strengths-based brief therapy approach presented in this book is managed care friendly and provides clinicians with the therapeutic armamentarium to do effective short-term work with children and their families. Managed care companies are constantly looking for therapists who work briefly with children and their families (Cummings, 2008; Oss & Stair, 1996; Poynter, 1994). Therefore, expertise in providing short-term goal-focused and strengths-based therapy with children will make a therapist highly marketable to major managed care companies and HMOs.

Garmezy (1971) has referred to resilient children as "the children of the dream" (p. 114). Resilient children have taught researchers a great deal about how to persevere and cope with growing up in high-stress family and social environments. The children's stories describe a combination of individual, familial, and social factors that had a steeling effect on them and empowered them to overcome adversity. Clinicians should familiarize themselves with these key protective factors and inquire with children and their parents about their past successes at overcoming adverse life events and how the child manages stressful situations and explore whether any of these protective factors are present and can be activated to help resolve the current presenting problems. In Chapter 6, I discussed 11 key qualities and skills that parents can cultivate and further develop in their children to help them to flourish in life and be more resilient. I also have developed a solution-oriented parenting group model (Selekman, 2005, 2009) for parents of adolescents, which also can be used with parents of younger children and can be used to teach them the importance of maintaining an optimistic attitude, how to capitalize on past problem-solving successes, and how to activate their children's strengths.

In this book, I have presented a collaborative strengths-based brief therapy approach for children and their families. The model is competency-based and collaborative and invites families to define the goals for treatment. A unique feature to this model is the use of children as expert consultants to their parents, to the therapist, and to involved helping professionals from larger systems. Children make excellent shamans. They can heal their parents in ways that therapists can never replicate. It is my hope that the therapeutic ideas discussed in this book will help therapists find the creative edge in their work, inject more playfulness into their sessions, and provide them with the therapeutic tools and strategies to do effective and efficient clinical work with children and their families.

References

Achenbach, T. (1990). Conceptualization of developmental psychopathology. In M. Lewis & S. M. Miller (Eds.), *Handbook of developmental psychopathology* (pp. 3–14). New York: Plenum Press.

Ahrons, C. R. (1994). *The good divorce.* New York: HarperCollins.

Ainsworth, M. (1978). *Patterns of attachment: A psychological study of the strange situation.* Hillsdale, NJ: Erlbaum.

Allgood, S. M., Parham, K. B., Salts, C. J., & Smith, T. A. (1995). The association between pretreatment change and unplanned termination in family therapy. *American Journal of Family Therapy, 23*(3), 195–202.

Almeida, R. V., Del-Vecchio, K. D., & Parker, L. (2008). *Transformative family therapy: Just families in a just society.* Boston: Allyn & Bacon.

Alvord, L. A., & Cohen-Van Pelt, E. (2000). *The scalpel and the silver bear: The first Navajo woman surgeon combines western medicine and traditional healing.* New York: Bantam Books.

American Psychiatric Association. (2000). *Diagnostic and statistical manual of mental disorders* (4th ed., text rev.). Washington, DC: Author.

Andersen, T. (1991). *The reflecting team: Dialogues and dialogues about the dialogues.* New York: Norton.

Andersen, T. (1995). Reflecting processes; acts of informing and forming: You can borrow my eyes, but you must not take them away from me. In S. Friedman (Ed.), *The reflecting team in action: Collaborative practice in family therapy* (pp. 11–38). New York: Guilford Press.

Anderson, H. (1996). A reflection on client–professional collaboration. *Family Systems and Health, 14*(2), 193–203.

Anderson, H. (1997). *Conversation, language, and possibilities: A post-modern approach to therapy.* New York: Basic Books.

Anderson, H., & Goolishian, H. (1988a). *Changing thoughts on self, agency, questions, narrative, and therapy.* Unpublished manuscript.

Anderson, H., & Goolishian, H. (1988b). Human systems as linguistic systems: Preliminary and evolving ideas about the implications for clinical theory. *Family Process, 27*(4), 371–395.

Anderson, H., & Goolishian, H. (1991a, October). *"Not knowing": A critical element of a collaborative language systems therapy approach.* Plenary address presented at the annual conference of the American Association for Marriage and Family Therapy, Dallas.

Anderson, H., & Goolishian, H. (1991b). Thinking about multiagency work with substance abusers and their families: A language systems approach. *Journal of Strategic and Systemic Therapies, 10*(1), 20–36.

Anthony, E. J. (1984). The St. Louis risk research project. In N. F. Watt, E. J. Anthony, L. C. Wynne, & J. Roth (Eds.), *Children at risk for schizophrenia: A longitudinal perspective* (pp. 105–148). Cambridge, UK: Cambridge University Press.

Anthony, E. J. (1987). Risk, vulnerability, and resilience: An overview. In E. J. Anthony & B. J. Cohler (Eds.), *The invulnerable child* (pp. 3–48). New York: Guilford Press.

Anthony, E. J., & Cohler, B. J. (Eds.). (1987). *The invulnerable child.* New York: Guilford Press.

Avis, J. M. (1986). Feminist issues in family therapy. In F. P. Piercy, D. H. Sprenkle, & Associates, *Family therapy sourcebook* (pp. 213–243). New York: Guilford Press.

Bailey, C. E. (Ed.). (2000). *Children in therapy: Using the family as a resource.* New York: Norton.

Barks, C. (2004). *The essential Rumi.* New York: Harper One.

Barrett, T. H. (1993). *Tao: To know and not be knowing.* San Francisco: Chronicle Books.

Berg, I. K., & de Shazer, S. (1991). Solution talk. In D. Sollee (Ed.), *Constructing the future* (pp. 15–29). Washington, DC: American Association for Marriage and Family Therapy.

Berg, I. K., & de Shazer, S. (1993). Making numbers talk: Language in therapy. In S. Friedman (Ed.), *The new language of change: Constructive collaboration in psychotherapy* (pp. 5–24). New York: Guilford Press.

Berg, I. K., & Gallagher, D. (1991). Solution-focused brief treatment with adolescent substance abusers. In T. C. Todd & M. D. Selekman (Eds.), *Family therapy approaches with adolescent substance abusers* (pp. 93–111). Needham Heights, MA: Allyn & Bacon.

Berg, I. K., & Miller, S. D. (1992). *Working with the problem drinker: A solution-focused approach.* New York: Norton.

Berg, I. K., & Steiner, T. (2003). *Children's solution work.* New York: Norton.

Berns, G. (2008). *Iconoclast: A neuroscientist reveals how to think differently.* Cambridge, MA: Harvard University Press.

Berra, Y. (1998). *The Yogi book: "I really didn't say everything I said!"* New York: Workman.

Bleuler, M. (1978). *The schizophrenic disorders.* New Haven, CT: Yale University Press.

Bodrova, E., & Leong, D. J. (2006). *Tools of the mind: The Vygotskian approach to early childhood education* (2nd ed.). Columbus, OH: Merrill/Prentice-Hall.

Bogdan, J. (1984). Family organization as an ecology of ideas. *Family Process, 23,* 375–388.

Bogdan, J. (1986, July/August). Do families really need problems? Why I am not a functionalist? *Family Therapy Networker, 10*(4), 31–69.

Bograd, M. (1990). Scapegoating mothers: Conceptual errors in systems formulations. In M. P. Mirkin (Ed.), *The social and political contexts of family therapy* (pp. 69–89). Needham Heights, MA: Allyn & Bacon.

Bohart, A. C., & Tallman, K. (1999). *How clients make therapy work: The process of active self-healing.* Washington, DC: American Psychological Association.

Bohm, D. (1985). *Unfolding meaning.* Loveland, CO: Foundation House.

Bohm, D. (1996). *On dialogue.* London: Routledge.

Bonny, H. L., & Savary, L. M. (1973). *Music and your mind.* New York: Harper & Row.

Boscolo, L., Cecchin, G., Hoffman, L., & Penn, P. (1987). *Milan systemic family therapy: Conversations in therapy and practice.* New York: Basic Books.

Bowlby, J. (1979). *The making and breaking of affectional bonds.* London: Tavistock.

Bowlby, J. (1988). *The secure base: Clinical applications of attachment theory.* London: Routledge.

Brazeau, C. M., Rovi, S., Yick, C., & Johnson, M. S. (2005). Collaboration between mental health professionals and family physicians: A survey of New Jersey family physicians. *Primary Care Companion to the Journal of Clinical Psychiatry, 7*(1), 12–14.

Briggs, J. (1992). *Fractals: The patterns of chaos.* New York: Simon & Schuster.

Briggs-Gowan, M. J., Horwitz, S. M., Schwab-Stone, M. E., Leventhal, J. M., & Leaf, P. J. (2000). Mental health in pediatric settings: Distribution of disorders and factors related to service use. *Journal of the American Academy of Child and Adolescent Psychiatry, 39,* 841–849.

Brookfield, S. D. (1987). *Developing critical thinkers.* San Francisco: Jossey-Bass.

Brooks, R., & Goldstein, S. (2007). *Raising a self-disciplined child: Help your child become more responsible, confident, and resilient.* New York: McGraw-Hill.

Brosco, J. (2003, June). *The future of primary prevention: Why integrate care?* Paper presented at the A Preview of the Future: Integrated Pediatric and Behavioral Healthcare for Children and Adolescents Conference, New York.

Brown, J., & Isaacs, D. (1997). Conversation as a core business process. *The Systems Thinker, 7*(10), 1–6.

Brown, J., & Isaacs, D. (2005). *The world café: Shaping our futures through conversations that matter.* San Francisco: Berret-Koehler.

Brunk, D. (2008, September). Survey addresses pediatricians' role in identifying and treating mental illness. *Clinical Psychiatry News, 36*(9), 27.

Bugental, J. F. (1987). *The art of the psychotherapist.* New York: Norton.

Buzan, T. (1984). *Make the most of your mind.* New York: Fireside.

Buzan, T. (1989). *Use both sides of your brain.* New York: Penguin Books.

Campbell, T. L., & Patterson, J. M. (1995). The effectiveness of family interventions in the treatment of physical illness. *Journal of Marital and Family Therapy, 21,* 545–584.

Campbell, T. W. (1996). Systemic therapies and basic research. *Journal of Systemic Therapies, 15*(3), 15–40.

Capra, F. (1988). *Uncommon wisdom: Conversations with remarkable people.* New York: Bantam Books.

Carter, B., & McGoldrick, M. (1988). *The changing family life cycle: A framework for family therapy.* New York: Gardner Press.

Casement, P. J. (1985). *Learning from the patient.* New York: Guilford Press.

Chang, J., & Phillips, M. (1993). Michael White and Steve de Shazer: New directions in family therapy. In S. Gilligan & R. Price (Eds.), *Therapeutic conversations* (pp. 95–112). New York: Norton.

Chodron, P. (1994). *Start where you are: A guide to compassionate living.* Boston: Shambhala.

Clark, R. E., Linville, D., & Rosen, K. H. (2009, April). A national survey of family physicians: Perspectives on collaboration with marriage and family therapists. *Journal of Marriage and Family Therapy, 35*(2), 220–230.

Compton, S., Burns, B., Egger, H., & Robertson, E. (2002). Review of the evidence base for treatment of childhood psychotherapy internalizing disorders. *Journal of Consulting and Clinical Psychology, 70*(6), 1240–1266.

Cooperrider, D. L., & Srivastva, S. (1987). Appreciative inquiry in organizational life. *Research in Organizational Change and Development, 1,* 129–169.

Cooperrider, D. L., Whitney, D., & Stavros, J. M. (2003). *Appreciative inquiry handbook: The first in a series of workbooks for leaders of change.* Bedford Heights, OH: Lakeshore.

Cottrell, L. S., & Foote, N. N. (1995). Sullivan's contributions to social psychology. In P. Mullahy (Ed.), *The contributions of Harry Stack Sullivan* (pp. 181–207). Northvale, NJ: Jason Aronson.

Cowan, P. A. (1978). *Piaget with feeling: Cognitive, social, and emotional dimensions.* New York: Holt, Rinehart & Winston.

Csikszentmihalyi, M. (1990). *Flow: The psychology of optimal experience.* New York: Harper & Row.

Csikszentmihalyi, M. (1997). *Finding flow.* New York: Basic Books.

Csikszentmihalyi, M., & Csikszentmihalyi, I. S. (Eds.). (2006). *A life worth living: Contributions to positive psychology.* New York: Oxford University Press.

Csikszentmihalyi, M., & Getzels, J. W. (1970). Concern for discovery: An attitudinal component of creative production. *Journal of Personality, 38*(1), 91–105.

Csikszentmihalyi, M., Rathunde, K., & Whalen, S. (1993). *Talented teenagers.* Cambridge, UK: Cambridge University Press.

Cummings, E. M., & Keller, P. S. (2007). How interparental conflict affects children. *Directions in Mental Health Counseling, 17*(8), 85–96.

Cummings, N. (2008, December). Upcoming national health reform: Is your practice ready? Plenary address presented at the Milton H. Erickson Brief Therapy Conference, San Diego, CA.

Dawes, R. M. (1994). *House of cards: Psychology and psychotherapy built on myth.* New York: Free Press.

DeBono, E. (1992). *Serious creativity.* New York: HarperCollins.

de Shazer, S. (1985). *Keys to solution in brief therapy.* New York: Norton.

de Shazer, S. (1988). *Clues: Investigating solutions in brief therapy.* New York: Norton.

de Shazer, S. (1991). *Putting difference to work.* New York: Norton.

de Shazer, S. (1994). *Words were originally magic.* New York: Norton.

de Shazer, S., Dolan, Y., Korman, H., Trepper, T., McCollum, E., & Berg, I. K. (2007). *More than miracles: The state of the art of solution-focused brief therapy.* New York: Haworth Press.

de Shazer, S., & White, M. (1996, October). *Narrative solutions/solution narratives.* Paper presented at conference sponsored by the Brief Therapy Center, Milwaukee, WI.

Diener, C. I., & Dweck, C. S. (1978). An analysis of learned helplessness: Continuous changes in performance, strategy, and achievement cognitions following failure. *Journal of Personality and Social Psychology, 36,* 451–462.

DiLeo, J. H. (1973). *Children's drawings as diagnostic aids.* New York: Brunner/Mazel.

Dillon, J. T. (1992). Problem-finding and solving. In S. J. Parnes (Ed.), *Sourcebook for creative problem-solving* (pp. 305–314). Buffalo, NY: Creative Education Foundation Press.

Dilts, R. B. (1994). *Strategies of genius* (Vol. II). Cupertino, CA: Meta.

Dinkmeyer, D., & McKay, G. D. (1989). *The parent's handbook.* Circle Pines, MN: American Guidance Service.

Doherty, W. J. (1995). The whys and levels of collaborative family healthcare. *Family Systems Medicine, 13*(3/4), 275–283.

Duncan, B. L., & Miller, S. D. (2000). *The heroic client: Doing client-directed, outcome-informed therapy.* San Francisco, CA: Jossey-Bass.

Durrant, M., & Coles, D. (1991). The Michael White approach. In T. C. Todd

& M. D. Selekman (Eds.), *Family therapy approaches with adolescent substance abusers* (pp. 135–175). Needham Heights, MA: Allyn & Bacon.

Dweck, C. S. (1975). The role of expectations and attributions in the alleviation of learned helplessness. *Journal of Personality and Social Psychology, 31,* 674–685.

Eastwood, M., Sweeney, D., & Piercy, F. (1987). The "no-problem problem": A family therapy approach for certain first-time adolescent substance abusers. *Family Relations, 36,* 125–128.

Emmons, R. A. (2007). *Thanks!: How the new science of gratitude can make you happier.* Boston: Houghton-Mifflin.

Engel, G. L. (1980). The clinical application of the biopsychosocial model. *American Journal of Psychiatry, 137,* 535–544.

Epston, D. (1989). Collected papers. Adelaide, South Australia: Dulwich Centre.

Epston, D. (1998). *Catching up with David Epston: Collection of narrative-based papers, 1991–1996.* Adelaide, South Australia: Dulwich Centre.

Erickson, M. H., & Havens, R. A. (1985). *The wisdom of Milton H. Erickson: Human behavior and psychotherapy* (Vol. II). New York: Irvington.

Erickson, M. H., & Rossi, E. (1983). *Healing in hypnosis.* New York: Irvington.

Festinger, T. (1983). *No one ever asked us.* New York: Columbia University Press.

Fisch, R., & Schlanger, K. (1999). *Brief therapy with intimidating cases: Changing the unchangeable.* San Francisco: Jossey-Bass.

Fisch, R., Weakland, J., & Segal, L. (1982). *The tactics of change.* San Francisco: Jossey-Bass.

Forehand, R., & Long, N. (2002). *Parenting the strong-willed child* (rev. ed.). New York: McGraw-Hill.

Fraser, J. S. (1995). Process, problems, and solutions in brief therapy. *Journal of Marital and Family Therapy, 21*(3), 265–279.

Fredrickson, B. L. (2006). The broaden-and-build theory of positive emotions. In M. Csikszentmihalyi & I. S. Csikszentmihalyi (Eds.), *A life worth living: Contributions to positive psychology* (pp. 85–104). New York: Oxford University Press.

Fredrickson, B. L. (2008). Promoting positive affect. In M. Eid & R. J. Larsen (Eds.), *The science of subjective well-being.* New York: Guilford Press.

Fredrickson, B. L. (2009). *Positivity: Groundbreaking research reveals how to embrace the hidden strength of positive emotions, overcome negativity, and thrive.* New York: Crown.

Freeman, J., Epston, D., & Lobovits, D. (1997). *Playful approaches to serious problems: Narrative therapy with children and families.* New York: Norton.

Freeman, J. C., & Lobovits, D. (1993). The turtle with wings. In S. Friedman

(Ed.), *The new language of change: Constructive collaboration in psychotherapy* (pp. 188–226). New York: Guilford Press.

Fruggeri, L. (1992). Therapeutic process as the social construction of change. In S. McNamee & K. J. Gergen (Eds.), *Therapy as a social construction* (pp. 40–54). London, UK: Sage.

Gandhi, M. K., Desai, M. H., & Bok, S. (1993). *Gandhi, an autobiography: The story of my experiments with truth*. Boston: Beacon Press.

Gardner, H. (1993). *Multiple intelligences: The theory in practice*. New York: Basic Books.

Gardner, H. (2004). *Changing minds: The art and science of changing our own and other people's minds*. Boston: Harvard Business School Press.

Garmezy, N. (1971). Vulnerability research and the issue of primary prevention. *American Journal of Orthopsychiatry, 41*(1), 101–116.

Garmezy, N. (1981). Children under stress: Perspectives on antecedents and correlates of vulnerability and resistance to psychopathology. In A. I. Rabin, J. Aronoff, A. M. Barclay, & R. Zucker (Eds.), *Further explorations in personality* (pp. 101–116). New York: Wiley.

Garmezy, N. (1991). Resiliency and vulnerability to adverse developmental outcomes associated with poverty. *American Behavioral Scientist, 34*, 416–430.

Garmezy, N. (1993). Children in poverty: Resilience despite risk. In D. Reiss, J. E. Richters, M. Radke-Yarrow, & D. Scharff (Eds.), *Children and violence* (pp. 127–136). New York: Guilford Press.

Garmezy, N. (1994). Reflections and commentary on risk, resilience, and development. In R. J. Haggerty, L. R. Sherrod, N. Garmezy, & M. Rutter (Eds.), *Stress, risk, and resilience in children and adolescents: Processes, mechanisms, and interventions* (pp. 1–19). Cambridge, UK: Cambridge University Press.

Gauron, E. F., & Dickson, J. K. (1969). The influence of seeing the patient first on diagnostic decision-making in psychiatry. *American Journal of Psychiatry, 126*, 199–205.

Gelb, M. J. (1995). *Thinking for a change*. New York: Harmony Books.

Getzels, J. W. (1992). Problem-finding and the inventiveness of solutions. In S. J. Parnes (Ed.), *Sourcebook for creative problem-solving* (pp. 301–305). Buffalo, NY: Creative Education Foundation Press.

Getzels, J. W., & Csikszentmihalyi, M. (1976a). From problem-solving to problem-finding. In I. A. Taylor & J. W. Getzels (Eds.), *Perspectives in creativity* (pp. 240–267). Chicago: Aldine.

Getzels, J. W., & Csikszentmihalyi, M. (1976b). *The creative vision: A longitudinal study of problem-finding in art*. New York: Wiley.

Gil, E. (1994). *Play in family therapy*. New York: Guilford Press.

Gingerich, W., & de Shazer, S. (1991). The BRIEFER project: Using expert systems as theory construction tools. *Family Process, 30*, 241–249.

Gingerich, W. J., de Shazer, S., & Weiner-Davis, M. (1988). Constructing change: A research view of interviewing. In E. Lipchik (Ed.), *Interviewing* (pp. 21–31). Rockville, MD: Aspen.

Gingerich, W. J., & Eisengart, S. (2000). Solution-focused brief therapy: A review of the outcome research. *Family Process, 39*(4), 477–498.

Glenn, M. L. (1987). *Collaborative healthcare: A family-oriented approach.* New York: Praeger.

Goleman, D. (2006). *Social intelligence: The new science of human relationships.* New York: Bantam Books.

Goodrich, T. J. (1991). Women, power, and family therapy: What's wrong with this picture? *Journal of Feminist Family Therapy, 3*(1/2), 5–38.

Goolishian, H. (1990). Family therapy: An evolving story. *Contemporary Family Therapy, 12*(3), 173–180.

Goolishian, H., & Anderson, H. (1988, November). *The therapeutic conversation.* A three-day intensive training sponsored by the Institute of Systemic Therapy, Chicago, IL.

Gordon, D., & Meyers-Anderson, M. (1981). *Phoenix: Therapeutic patterns of Milton H. Erickson.* Cupertino, CA: Meta.

Gordon, T. (1970). *P.E.T.: Parent effectiveness training.* New York: Plume.

Gordon, W. J. (1992). On being explicit about creative process. In S. J. Parnes (Ed.), *Sourcebook for creative problem-solving* (pp. 164–168). Buffalo, NY: Creative Education Foundation Press.

Gordon, W. J., & Poze, T. (1981). Conscious/subconscious interaction in a creative act. *Journal of Creative Behavior, 15*(1), 55–65.

Greenspan, S. I. (1995). *The challenging child: Understanding, raising, and enjoying the five "difficult" types of children.* Reading, MA: Addison-Wesley.

Hacker, K., Weidner, D., & McBride, J. (2004, August). Integrating pediatrics and mental health: The reality is in the relationships. *Archives of Pediatric Adolescent Medicine, 158,* 833–834.

Haggerty, R. J., Sherrod, L. R., Garmezy, N., & Rutter, M. (1994). *Stress, risk, and resilience in children and adolescents: Processes, mechanisms, and interventions.* Cambridge, UK: Cambridge University Press.

Haley, J. (1986). *Uncommon therapy: The psychiatric techniques of Milton H. Erickson, M.D.* (2nd ed.). New York: Norton.

Haley, J. (1987). *Problem-solving therapy* (2nd ed.). San Francisco: Jossey-Bass.

Hall, D. (1995). *Jump start your brain: A proven method for increasing creativity up to 500%!* New York: Warner Books.

Hanh, T. N. (1991). *Peace is every step: The path of mindfulness in everyday life.* New York: Bantam Books.

Hanh, T. N. (1997). *Teachings on love.* Berkeley, CA: Parallax Press.

Hanh, T. N. (1998). *The heart of Buddha's teachings: Transforming suffering into peace, joy, and liberation.* Berkeley, CA: Parallax Press.

Hanh, T. N. (2003). *Creating true peace: Ending violence in yourself, your family, your community, and the world.* New York: Free Press.

Hanh, T. N. (2007). *The art of power.* New York: Harper One.

Hauser, S. T., Allen, J. P., & Golden, E. (2006). *Out of the woods: Tales of resilient teens.* Cambridge, MA: Harvard University Press.

Havens, R. A. (2003). *The wisdom of M. H. Erickson: The complete volume.* Williston, CT: Crown House.

Hawking, S. W. (1998). *A brief history of time: Updated and expanded tenth anniversary edition.* New York: Bantam Books.

Heneghan, A., Gardner, A. S., Storfer-Isser, A., Kortepeter, K., Stein, R. E. K., & Horowitz, S. M. (2008, August). Pediatricians' role in providing mental health care for children and adolescents: Do pediatricians and psychiatrists agree? *Developmental Behavioral Pediatrics, 29*(4), 262–269.

Henggeler, S. W., Schoenwald, S. K., Borduin, C. M., Rowland, M. D., & Cunningham, P. B. (2009). *Multisystemic therapy for antisocial behavior in children and adolescents* (2nd ed.). New York: Guilford Press.

Hoffman, L. (1990). Constructing realities: An art of lenses. *Family Process, 29,* 1–12.

Hoffman, L. (2002). *Family therapy: An intimate journey.* New York: Norton.

Horigan, V. E., Suarez-Morales, L., Robbins, M. S., Zarate, M., Mayorga, C. C., Mitrani, V. B., & Szapocznik, J. (2005). Brief strategic family therapy for adolescents with behavior problems. In J. L. Lebow (Ed.), *Handbook of clinical family therapy* (pp. 73–103). New York: Wiley.

Hubble, M. A., Duncan, B. L., & Miller, S. D. (1999). *The heart and soul of change: What works in therapy.* Washington, DC: American Psychological Association.

Hurson, T. (2008). *Think better: An innovator's guide to productive thinking.* New York: McGraw-Hill.

Isaacs, W. (1993). Dialogue: The power of collective thinking. *The Systems Thinker, 4*(3), 1–4.

Isenberg, B. (2009). *Conversations with Frank Gehry.* New York: Knopf.

Jansson, T. (1962). *Moomin's invisible friend.* London: Heinemann.

Jellinek, M. S., & Murphy, J. M. (1988). Screening for psychological disorders in pediatric practice. *American Journal of Disease and the Child, 142,* 117–153.

Jellinek, M. S., Murphy, J. M., Little, M., Pagano, M. E., Comer, D. M., & Kelleher, K. J. (1999). Use of a pediatric symptom checklist to screen for psychosocial problems in pediatric primary care: A national feasibility study. *Archives of Pediatric Adolescent Medicine, 153,* 254–260.

Jenkins, A. (1994). Therapy for abuse or therapy as abuse? *Dulwich Centre Newsletter, 1,* 11–19.

Kagan, J. (1994). *The nature of the child: Tenth anniversary edition.* New York: Basic Books.

Kashdan, T. (2009). *Curious?: Discover the missing ingredient to a fulfilling life.* New York: Morrow.

Kauffman, C., Grunebaum, H., Cohler, B., & Gamer, E. (1979). Superkids:

Competent children of psychotic mothers. *American Journal of Psychiatry, 136*, 1398–1402.

Kazdin, A. E. (2008). *The Kazdin method for parenting the defiant child with no pills, no therapy, no contest of wills.* New York: First Mariner Books.

Kearns-Goodwin, D. (2005). *Team of rivals: The political genius of Abraham Lincoln.* New York: Simon & Schuster.

Kegan, R., & Lahey, L. L. (2009). *Immunity to change: How to overcome it and unlock the potential in yourself and your organization.* Boston, MA: Harvard School Business Press.

Keith, D. V., & Whitaker, C. A. (1994). Play therapy: A paradigm for work with families. In C. Schaefer & L. Carey (Eds.), *Family play therapy* (pp. 185–202). Northvale, NJ: Jason Aronson.

Keyes, C. L., & Haidt, J. (2003). *Flourishing: Positive psychology and the life well-lived.* Washington, DC: American Psychological Association.

Kohn, A. (2005). *Unconditional parenting: Moving from rewards and punishments to love and reason.* New York: Atria.

Kohut, H. (1971). *The analysis of the self.* New York: International Universities Press.

Kwiatkowska, H. Y. (1978). *Family therapy and evaluation through art.* Springfield, IL: Thomas.

Landau-Stanton, J. (1990). Issues of methods of treatment for families in cultural transition. In M. P. Mirkin (Ed.), *The social and political contexts of family therapy* (pp. 251–275). Needham Heights, MA: Allyn & Bacon.

Lantieri, L., & Goleman, D. (2008). *Building emotional intelligence: Techniques to cultivate inner strength in children.* Boulder, CO: Sounds True.

Leake, G. J., & King, A. S. (1977). Effect of counselor expectations on alcoholic recovery. *Alcohol Health and Research World, 1*(3), 16–22.

Lebow, J. (Ed.). (2005). *Handbook of clinical family therapy.* New York: Wiley.

Lebow, J., & Gurman, A. S. (1996). Making a difference: A new research review offers good news to couples and family therapists. *Family Therapy Networker, 20*(1), 69–76.

Levin, R. (1987). Liner notes for *Outward bound: The music of the Eric Dolphy quintet.* Prestige/New Jazz 8236.

Lipchik, E. (1988). Purposeful sequences for beginning the solution-focused interview. In E. Lipchik (Ed.), *Interviewing* (pp. 105–116). Rockville, MD: Aspen.

Luepnitz, D. (1988). *The family interpreted.* New York: Basic Books.

Macdonald, A. (2007). *Solution-focused therapy: Theory, research, and practice.* London, UK: Sage.

Mackworth, N. H. (1965). Originality. *American Psychologist, 20*, 51–66.

Madanes, C. (1981). *Strategic family therapy.* San Francisco: Jossey-Bass.

Madanes, C. (1984). *Behind the one-way mirror: Advances in the practice of strategic therapy.* San Francisco: Jossey-Bass.

Malchiodi, C. A. (Ed.). (2003). *Handbook of art therapy*. New York: Guilford Press.

Margulies, N. (2002). *Mapping inner space: Learning and teaching visual mapping*. Chicago: Zephyr Press.

Masten, A., Best, K. M., & Garmezy, N. (1990). Resilience and development: Contributions from the study of children who overcome adversity. *Development and Psychopathology, 2*, 425–444.

Masten, A., & Garmezy, N. (1985). Risk, vulnerability, and protective factors in developmental psychopathology. In B. B. Lahey & A. E. Kazdin (Eds.), *Advances in clinical child psychology* (pp. 1–52). New York: Plenum Press.

Mauksch, L. B., & Leahy, D. (1993). Collaboration between primary care medicine and mental health in an HMO. *Family Systems Medicine, 11*, 121–135.

McDaniel, S. H., Campbell, T. L., Hepworth, J., & Lorenz, A. (2005). *Family-oriented primary care* (2nd ed.). New York: Springer.

McDaniel, S. H., Campbell, T. L., & Seaburn, D. B. (1995). Principles for collaboration between health and mental health providers in primary care. *Family Systems Medicine, 13*(3/4), 283–299.

McDermott, D., & Snyder, C. R. (1999). *Making hope happen: A workbook for turning possibilities into reality*. Oakland, CA: New Harbinger.

McLuhan, M. (1964). *Understanding the media: The extensions of man*. New York: McGraw-Hill.

Miller, S. D., & Berg, I. K. (1995). *The miracle method: A radically new approach to problem drinking*. New York: Norton.

Miller, S. D., Mee-Lee, D., Plum, W., & Hubble, M. A. (2005). Making treatment count: Client-directed, outcome-informed clinical work with problem drinkers. In J. L. Lebow (Ed.), *Handbook of clinical family therapy* (pp. 281–309). New York: Wiley.

Minuchin, S. (1974). *Families and family therapy*. Cambridge, MA: Harvard University Press.

Minuchin, S., & Fishman, H. C. (1981). *Family therapy techniques*. Cambridge, MA: Harvard University Press.

Minuchin, S., Rosman, B. I., & Baker, L. (1978). *Psychosomatic families: Anorexia nervosa in context*. Cambridge, MA: Harvard University Press.

Mitchell, S. (1988). *Tao Te Ching: A new English version*. New York: Harper-Collins.

Moore, M. T. (1985). The relationship between the originality of essays and variables in the problem-discovery process: A study of creative and non-creative middle school students. *Research in the Teaching of English, 19*(1), 84–95.

Moskovitz, S. (1983). *Love despite hate*. New York: Schocken Books.

Murphy, J. J., & Duncan, B. L. (2007). *Brief intervention for school problems: Outcome-informed strategies* (2nd ed.). New York: Guilford Press.

Murray, B., & Fortinberry, A. (2006). *Raising an optimistic child: A proven plan for depression-proofing young children—for life.* New York: McGraw-Hill.

Newfield, N. A., Kuehl, B. P., Joanning, H. P., & Quinn, W. H. (1991). We can tell you about "psychos" and "shrinks": An ethnography of the family therapy of adolescent drug abuse. In T. C. Todd & M. D. Selekman (Eds.), *Family therapy approaches with adolescent substance abusers* (pp. 275–307). Needham Heights, MA: Allyn & Bacon.

Nichols, M. P. (1995). *The lost art of listening.* New York: Guilford Press.

Nisker, W. S. (1990). *Crazy wisdom.* Berkeley, CA: Ten Speed.

Norcross, J. C. (2008, December). *Psychotherapy relationships that work: Tailoring the relationship to the individual client.* Workshop presented at the Milton H. Erickson Brief Therapy Conference, San Diego, CA.

O'Hanlon, W. H. (1987). *Taproots: Underlying principles of Milton Erickson's therapy and hypnosis.* New York: Norton.

O'Hanlon, W. H., & Weiner-Davis, M. (1989). *In search of solutions: A new direction in psychotherapy.* New York: Norton.

Omer, H. (2004). *Nonviolent resistance: A new approach to violent and self-destructive children.* Cambridge, UK: Cambridge University Press.

Osborn, A. F. (1993). *Applied imagination: Principles and procedures of creative problem-solving* (3rd ed.). Buffalo, NY: Creative Education Foundation Press.

Oss, M. E., & Stair, T. (1996). *Managed behavioral health market share in the United States, 1996–1997.* Gettysburg, PA: Behavioral Health Industry News.

Oster, G. D., & Gould, P. (1987). *Using drawings in assessment and therapy.* New York: Brunner/Mazel.

Ostrander, S., Schroeder, L., & Ostrander, N. (1994). *Superlearning 2000.* New York: Dell.

Palazzoli, M. S., Boscolo, L., Cecchin, G., & Prata, G. (1980). Hypothesizing—circularity—neutrality: Three guidelines for the conductor of the session. *Family Process, 19*(1), 3–13.

Papp, P. (1983). *The process of change.* New York: Guilford Press.

Park, E. S. (1997). An application of brief therapy to family medicine. *Contemporary Family Therapy, 19,* 81–88.

Parnes, S. J. (1992). *Visionizing.* Buffalo, NY: Creative Education Foundation Press.

Peek, C. J., & Heinrich, R. L. (1995). Building a collaborative healthcare organization: From idea to invention to innovation. *Family Systems Medicine, 13*(3/4), 327–343.

Peele, S. (1985). *The meaning of addiction: Compulsive experience and its interpretation.* Lexington, MA: Lexington Books.

Peterson, C. (2006). *A primer in positive psychology.* New York: Oxford University Press.

Peterson, C., & Seligman, M. E. P. (2004). *Character strengths and virtues: A handbook and classification.* New York: Oxford University Press.

Phillips, J. (1986, May/June). Language, communication, and the therapeutic context: A review. *Family Therapy Newsletter,* pp. 5–7.

Piattelli-Palmarini, M. (1994). *Inevitable illusions: How mistakes of reason rule our minds.* New York: Wiley.

Pinderhughes, E. (1990). Legacy of slavery: The experience of black families in America. In M. P. Mirkin (Ed.), *The social and political contexts of family therapy* (pp. 289–305). Needham Heights, MA: Allyn & Bacon.

Pollack, S. (2005). *Sketches of Frank Gehry* [film]. Sony Pictures.

Popkin, M. H. (2007). *Taming the spirited child: Strategies for parenting challenging children without breaking their spirits.* New York: Fireside.

Poynter, W. L. (1994). *The preferred provider's handbook: Building a successful private therapy practice in the managed care marketplace.* New York: Brunner/Mazel.

Prince, G. M. (1992). The mindspring theory: A new development from synectics research. In S. J. Parnes (Ed.), *Sourcebook for creative problem-solving* (pp. 177–193). Buffalo, NY: Creative Education Foundation Press.

Prochaska, J. O., Norcross, J. C., & DiClemente, C. C. (1994). *Changing for good.* New York: Morrow.

Rhyne, J. (1996). *The gestalt art experience: Patterns that connect.* Chicago: Magnolia Street.

Riley, S., & Malchiodi, C. A. (1994). *Integrative approaches to family art therapy.* Chicago: Magnolia Street.

Roberto, M. A. (2009). *Know what you don't know: How great leaders prevent problems before they happen.* Upper Saddle River, NJ: Pearson Education.

Rolland, J. (1998). *Families, illness, and disability.* New York: HarperCollins.

Ruddy, N., Borreson, D., & Gunn, W. (2008). *The collaborative psychotherapist.* Washington, DC: American Psychological Association.

Salamon, E., & Grevelius, K. (1996, June). *Who has got a problem with what?: Why social workers and therapists in Sweden have got a drinking problem.* A workshop presented at the Conference on NLP and other Solution-Oriented Approaches, Jyvaskyla, Finland.

Schaefer, C. E., & DiGeronimo, T. F. (1995, February). Making sense of make-believe: Understanding and encouraging your child's imagination. *Child,* pp. 29–33.

Schafer, R. (1994). *Re-telling a life: Narration and dialogue in psychoanalysis.* New York: Basic Books.

Scharmer, C. O. (2007). *Theory U: Leading from the future as it emerges.* Cambridge, MA: The Society for Organizational Learning.

Schon, D. A. (1983). *The reflective practitioner: How professionals think in action.* New York: Basic Books.

Schrage, M. (1990). *Shared minds: The new technologies of collaboration.* New York: Random House.

Selekman, M. D. (1995). "Help me out ... I'm confused": The Columbo approach with difficult youth. *Newsletter of the Brief Therapy Network, 1*(4), 1–4.

Selekman, M. D. (1996). Turning out the light on a seasonal affective disorder. *Journal of Systemic Therapies, 15*(3), 40–51.

Selekman, M.d. (2005). *Pathways to change: Brief therapy with difficult adolescents* (2nd ed.). New York: Guilford Press.

Selekman, M. D. (2006). *Working with self-harming adolescents: A collaborative strengths-based therapy approach.* New York: W. W. Norton & Co.

Selekman, M. D. (2009). *The adolescent and young adult self-harming treatment manual: A collaborative strengths-based brief therapy approach.* New York: Norton.

Selekman, M. D., & Shulem, H. (2007). *The self-harming adolescents and their families expert consultants research project: A qualitative study.* Unpublished manuscript.

Seligman, M. E. P. (2002). *Authentic happiness.* New York: Free Press.

Seligman, M. E. P., & Dean, B. (2003). *Nine-month vanguard master class in authentic happiness coaching and positive psychology.* Bethesda, MD.

Seligman, M. E. P., Reivich, K., Jaycox, L., & Gillham, J. (1995). *The optimistic child: A revolutionary program that safeguards children against depression and builds lifelong resilience.* Boston: Houghton Mifflin.

Senge, P., Scharmer, C. O., Jaworski, J., & Flowers, B. S. (2005). *Presence: An exploration of profound change in people, organizations, and society.* New York: Currency/Doubleday.

Senge, P. M., Kleiner, A., Roberts, C., Ross, R. B., & Smith, B. J. (1994). *The fifth discipline fieldbook: Strategies and tools for building a learning organization.* New York: Currency/Doubleday.

Seuss, D. (1961a). *The Sneetches.* New York: Random House.

Seuss, D. (1961b). *The Zax.* New York: Random House.

Sexton, T. L., & Alexander, J. F. (2005). Functional family therapy for externalizing disorders in adolescents. In J. L. Lebow (Ed.), *Handbook of clinical family therapy* (pp. 164–195). New York: Wiley.

Siegel, D. J. (2007). *The mindful brain: Reflection and attunement in the cultivation of well-being.* New York: Norton.

Siegel, D. J., & Hartzell, M. (2003). *Parenting from the inside out: How a deeper self-understanding can help you raise children who thrive.* New York: Tarcher.

Sluzki, C. E. (1979). Migration and family conflict. *Family Process, 18*(4), 379–390.

Snyder, C. R., & Lopez, S. J. (Eds.). (2007). *Positive psychology: The scientific and practical explorations of human strengths.* Thousand Oaks, CA: Sage.

Sobol, B. (1982). Art therapy and strategic family therapy. *American Journal of Art Therapy, 21,* 23–31.

Spence, D. (1982). *Narrative truth and historical truth.* New York: Norton.

Stein, R. E. K., Horwitz, S. M., Storfer-Isser, A., Heneghan, A., Olson, L., & Hoagwood, K. E. (2008, January–February). Do pediatricians think they are responsible for identification and management of child mental health problems?: Results of the AAP periodic survey. *Ambulatory Pediatrics, 8*(1), 11–17.

Stinnett, N., & O'Donnell, M. (1996). *Good kids: How you and your kids can successfully navigate the teen years.* New York: Doubleday.

Stith, S. M., Rosen, K. H., McCollum, E. E., Coleman, J. U., & Herman, S. A. (1996). The voices of children: Preadolescent children's experiences in family therapy. *Journal of Marital and Family Therapy, 22*(1), 69–86.

Taffel, R. (2009). *Childhood unbound: Saving our kids' best selves—confident parenting in a world of change.* New York: Free Press.

Talmon, M. (1990). *Single session therapy.* San Francisco: Jossey-Bass.

Taras, H. L., Frankowski, B. L., McGrath, J. W., & Mears, C. J. (2004). School-based mental health services. *Pediatrics, 113*(6), 1839–1845.

Thomas, E., Polansky, N., & Kounin, J. (1955). The expected behavior of a potentially helpful person. *Human Relations, 8,* 165–174.

Thomas, P. (2003). *The power of relaxation.* St. Paul, MN: Red Leaf Press.

Tinnin, L. (1990). Biological processes in nonverbal communication and their role in the making and interpretations of art. *American Journal of Art Therapy, 29,* 9–13.

Tolan, P., & Dodge, K. A. (2005). Child mental health as a primary care and concern: A system for comprehensive support and service. *American Psychologist, 60,* 601–614.

Tomm, K. (1987). Interventive interviewing: Part II. Reflexive questioning as a means to enable self-healing. *Family Process, 26,* 167–183.

Tomm, K., & White, M. (1987, October). *Externalizing problems and internalizing directional choices.* Training Institute presented at the annual conference of the American Association for Marriage and Family Therapy, Chicago.

Trepper, T. S., & Barrett, M. J. (1989). *Systemic treatment of incest.* New York: Brunner/Mazel.

Unwin, D. (2005). SFGP! Why a solution-focused approach is brilliant in primary care. *Solution News, 1,* 10–12 (available at *www.solution-news.co.uk*).

U.S. Public Health Service (2000). *Report of the Surgeon General's Conference on Children's Mental Health: A national action agenda.* Washington, DC: U.S. Department of Health and Human Services.

Vandenberg, J. (1993). Integration of individualized mental health services into the system of care for children and adolescents. *Administration and Policy in Mental Health, 20*(4), 91–112.

Van Gundy, A. B. (1988). *Stalking the wild solution: A problem-finding approach to creative problem-solving.* Buffalo, NY: Bearly Limited.

Van Gundy, A. B. (1992). *Idea power.* New York: AMACOM.

Viswanathan, P., Brucia, L., & Daymont, C. (2006, November). The role of pediatricians in children's mental health. *PCCY Philadelphia Citizens for Children and Youth Newsletter,* pp. 1–8.

Wachtel, E. F. (1994). *Treating troubled children and their families.* New York: Guilford Press.

Wallerstein, J., & Lewis, J. (1998). The long-term impact of divorce on children: A first report from a 25-year study. *Family and Conciliation Courts Review, 36,* 368–383.

Walsh, F., & Scheinkman, M. (1989). Female: The hidden gender dimension in models of family therapy. In M. McGoldrick, C. M. Andersen, & F. Walsh (Eds.), *Women in families: A framework for family therapy* (pp. 16–42). New York: Norton.

Watzlawick, P., Weakland, J., & Fisch, R. (1974). *Change: Principles of problem formation and problem resolution.* New York: Norton.

Weiner-Davis, M., de Shazer, S., & Gingerich, W. (1987). Building on pretreatment change to construct the therapeutic solution: An exploratory study. *Journal of Marital and Family Therapy, 13*(4), 359–363.

Weissbourd, R. (2009). *The parents we mean to be: How well-intentioned adults undermine children's moral and emotional development.* Boston: Houghton Mifflin Harcourt.

Weisz, J. R., McCarty, C. A., & Valeri, S. M. (2006). Effects of psychotherapy for depression in children and adolescents: A meta-analysis. *Psychological Bulletin, 132*(1), 132–149.

Wenger, W. (1985). *A method of personal growth and development.* Gaithersburg, MD: Psychogenics Press.

Wenger, W., & Poe, R. (1996). *The Einstein factor.* Rocklin, CA: Prima.

Werner, E. E. (1987a). Resilient children. In E. M. Hetherington & R. D. Parke (Eds.), *Contemporary readings in child psychology.* New York: McGraw-Hill.

Werner, E. E. (1987b). Vulnerability and resiliency in children at risk for delinquency: A longitudinal study from birth to young adulthood. In J. D. Burchard & S. N. Burchard (Eds.), *Prevention in delinquent behavior* (pp. 44–60). Newbury Park, CA: Sage.

Werner, E. E., & Smith, R. S. (1982). *Vulnerable but invincible.* New York: McGraw-Hill.

Werner, E. E., & Smith, R. S. (1992). *Overcoming the odds.* Ithaca, NY: Cornell University Press.

Whipple, V. (1996). Developing an identity as a feminist family therapist: Implications for training. *Journal of Marital and Family Therapy, 22*(3), 381–396.

White, M. (1988, Winter). The process of questioning: A therapy of literary merit? *Dulwich Centre Newsletter,* pp. 8–14.

White, M. (1995). *Re-authoring lives: Interviews and essays.* Adelaide, South Australia: Dulwich Centre Publications.

White, M. (2007). *Maps of narrative practice.* New York: Norton.

White, M., & Epston, D. (1990). *Narrative means to therapeutic ends.* New York: Norton.

Williams, J., Palmes, G., Klinepeter, K., Pulley, A., & Meschan, J. (2005, May). Referral of pediatricians of children with behavioral health disorders. *Clinical Pediatrics, 44,* 343–349.

Winnicott, D. W. (1971a). *Playing and reality.* New York: Basic Books.

Winnicott, D. W. (1971b). *Therapeutic consultations in child psychiatry.* New York: Basic Books.

Winnicott, D. W. (1985). *Deprivation and delinquency.* London: Tavistock/Routledge.

Wittgenstein, L. (1963). *On certainty.* Oxford, UK: Basil/Blackwell.

Wolin, S., O'Hanlon, W. H., & Hoffman, L. (1995, October). *Three strength-based therapies.* Workshop presented at the annual conference of the American Association for Marriage and Family Therapy, Baltimore.

Wolin, S. J., & Wolin, S. (1993). *The resilient self: How survivors of troubled families rise above adversity.* New York: Villard Books.

Wood, N., & Howell, F. (1993). *Spirit walker.* New York: Doubleday.

Wujec, T. (1995). *Five star mind.* New York: Doubleday.

Yager, J. (1977). Psychiatric eclecticism: A cognitive view. *American Journal of Psychiatry, 134,* 736–741.

Zilbach, J., Bergel, E., & Gass, C. (1972). The role of young children in family therapy. In C. J. Sager & H. S. Kaplan (Eds.), *Progress in group and family therapy* (pp. 385–399). New York: Brunner/Mazel.

Index